JOHN COOKSON

CORNELIUS KATONA

DAVID TAYLOR

USE OF DRUGS IN PSYCHIATRY

THE EVIDENCE FROM PSYCHOPHARMACOLOGY

FIFTH EDITION

© The Royal College of Psychiatrists 2002

Gaskell is an imprint of the Royal College of Psychiatrists
17 Belgrave Square, London SW1X 8PG

All rights reserved. No part of this book may be reprinted
or reproduced or utilised in any form or by any electronic,
mechanical or other means, now known or hereafter invented,
including photocopying and recording, or in any information
storage or retrieval system, without permission in writing from the
publishers.

British Library Cataloguing-in-Publication Data
A catalogue record for this book is available from
the British Library.
ISBN 1-901242-29-3

Distributed in North America
by Balogh International Inc.

The views presented in this book do not necessarily reflect those
of the Royal College of Psychiatrists, and the publishers are not
responsible for any error of omission or fact.

Gaskell is a registered trademark of the Royal College of
Psychiatrists.

The Royal College of Psychiatrists is a registered charity
(no. 228636).

Printed by Cromwell Press Limited, Trowbridge, UK.

CONTENTS

Part 3:   The drugs

John Cookson BM, DPhil, FRCP, FRCPsych

John Cookson studied at Oxford, winning the Theodore Williams scholarship in physiology, and obtaining a doctorate in pharmacology. He trained in clinical medicine at University College Hospital in London, and in psychiatry at St Bartholomew's Hospital and the Maudsley Hospital. He has been a consultant at The Royal London Hospital, St Clements, since 1981, and his duties have included an inner-city catchment area, a psychiatric intensive care unit, and responsibility for a specialist drug dependency unit. His main areas of research have been in psychopharmacology, and he has been involved in the early stages of clinical development of several new drug treatments. He was a founding member of the editorial board of *Advances in Psychiatric Treatment*.

Cornelius Katona MD, FRCPsych

Cornelius Katona studied medicine at Cambridge and The Royal London Hospital, and trained in psychiatry in Cambridge and at St George's Hospital. He won the Gaskell medal in 1984. He has been an academic and honorary consultant since 1986, and professor of psychiatry of the elderly since 1991 at University College London. He has a clinical role in the North Essex Mental Health Partnership Trust. He has conducted neuropharmacology research and clinical trials in depression and dementia. He is editor-in-chief of the *Journal of Affective Disorders*, and in 1998 was elected Dean of the Royal College of Psychiatrists. He is chair of the affective disorders section of the World Psychiatric Association.

David Taylor BSc, MSc, MRPharmS

David Taylor studied pharmacy at Brighton and later gained a master's degree in clinical pharmacy. Having first worked in general hospital pharmacy and academia, he joined the Maudsley hospital in 1993. He is now Head of Pharmacy at the South London and Maudsley NHS Trust and honorary senior lecturer at the Institute of Psychiatry. He is a former chairman of the UK Psychiatric Pharmacy Group and foundation president of the College of Mental Health Pharmacists. His research interests include pharmacokinetics, pharmacoeconomics, and prescribing quality.

This is a practical book, for use in the clinic, ward or surgery. It advises when and how to use medication to help people with psychological disturbances. Drug prescriptions are described in the context of the general management of the individual patient. Where possible, treatments are based on established evidence; otherwise they represent our own experience and what we teach as good practice. It is not necessarily the only successful way of doing things, but one we can recommend in the present state of knowledge. It is based on our belief that taking pains over the choice, introduction and dose schedule of drugs results in better therapeutic results and fewer side-effects and reduced toxicity. We have introduced a particular method to display evidence resulting from randomised controlled trials, using the concept of 'number needed to treat'; we hope that this proves a helpful and user-friendly approach. We have also included a large number of references for further reading.

In the past, many psychiatrists have been prepared to take great trouble over their psychotherapeutic handling of patients, but used drugs in a less thoughtful way. They have sometimes been frightened of proper doses, or combinations, or persisting for long enough with medical treatment. We believe that psychological treatment must often be combined with drug treatment, in a balanced way, to relieve and to cure.

The book is divided into three sections. The first is a general introduction to the social and neurobiological background and to psychological and social factors to be borne in mind in good prescribing. It can be read as a whole, or in parts, at any time. Brain structure, neurotransmitters and receptors are described, focusing on aspects that seem of most relevance to the drugs in current use. The second section is a series of essays on the role of drugs in different psychiatric conditions and the third an account of the drugs currently available in Britain for psychiatric treatment. These two sections work together, the former describing the factors affecting the choice of particular drugs for the condition and the latter giving more detail about the mechanisms of action of the drugs and their side-effects. In everyday use one may dip into the book by looking up an individual drug through the index of trade and approved names, or use the symptom index to see what the book says about treatment of a particular symptom or syndrome. One can also take the patient's diagnosis, read the appropriate part of the management chapter and look up the mentioned drugs in the third section.

While, simply for information, we give the names of all available drugs, we do not give details about all of them. In some groups we give one at length that we regard as typical of the group and well established, and follow it with shorter entries on others of the same group that we regard as useful. When describing side-effects we try to name the commonest and most important first, the lesser ones later;

and we do not list all the side-effects ever reported because to do so would be to blur the impact of the important with excessive information about the rare. The doses described here are intended to be consistent with those in the *British National Formulary* (*BNF*) and the manufacturers' data sheets or summaries of product characteristics, but they refer mainly to the treatment of adults who are not elderly. In treating the elderly, lower doses are often required. We do not list all possible interactions and further information on these should be sought in Appendix I of the *BNF*.

This is a book for trainees in psychiatry and is based specifically on the curriculum of the Membership examination of the Royal College of Psychiatrists. It should also be helpful to medical students, general practitioners and casualty officers, and perhaps also to nurses, social workers and clinical psychologists. It should also be useful to their trainers. It is not a comprehensive textbook of psychopharmacology, but it does attempt to lay the foundations upon which a more detailed understanding of the subject may be built.

At present biological science helps up to understand something of how drugs work and their side-effects, but casts little light on the underlying pathophysiology of mental illness. We should use the drugs we do on the basis of systematic clinical study and experience with many patients of different types, and not because of any hypotheses about the nature of mental illness. Our book reports some of this experience and study, and describes how drug therapy fits into the wider context of psychiatric treatment. Everyday practice is our touchstone.

ACKNOWLEDGEMENTS

We should like to acknowledge the assistance received from many people in the preparation of these chapters: senior registrars, including Richard Duffett and Martin Feakins; trainees, including Karl Marlowe, Ali Novitt, Christabel Hill, Dimitris Samellas; chapter 18 was revised by Dr Wai Chen; chapter 34 was revised by Dr David Branford, Dr Harry McConnell, Ms Lucy Reeves and Dr Janie Sheridan; chapter 35 was revised by Ms Lucy Reeves.

We are grateful for comments on individual chapters from Professor Thomas Barnes (chapters 17 and 29), Dr Eleni Palazidov (Chapter 11), Dr Michael Farrell (chapter 21), Dr Angela Hassiotis (chapter 19), Dr Peter McCarthy (chapters 1 and 7), Lee McCarthy (herbal medicine), Dr Harry McConnell (chapters 19, 32 and 34), Professor Richard Morriss (chapters 3 and 5) and Dr Rob Wood (chapter 9).

Dr Ian Anderson kindly provided references on guidelines.

We owe gratitude to previous authors of this book; Brian Barraclough, who had the idea and recruited John Crammer and Bernard Heine for the first edition in 1978. Bernard Heine invited John Cookson to help him revise the fourth edition (1993).

ADH antidiuretic hormone, vasopressin

ADR adverse drug reactions

AED antiepileptic drug (anticonvulsant)

BNF British National Formulary

c-AMP cyclic-adenosine monophosphate

CBT cognitive–behavioural therapy

CGI Clinical Global Impression

COMT catechol-ortho-methyl transferase

CPN community psychiatric nurse

CSF cerebrospinal fluid

D- dopamine receptor subtype

DAT dopamine transporter

DLB dementia with Lewy bodies

DOPA dihydroxyphenylalanine

DRI dopamine reuptake inhibitor

DST dexamethasone suppression test

ECT electroconvulsive therapy

EMEA European Medicines Evaluation Agency

EPS extrapyramidal side-effects

FDA Food and Drug Administration

GABA gamma-amino butyric acid

GP general practitioner

H- histamine receptor subtype

5-HIAA 5-hydroxindole acetic acid

5-HT 5-hydroxytryptamine, serotonin

HVA homovanillic acid

IPT Interpersonal psychotherapy

LTP long-term potentiation

LSD lysergic acid diethylamide

OCD obsessive–compulsive disorder

M- acetylcholine muscarinic receptor subtype

mCPP metachlorophenylpiperazine

MHA Mental Health Act

MAOI monoamine oxidase inhibitor

MARI monoamine reuptake inhibitor

MDMA ecstacy

MHPG methoxy-hydroxyphenylglycol

NaSSA noradrenergic and specific serotonergic antidepressant

NAT noradrenaline transporter

NO nitric oxide

NMS neuromalignant syndrome

NNT number needed to treat

NRI noradrenaline reuptake inhibitor

PCP phencyclidine

PET positron emisson tomography

PRA pluripotent receptor antagonist

PTSD post-traumatic stress disorder

RCT randomised controlled trial

RIMA reversible inhibitor of monoamine oxidase

m-RNA messenger ribonucleic acid

SARI serotonin antagonist and reuptake inhibitor

SDA serotonin and dopamine receptor antagonist

SERT serotonin reuptake transporter

SNRI serotonin and noradrenalin reuptake inhibitor

SSRI selective serotonin reuptake inhibitor

TCA tricyclic antidepressant

TRH thyrotropin releasing hormone

TSH thyroid stimulatory hormone (thyrotropin)

V- vasopressin receptor subtype

The modern era of drug treatment in psychiatry began half a century ago with the discovery in 1948 by John Cade, in Australia, of the use of lithium in mania (Mitchell *et al*, 1999), and by French scientists in 1952 of the use of the synthetic phenothiazine, chlorpromazine, as an antipsychotic. However, many lessons can be learned about treatment from the earlier history of psychiatry; furthermore the use of drug treatment should be seen in the context of contemporary psychological approaches and psychiatric services. Edward Shorter's *A History of Psychiatry* (1997) and Porter's work (1997) provide rich detail of much of the following.

ANCIENT AND CLASSICAL TIMES

Prehistoric neolithic fossil skulls show evidence of trephination, which was carried out in ancient times on live patients to release evil spirits or to relieve skull fractures, headaches, convulsions or insanity. It must often have been fatal, but some skulls show healing, indicative of survival. We know little of what other desperate remedies were attempted by Stone Age man, as herbal medicine began its evolution.

The opium poppy is an ancient medicinal plant, included among 700 remedies in the Ebers Papyrus of about 1550 BC Egypt.

Hippocrates (460–377 BC) of Greece challenged the view that disease was punishment sent from the gods, and linked epilepsy to brain function. The Oath that later was given his name refers to the importance of maintaining confidentiality of information divulged by patients, and of avoiding sexual relations with them. Hippocratic texts propounded the notion of four humors (including the black bile of melancholia), according to which, disease results from an imbalance of these. This broad explanatory scheme (elaborated by Galen, a Greek of the first century AD) survived to some extent until the 19th century and probably impeded scientific advance.

Mania, melancholia and paranoia were prominent categories in Greek medicine. However, it is very difficult to relate ancient accounts of illness or even those from a hundred years ago to their counterparts in modern diagnostic systems.

THE MIDDLE AGES

Mad people were the responsibility of their family or community and might become excluded. Mental illness was widely regarded as a spiritual affliction associated with witchcraft or possession by the Devil. Religious institutions developed a tradition of caring for mad people, and exorcism might be attempted. 'Shock' was also used in various forms.

The Renaissance and the Reformation

The French philosopher and anti-psychiatrist Foucault (1926–1984) has written of the alienation and plight of the insane in these periods, although the historical basis for his statements seems slender.

In the 17th century 'madness' began to rank as one of the problems of the cities. Places of confinement were developed that grouped the poor and the unemployed with criminals and the insane. The Poor Laws of 1572 and1601, the savage ancestors of the modern welfare state, made local parishes responsible for electing overseers to provide relief for the sick and work for the able-bodied poor, in workhouses. An Act of 1670 gave an increasing sense of a duty of assistance, coupled with the view that work was the cure for idleness and poverty. Within such places, when the insane became dangerous their rages were dealt with by mechanical restraint, iron chains, cuffs and bars – leading Foucault to conclude that they were treated as animals, or wild beasts.

The Asylum and Moral Therapy

The history of psychiatry began with the custodial asylum – an institution to confine raging individuals who were dangerous or a nuisance. The discovery that the institution itself could have a therapeutic function led to the birth of psychiatry as a medical specialism. This notion can be traced to the late 18th century to scattered clinicians such as William Battie (St Luke's), Chiarugi (Florence) and Pinel (Paris) and lay-people such as William Tuke, a Quaker tea-merchant who founded the Retreat in York.

Pinel (at the Salpêtrière for women and the Bicêtre for men), in particular, anticipated several trends, abolishing the use of restraining chains and recognising a group of curable lunatics (mainly with melancholia or mania without delusions), for whom a more humanitarian approach in an 'institution morale' might be therapeutic.

The term 'psychiatry' was first used by Reil, a professor of medicine in Germany, in 1808 to describe the evolving discipline, but its practitioners remained known as alienists (treaters of mental alienation) until the 20th century.

During the 18th century there had been a growing trade in lunacy throughout Europe; in Britain in particular the insane were handed to private madhouses. Physicians would have limited input to these. In 1788, King George III suffered a bout of mental illness for which eventually he received attention from Francis Willis, a mad-doctor renowned for his piercing stare and mastery. The constitutional implications were considerable, and subsequently Parliament instituted a Committee to enquire into this and into the care of the mentally ill generally.

The therapeutic asylums that sprang up in the 19th century had in common a routine of work and activity, and an approach by the staff encompassed in the term 'moral therapy': "a mildness of manner and expression, an attention to their narrative and seeming acquiescence in its truth" (Haslam, Bedlam); "the soothing voice of friendship" (Burrows, London); "encouraging esteem... conducive to a salutary habit of self-restraint" (Samuel Tuke, York) (See Shorter, 1997, chapter 2). Uplifting architecture was valued, as well as access to sunlight and the opportunity to work in the open air.

Many of these institutions had charismatic directors and employed attendants who could be trusted not to beat the patients. Reil (1803) described the qualities of a good psychiatrist as having "perspicacity, a talent for observation, intelligence, good-will, persistence, patience, experience, an imposing physique and a countenance that commands respect" (See Shorter, 1997, chapter 2). These are recognisable ingredients contributing to a placebo effect (see chapter 5), and most of the physical treatments at their disposal were largely that: purgatives, enemas, bloodletting (advocated for example for mania by Benjamin Rush, the founding father of American medicine) and emetics, aimed to draw out nervous irritants (catharsis, a term first used by Aristotle to describe the emotional release of the audience in Greek theatre).

During the 19th century the confining of patients to an asylum passed from an unusual procedure born of grave necessity, to societies' first response in dealing with psychotic illness. Therapeutic asylums were built on a vast scale as politicians responded to the claims of the early enthusiasts. Unfortunately, while the doctors had no effective treatments, the asylums were destined to accumulate more and more incurable patients, leaving the staff overwhelmed, demoralised and with insufficient time or conviction to sustain their moral approach. The situation was exacerbated by an increase in the numbers of people with mental illness, especially through neurosyphilis and alcoholism, and by the increasing reluctance of families in industrialised society to tolerate madness.

In 1894 the American neurologist Silas Weir Mitchell told asylum physicians that they had lost contact with the rest of medicine, and that their treatments were "a sham". In Britain, apart from the Maudsley Hospital, which opened in 1923 for teaching and research and for the treatment of recently ill patients, asylum psychiatry remained virtually divorced from the rest of medicine until the 1930s.

ACADEMIC PSYCHIATRY

During the 19th century many developments occurred in the academic centres, particularly in Germany where the new techniques of neuroanatomy (Wernicke), histology (Meynert) and pathology (Alzheimer's) were brought to bear in centres where observation and description of phenomena were also emphasised. Griesinger wrote an influential textbook (1861) and strove to link psychiatry with general medicine. Griesinger's view was that "psychological diseases are diseases of the brain" (p. 3). The old humoral theories began to be replaced with new ideas about the connection between mental illness and brain function. The pursuit of these links was successful for neurosyphilis, cretinism and dementia. By 1900 German academic centres had set a model for psychiatry to be taught alongside medicine.

But despite these developments, the scene was set for a period of therapeutic nihilism, and the rise of the new ideology of psychoanalysis.

By the turn of the century many leading clinicians believed that psychiatric illness was largely incurable, and therefore dedicated themselves to research rather than patient care. Kraepelin had concluded that mental illness should be defined by its prognosis rather than its cause, and that brain sciences were as yet too premature to provide an understanding of mental illness. This line of thought nullified the premise that enthusiasm for research is a hallmark of better clinical care. It also failed to recognise that better treatments can be developed without a knowledge of aetiology provided one retains confidence that the illness has a biological basis. Wernicke did attempt to link psychiatric symptoms to brain localisation; although successful for aphasia and the speech areas, this approach led to a confusing attempt at classification that Karl Jaspers later described as brain mythology. Furthermore, the attitude of many clinicians was affected by the doctrine of degeneracy promulgated by Morel (1857) and the early sexologist Krafft-Ebing (1879), according to whom severe mental illness represents the action of hereditary processes progressing over generations, and constituting a threat to society. In France the excessive emphasis by Charcot (1825–93) on hysteria shows us, in retrospect, that illness behaviour may produce the very symptoms that the doctor is keen to treat – through the mechanism of suggestibility.

In the first half of the 20th century, American psychiatry became dominated by the ideas of Adolf Meyer (Johns Hopkins University) which elevated history-taking, investigations and note-keeping above treatment. Furthermore, academic psychiatrists began to devote more attention to the less severe mental conditions encountered outside the asylum.

A notable voice retaining enthusiasm for developing better treatments was that of Thomas Clouston, in Edinburgh, whose textbook (1896) described clearly the shortcomings of available physical treatments and the hope for better treatments.

NERVOUS ILLNESS, REST CURES AND PSYCHOANALYSIS

By 1900 the public was so frightened of psychiatry that care often had to be delivered under the guise of nervous illness, and avoided accurate diagnostic terms.

The less severely ill and the better-off sought help in less stigmatising nerve clinics or hydros (spas offering spring mineral water, showers and baths in pleasant resorts). In 1869 George Beard (New York) invented the term neurasthenia to encompass many non-psychotic or psychosomatic disorders, attributed to exhaustion of nerves. In 1875 Weir Mitchell – despite his subsequent debunking of sham treatments – devised a rest cure consisting of seclusion, enforced bed rest, a diet of milk products, electrical treatments and massage. It transpired that the essence of the cure was in fact the physician's authority and the patient's submission to it. Its effectiveness in some cases illustrated the importance of the one-to-one relationship between doctor and patient, and what might be achieved psychologically through it. The method remained in widespread use by neurologists and psychiatrists until the 1940s.

THE HISTORY OF DRUG TREATMENT IN PSYCHIATRY

The introduction of psychoanalysis – with its concepts of transference and countertransference – made doctors more aware of the active nature of the therapeutic relationship. It helped also understanding of the content, though not the form, of mental symptoms. Its depth made psychiatrists rather than neurologists the appropriate specialists to deal with nervous illness. However, despite its initial promise of hope for the treatment of psychosis and other diagnostic groups, this proved unjustified; worse still, with concepts such as that of the schizophrenogenic mother (Frieda Fromm-Reichmann) it was dogmatic, misleading and inappropriate for understanding the causes of psychosis.

HERBAL MEDICINE AND PLANT ALKALOIDS

Dioscordes (57AD), Nero's surgeon, compiled a list – materia medica – of medicines, including almost 500 derived from plants. Paracelsus (b. 1493, Switzerland) is regarded as the grandfather of pharmacology; he taught that each drug (or plant) should be used alone, that chemistry was the science to produce medicines, and that it is only the dose that makes a thing a poison.

Plants with medicinal uses affecting the mind include *Papaver somniferum* (poppy; opium and morphine), *Hellebore* (veratrum), *Rauwolfia serpentina* (reserpine), the *Solanacea* henbane (hyoscine), *Atropa belladona* (atropine) and *Hypericum perforatum* (St John's wort; hypericum alkaloids). *Valeriana officianalis* (valerianic acid) is used for insomnia, as are *Passiflora* and Chamomile (*Chamaemilum nobile*, *Matricaria recutita*). Kava root (*Piper methysticum*) from South Pacific islands has at least 15 chemical ingredients and effects including relaxation and sedation. *Gingko biloba* may help dementia; hops (for beer) increase depression. In 1896, Clouston described *Cannabis indica* being used in combination with potassium bromide as a treatment for manic excitement.

Plants are difficult to identify, although the classification introduced by Linnaeus (1707–78) helped in this. In their natural form the medicines derived from plants lacked purity and varied in strength; they were consequently dangerous to administer, with the risk of overdose. Chemical techniques of the 19th century enabled the active alkaloid ingredients to be extracted, purified and identified.

Morphine was isolated in 1806 (Serturner, Germany) and used orally and (with the introduction of the hypodermic syringe by the Scottish physician Alexander Wood in 1855) by subcutaneous injection as a sedative, until it was realised how addictive it was. Henbane and later hyoscine (isolated in 1880) were used to calm agitated and manic patients, as was atropine. *R. serpentina* was used in India more than 2 000 years ago for Oonmaad (insanity). Reserpine was isolated from it in 1953, synthesised and introduced as an antipsychotic in 1954; it provided insights into the role of dopamine, noradrenaline and setononin (5-HT) in the brain, and the mechanisms of antidepressant drug actions. Veratrum was the source of modern calcium antagonists, some of which may have antimanic properties. St Johns wort has recently been confirmed to have antidepressant activity, and its ingredients

5

(hypericin and hyperforin) share biochemical properties with modern monoamine reuptake inhibitors and 5-HT agonists.

Heroin (diacetylmorphine) was synthesised in Bayer laboratories in 1896 and promoted as a cough remedy. Its name arose because it was said to make factory workers feel heroic. At about that time chemists at Bayer (Hoffmann and the Jewish Eichengrun, whose name was later omitted from the 'official' story) were creating aspirin; this they did by acetylating salicylic acid, the active ingredient of myrtle, meadow-sweet and willow bark; a drug was thus made that was more stable and less bitter.

Such was the success of Bayer in making vast sums from healing common ailments that at the Treaty of Versailles, the allies expropriated the Bayer trademark – and with it aspirin – as part of World War One reparations. Only in the 1970s did Vane discover the actions of aspirin blocking prostaglandin production; this was work for which he received a Nobel prize, and which led to further uses for aspirin, including stroke.

The French physiologist Claude Bernard had predicted that certain drugs (such as curare from South American arrow poison) could be used as physiological scalpels to dissect the workings of neuro-transmission. This proved prophetic with regard to biochemical theories of depression and schizophrenia, which arose from knowledge of the mechanism of action of antidepressants and antipsychotics, and Bernard's ideas anticipated the search for drugs with selective actions at particular receptors.

SEDATIVES, ANTICONVULSANTS AND BROMIDES

The synthesis by chemists, particularly in Germany, of sedative drugs in the 19th century, began the modern pharmaceutical industry. Chloral (1832), synthesised by von Liebig (the founder of organic chemistry), was found to be a sedative (1869) and was produced by the pharmaceuticals division formed by Bayer (1888). It became widely used in psychiatry, although prone to abuse and addiction; there were also cases of sudden death on chloral (for overview see Shorter, 1997).

Paraldehyde was introduced into medicine in 1882, and used as an anticonvulsant and sedative, being regarded as relatively safe, although unpleasant.

Bromide salts were produced by French chemists in the 19th century and found to be sedative. In 1857 Locock (London) reported the use of potassium bromide in epilepsy and hysteria; bromides became popular and remained in use as cheap alternatives to chloral for sedation until the 1940s. In higher doses they produce bromism, a toxic confusional state, beautifully described from personal experience by Evelyn Waugh (1957). McLeod used high doses of bromides to induce long periods of deep sleep in patients with mania, with reportedly good results.

Barbituric acid was first synthesised in 1864 but its first useful hypnotic and anticonvulsant derivative, diethyl babituric acid ('Veronal'), was produced much later, in 1904. Many other barbiturates followed, including phenobarbitone. These drugs induced sleep and relieved agitation; they also led the way to deep sleep therapy or prolonged narcosis. Patients would be induced to sleep for 16 hours a day for several days, with drowsy intervals to eat and drink. Although widely used, and much appreciated by the staff, the long-term efficacy of this treatment was never proven in a controlled trial. It also carried a significant risk of respiratory and cardiovascular depression, pneumonia and death. The subsequent use of benzodiazepines for prolonged sedation was safer. The first benzodiazepine, chlordiazepoxide (librium) was introduced in 1961. Valium (diazepam) became the most commonly prescribed drug in the world; but the risk of dependence on therapeutic doses of benzodiazepines was not widely recognised until 1981.

Sedatives were used to assist catharsis or abreaction in victims of shell shock in World War One.

MALARIA, INSULIN COMA AND ECT

Wagner von Jauregg, an Austrian, had noted in 1883 that a psychotic patient recovered her sanity after developing a streptococcal fever with erysipelas. In 1887 he proposed fever treatment with malaria for psychosis. We know now that high fever is specifically effective for neurosyphilis (because it kills the treponemata) but not against other psychoses. In 1917 he returned to the subject, treating advanced neurosyphilis patients successfully by the injection of blood, infected with malaria; he induced a series of fevers, which were later terminated by the use of quinine. In 1927 he was awarded a Nobel Prize for this (for overview see Shorter, 1997). Subsequently penicillin, discovered by Fleming in 1929 and available clinically from 1944, virtually put an end to neurosyphylis in the developed world. These discoveries had important lessons for psychiatry: that a mental illness could be cured, and that heroic methods might at first be justified.

Insulin was isolated by Banting and Best in 1922. Sakel thought that insulin-induced hypoglycaemic coma could relieve opiate withdrawal problems, and suggested its use in schizophrenia, claiming success in 1934. Insulin units were set up in many hospitals; in some centres insulin coma was repeated in increasing doses until convulsions occurred. By 1944 insulin coma therapy was the main physical treatment recommended for acute schizophrenia, for instance by Sargant and Slater in London. However, in 1953 Bourne, a junior psychiatrist, challenged its efficacy (Bourne, 1953); several academic psychiatrists wrote in its defence, but the controlled trial that followed failed to demonstrate any advantage of insulin coma therapy over sedation with barbiturates (Ackner, 1957). The use of this dangerous and ineffective treatment then gradually ended and the antipsychotic drugs took its place.

Camphor was used to induce convulsions and claimed to treat melancholia in the 18th century. The method could result in fractured bones. Convulsions induced by the chemical metrazol ('Cardiazol'), were proposed by von Meduna to relieve schizophrenia. However, the procedure itself was extremely unpleasant. A more controlled means of inducing convulsions was devised by Cerletti and Bini (Rome), using brief electrical currents applied through electrodes on the temples.

GOOD PRESCRIBING

Electroconvulsive therapy (ECT) was found to alleviate schizophrenia temporarily. The treatment was introduced at St Bartholomew's Hospital in London by Strauss in 1940; Felix Post (1978) has subsequently described its dramatic impact on the practice of psychiatry at the Bethlem Hospital in relation to depressive psychosis during the 1940s. Later the use of anaesthetics and muscular relaxants reduced many of its dangers. By demonstrating its effectiveness in double-blind controlled trials, its efficacy was established scientifically by the 1980s.

DIAGNOSTIC PRECISION

Accurate diagnosis becomes more important when treatments are discovered that are specifically effective in particular conditions.

There is a tendency to overdiagnose conditions for which a new treatment is found. This occurred in the USA with bipolar disorder after the introduction of lithium. When Baldessarini (1970) compared the frequency of affective illness and schizophrenia in patients discharged from hospital before and after the introduction of lithium, a reciprocal pattern was noted, with increasingly frequent diagnosis of bipolar illness and decreasing frequency of schizophrenia.

Subsequently the general acceptance of criteria-based diagnostic systems, particularly the third edition of the American Psychiatric Association's Diagnostic and Statistical Manual (DSM–III) in 1980, introduced greater diagnostic reliability. However, in this edition the definition of bipolar mood disorder was broadened to include patients with mood-incongruent psychotic features, who would previously have been regarded as having schizoaffective disorder or schizophrenia. Thus, the availability of lithium and the wider use of standard diagnostic systems have led patients to receive a diagnosis of bipolar disorder who might previously have been diagnosed with schizophrenia, at least in the USA.

PSYCHOTHERAPIES

Sigmund Freud (1856–1939) was a Viennese neurologist who studied with Charcot in 1885. However, he abandoned hypnosis in favour of free association and the interpretation of dreams, as means to attain catharsis and to understand symptoms in psychoanalysis. He described the dangers and the therapeutic potential of transference – the feelings directed towards the doctor by a patient bringing experiences from earlier influential relationships. Since the 1960s, the application of psychoanalysis for the treatment of severe mental illness has been progressively eroded. Other forms of psychotherapy have been developed with firmer foundations, in terms of evidence of efficacy and practicability. These include cognitive therapies, behavioural therapies and more time-limited and focused forms, such as interpersonal psychotherapy. Some of the ideas arising from psychoanalysis are now ubiquitous, and some are part of the armamentarium of everyday clinical practice; they help to make sense of complex behaviour.

THE SLOW EMERGENCE OF DRUG TREATMENT (SEE BOX 1.1)

By the end of the 19th century drugs were available to calm the manic or agitated, including chloral and paraldehyde, as well as the bromides and hyoscine. However, there were no specific drugs known for depression or for paranoid psychoses.

Fifty years later, the first edition of Sargant & Slater's book (1946) on physical methods of treatments in psychiatry still referred to the Weir Mitchell method, but recommended ECT for melancholia and mania, insulin coma for schizophrenia, and malaria treatment for general paralysis of the insane (neurosyphilis). For chemical sedation, paraldehyde and barbiturates were the main drugs; bromides were regarded as relatively ineffective and unsafe but were still being used. The authors stated that "most people would rather have their relatives dead than linger on for years, depressed or demented in a mental hospital" (p. 2). By the time of the second edition in 1948 the authors said "apathy has given way to enthusiasm in mental hospitals", as facilities for ECT, deep insulin treatment and leucotomy (first proposed by Moniz, Lisbon) became more accessible. The fourth edition in 1963

Box 1.1 The history of psychotropic agents

1831	Atropine isolated
1857	Bromides synthesised
1869	Chloral as sedative
1880	Hyoscine isolated
1882	Paraldehyde
1903	Barbiturates ('Veronal')
1917	Malaria for neurosyphilis
1930	Insulin coma for schizophrenia
1935	Amphetamine (narcolepsy)
1938	Phenytoin introduced, electroconvulsive therapy
1942	Antihistamines
1948	Lithium in mania (Cade)
1949	Hexamethonium and decamethonium (Paton and Zaimis)
1952	Chlorpromazine (Delay and Deniker)
1954	Lithium (Schou)
1957	Iproniazid, psychic energiser – MAOIs
1958	Haloperidol (Janssen), imipramine (Kuhn): TCAs, MARIs.
1961	Chlordiazepoxide: benzodiazepines
1968	Depot antipsychotic injections: 'Modecate'
1968	Lithium prophylaxis
1973	Carbamazepine in mania
1982	Zimelidine: SSRIs
1987	Fluoxetine ('Prozac') approved
1988	Clozapine: Kane et al
1988	SSRIs in panic disorder
1993	Risperidone: new atypical antipsychotics
1994	Valproate in mania (Bowden et al)

MAOIs, monoamine-oxidase inhibitors; TCAs, tricyclic antidepressants; MARIs, monoamine reuptake inhibitors; SSRIs, selective serotonin reuptake inhibitors

GOOD PRESCRIBING

described the advent of many new drugs that had allowed a "therapeutic community approach and open doors" in hospitals, "and it is through the use of these (physical) methods that community care becomes possible" (p. 1).

The discovery by Bradford Hill of the experimental design known as the randomised controlled trial (RCT) was such a potentially powerful one that it was guarded as part of the British war effort. Its importance continues to be appreciated as evidence-based medicine (see chapter 5) gathers momentum, through the Cochrane project.

LITHIUM AND MOOD STABILISERS

John Cade in Australia was interested in the effects of injecting the urine of manic patients into guinea pigs, when he noticed the calming effect of lithium (as its uric acid salt). He decided to inject lithium into psychotic patients and discovered the effect of lithium in mania. It remained to Mogens Schou, an academic psychiatrist in Aarhus, Denmark, to confirm this in a controlled trial. The prophylactic efficacy of lithium in manic–depressive illness was established by 1968. Thus, from about 1950 psychiatrists stopped giving their patients chemical sedation with the large anion bromide, and began to administer the small cation lithium, on a surer scientific footing.

The anticonvulsant carbamazepine was first recognised as useful in bipolar patients by Okuma *et al* (Japan). Independently, Post and Ballenger surmised that certain anticonvulsants might be useful by preventing the kindling of electrical excitability in limbic areas of the brain. A seminal report by Bowden *et al* (1994, see chapter 12) proved the efficacy of another anticonvulsant valproate in mania.

ANTIHISTAMINES, CHLORPROMAZINE AND THE ANTIPSYCHOTICS

More than a quarter of a century elapsed between the description of the actions of histamine by Dale and Laidlaw and the discovery of the first clinically useful antihistamine in 1942. By the late 1940s drug manufacturers were in a frenzy to synthesise new antihistamines. However, although sedative, these drugs were not otherwise advantageous in schizophrenia.

The possibility of synthesising exciting new drugs acting on the nervous system was reinforced in 1949 when Paton and Zaimis in London described a series of compounds based on quaternary ammonium (related to acetylcholine), which included an autonomic ganglion blocker (hexamethonium) and a depolarising skeletal muscle relaxant (decamethonium).

Chlorpromazine was synthesised in France as a variant of an antihistamine, promethazine. Following Laborit's description of its effects in anaesthesia (1951), the psychiatrists Delay and Deniker reported its effects in psychosis, calming patients without deep sedation and relieving psychotic symptoms in only a few weeks. The use of the drug spread rapidly, beginning a psychopharmacological revolution. Many other phenothiazines were synthesised. In 1958 the creative genius of Paul Janssen, the Belgian clinician and chemist, led to the introduction of haloperidol, a butyrophenone with antipsychotic properties. This had been synthesised as a variant of the pethidine molecule and it was observed to antagonise the effects of amphetamines in animals. The fact that amphetamines were being associated with psychotic reactions in cyclists, who were taking them to enhance their performance, led Janssen to study the effects of haloperidol in schizophrenia and mania.

The occurrence of neurological (Parkinsonian) side-effects indicated that these drugs affected neurons, and the name neuroleptic (seizes neurons) was used to describe them; the term 'antipsychotic' is now preferred. Later, newer drugs would be developed to avoid these side-effects (the atypical antipsychotics).

The antipsychotic drugs enabled many patients to be discharged from hospital, or to avoid hospitalisation. The number of in-patients with schizophrenia declined rapidly, by 80% between 1955 and 1988. This continued a slight downward trend that had occurred in the 1940s when the ideas of social and community psychiatry offered alternatives to in-patient care, such as day hospitals and group therapy.

The first depot injectable forms of antipsychotic medication, fluphenazine enanthate ('Moditen') and decanoate ('Modecate') were introduced in 1968 and stimulated the development of community psychiatric nursing services, in which nurses giving injections became keyworkers for patients with psychosis outside hospital.

A further breakthrough was the proof in a controlled trial by Kane *et al* (1988) that clozapine was effective in schizophrenia that had been resistant to all other types of antipsychotic. Clozapine had been studied from 1960 and had been widely rejected because of its many side-effects (including agranulocytosis), but the confirmation of its value in treatment-resistant patients has stimulated a search for other, better drugs. Among these risperidone was developed (and marketed from 1993) because it was known to share with clozapine the ability to block potently the effects of both dopamine and 5-HT; olanzapine and quetiapine are also potent in these actions and were developed because of their structural similarity to clozapine (see chapter 30).

IMIPRAMINE AND THE ANTIDEPRESSANTS

Imipramine was also synthesised (in Geigy, Switzerland) as an antihistamine, and was tried clinically at first on schizophrenia. Its activating effects led Ronald Kuhn to give it to depressed patients. In 1958 he reported its dramatic effects in some patients with depression, thus heralding the tricyclic antidepressants.

Another group of antidepressants, the monoamine oxidase inhibitors, evolved from antituberculous therapy. Iproniazid – in contrast to isoniazid – was devoid of antibiotic effects but improved the mood of the patients with tuberculosis. Iproniazid (introduced in 1957) was at first called a psychic energiser, later an antidepressant.

The discovery that both classes of antidepressants acted to enhance noradrenaline and serotonin (5-HT) transmission led to strategies for developing drugs aimed specifically at those neurotransmitters. The first of the selective 5-HT reuptake inhibitors (SSRIs) was zimelidine, developed under the guidance of Arvid Carlsson and launched by Astra (Sweden) in 1981, but soon withdrawn because of rare toxic-allergic side-effects (Guillain-Barré syndrome) and 'flu-like symptoms, fluvoxamine followed. A more successful SSRI, fluoxetine ('Prozac'), was approved in 1987. This drug caught the public imagination perhaps more than any other psychotropic drug. Books were written about it, mostly praising but some vilifying it. Its huge financial success continues to act as a spur to pharmaceutical companies to develop better psychotropic medications.

The pharmaceutical industry recognises the value of promoting drugs directly to the public, and uses various means of health awareness to achieve this. Such campaigns became so prevalent that in 1997 the US Food and Drug Administration (FDA) made direct-to-consumer advertising of prescription drugs legal.

DRUGS AND BIOLOGICAL PSYCHIATRY

Many of the theories of biological psychiatry have been developed from knowledge of the mechanisms of action of psychotropic drugs. The discovery that reserpine, which can cause depression as a side-effect, depletes neurons of 5-HT (and noradrenaline and dopamine) contributed to the monoamine hypothesis of affective disorders. The deduction by Carlsson and Linquist that antipsychotics work largely by blocking DA receptors led them to propose the dopamine hypothesis of schizophrenia. In 2000 Arvid Carlsson was awarded the Nobel prize for medicine (see Box 1.2 for list of Nobel Prize winners associated with psychiatry).

The development of an effective treatment could generate an explosion of interest in a previously poorly studied area, as well as funds for further investigations. In 1964 Donald Klein in New York showed that panic was an illness distinct from other forms of anxiety and treatable with imipramine; this distinction was recognised in 1980 by the inclusion of panic disorder in DSM–III. The surprising finding

---

Box 1.2 Nobel Prize winners associated with psychiatry

Wagner von Jauregg	1927	Malarial treatment of neurosyphilis
Egas Moniz	1949	Prefrontal leucotomy for schizophrenia
Julius Axelrod	1970	Noradrenaline reuptake mechanisms for antidepressants
Arvid Carlsson	2000	Dopamine as a central neurotransmitter; dopamine hypothesis of schizophrenia and antipsychotics
Paul Greengard	2000	Second messenger systems in neurotransmitter actions
Eric Kandel	2000	Synaptic molecular mechanisms in the formation of memories

Note: only von Jauregg and Kandel were psychiatrists.

that the SSRI fluvoxamine is effective in panic disorder (Den Boer & Westenberg, 1988) – and also in obsessive–compulsive disorder – focused attention on the role of 5-HT in anxiety, and stimulated further research in these areas.

DRUG DEPENDENCE

Drug misuse and dependence is an important accompaniment of drug discovery. Problems were recognised with opium, chloral and barbiturates but assumed greater significance with heroin. The report of the Rolleston Committee led to the British System of treating opiate addicts with maintenance substitutes (see chapter 21). The ideas were revised in the reports of Russell Brain, with more emphasis on strategies of reduction. Methadone was introduced as an oral substitute in 1965. However, in 1989 the Advisory Council on the Misuse of Drugs stated that "the spread of HIV is a greater danger to individual and public health than drug misuse". This changed prescribing practice back towards maintenance rather than reduction strategies.

ANTIPSYCHIATRY

It may be no coincidence that following a decade of genuine innovation and progress in treatment in the 1950s, the following decade became known as the era of antipsychiatry. It was also a time of liberal thinking, student socialism, experimentation with mind-altering drugs (such as lysergic acid diethylamide; LSD) and the beginning of widespread misuse of illicit addictive drugs (from cannabis to heroin) that later expanded in epidemic proportions. Misuse of the new psychopharmacological agents by prescribers was also seen in the almost indiscriminate use of benzodiazepines in general practice, and the use of inappropriately high doses of antipsychotic drugs in hospitalised patients who seemed resistant to treatment.

The success of effective psychiatric treatments, which had led to open-door policies and the rundown of psychiatric beds, left the mental hospitals even more vulnerable to criticism. Indeed, they were blamed for causing the very condition of the patients, who were now left in, or leaving them, having acquired the deficits of chronic schizophrenia. The influential 'three hospitals' study, by Wing and Brown, appeared in1961. This seemed to show that patients deteriorated more in a hospital where they were given less individual attention, had fewer personal possessions and were generally treated less well than they would be in a family – the antithesis of moral therapy. This finding in a non-randomised study was often misinterpreted. The terms institutionalism and institutionalisation were misapplied as descriptions of, and an explanation for, the social impoverishment of chronic schizophrenia, even though the same phenomenon could be seen in patients who had little exposure to psychiatric wards, let alone spending years in a mental hospital.

The asylum was rightly criticised, in its 20th century embodiment, by Goffman, as a total institution that could degrade its inmates. At the same time, however, more sinister and insidious attacks were made upon the very concept of mental illness, and upon the claims of doctors to be able to treat it. Those articulating these ideas included Szasz and Scheff in the US, R. D. Laing in Britain, and Foucault in France. Gradually their claims were exposed and discredited by thoughtful argument, based on well-conducted studies of the epidemiology, genetics and psychopharmacological responses of the major mental disorders. Vestiges are still occasionally encountered, usually among those who were acquainted with sociology during the 1960s, and those with bad personal experiences of psychiatric services.

INTEGRATING TREATMENT APPROACHES

Accompanying the clinical and financial success of modern drug treatments, there has been a tendency to polarise treatment approaches into the organic or biological and the psychological. The polarisation can also be extended to the doctors who favour one or other approach. Such a division may be valid for focusing research interests, but is unhelpful for clinicians. Doctors should avoid becoming identified as solely organic; it may give a sense of knowledge and authority, but it undermines the basis of the doctor–patient relationship, which has been important as long as psychiatry, and indeed medicine, has existed. The expanding knowledge base of psychopharmacology places an additional strain upon the therapeutic relationship, which is one that entails a degree of trust. The doctor is expected to be knowledgeable about the treatments being used. Patients may easily acquire detailed information that can seem to expose gaps in their doctor's knowledge, rather than supporting a constructive dialogue. There is also a growing expectation of what the doctor should tell the patient about his or her illness and treatment; again, the patient's trust in the doctor can be eroded if the patient feels he or she has not been given accurate or sufficient information.

COMPLEMENTARY THERAPIES

Perhaps as a reaction against scientific rationalism, or in disappointment with its results, people have turned increasingly since the 1970s to treatments that have less clearly established mechanisms of action or efficacy, often provided by practitioners outside mainstream medicine. These include herbal medicine and homoeopathy. A British Medical Association report in 1986 listed 116 different types, ranging from acupuncture to yoga. While some have specific therapeutic ingredients, most rely heavily if not exclusively upon the self-healing power of the body, and their practitioners maximise the potential of placebo effects.

REGULATORY AUTHORITIES

Disasters with drugs, such as that associated with thalidomide and foetal malformations in 1961, have led to legislation to regulate the marketing of medicines, for instance the Medicines Act of 1968 in the UK. The agencies, the FDA in the USA and the European Medicines Evaluation Agency (EMEA), now set standards for the approval of new drugs and dictate much of the research that is done.

Conclusions

At the end of the 20th century the physical treatments available in psychiatry included an increasing number of highly crafted molecules with selective actions on neurochemical systems. They also included three older treatments that are relatively crude in their mechanism of action – two drugs, lithium and clozapine, that have extensive biological actions and side-effects, and ECT. Although relatively crude, these treatments are still used because they are of proven efficacy. As our understanding of the mechanisms of action of drugs develops, so too does the possibility of developing more sophisticated treatments, with greater efficacy and with fewer side-effects. Psychopharmacology is so fascinating because it spans the spectrum from molecules to the mind of the patient.

Experimental techniques play a crucial role in advancing scientific knowledge. The new techniques of computerised tomography, pioneered by Hounsfield, combined with isotope-labelled drugs with known sites of action, provide powerful tools with which to explore the brain in health and disease, and to expand our understanding of treatments. Together with the new science of molecular genetics, they offer hope that the era of effective treatments in psychiatry will advance much further.

Further reading

Highly recommended further reading

Shorter, E. (1997) *A History of Psychiatry. From the Era of the Asylum to the Age of Prozac*. New York and Chichester: John Wiley & Sons.

Further reading

Ackner, B. (1957) Insulin treatment of schizophrenia: a controlled study. *Lancet*, **2**, 607–611.
American Psychiatric Association (1980) *Diagnostic and Statistical Manual of Mental Disorders* (3rd edn) (DSM–III). Washington, DC: AMA.
Baldessarini, R. J. (1970) Frequency of diagnoses of schizophrenia versus affective disorders from 1944 to 1968. *American Journal of Psychiatry*, **127**, 757–763.
Bourne, H. (1953).The insulin myth. *Lancet*, **2**, 964–969.
Clouston, T. S. (1896) *Clinical Lectures on Mental Diseases* (4th edn). London: J. & A. Churchill.
Davidson, J. R. T. & Connor, K. M. (2000) *Herbs for the Mind: What Science Tells us about Nature's Remedies for Depression, Stress, Memory Loss and Insomnia*. New York and London: Guilford Press.
den Boer, J. A. & Westenberg, H. G. (1988) Effect of a serotonin and noradrenaline uptake inhibitor in panic disorder; a double-blind comparative study with fluvoxamine and maprotiline. *International Clinical Psychiatry*, **3**, 59–74.
Griesinger, W. (1867) *Mental Pathology and Therapeutics* (2nd edn) (C. Lockart Robertson & J. Rutherford, trans.). London: New Sydenham Society, vol. 23.

Healy, D. (1996) *The Psychopharmacologists I. Interviews by David Healy*. Altman: London.

— (1998a) *The Psychopharmacologists II. Interviews by David Healy*. Altman: London.

— (1998b) *The Antidepressant Era*. London: Harvard University Press.

Kane, J., Honigfeld, G., Singer, J., *et al* (1988) Clozapine for the treatment-resistant schizophrenic: a double-blind comparison with chlorpromazine. *Archives of General Psychiatry*, **45**, 789–796.

Krafft-Ebing, R. (1879) *Psychopathia Sexualis. A Medico-Forensic Study*. New York: Pioneer.

Mitchell, P. B., Hadzi-Pavlovic, D. & Manji, H. K. (eds) (1999) Fifty years of treatments for bipolar disorder: a celebration of John Cade's discovery. *Australia and New Zealand Journal of Psychiatry*, **33** (suppl), S1–S122.

Morel, B. A. (1857) *Traité des Dégénérescences Physiques, Intellectuelles et Morales de l'Espéce Humaine, et des Causes qui Produisent ces Variétés Maladives*. Paris: Nancy.

Porter, R. (1997) Psychiatry. In *The Greatest Benefit to Mankind: A Medical History of Humanity from Antiquity to the Present*, pp. 493–524. London: HarperCollins.

Post, F. (1978) Then and now. *British Journal of Psychiatry*, **133**, 83–86.

Sargant, W. & Slater, E. (1946) *An Introduction to Physical Methods of Treatment in Psychiatry*. Edinburgh: Livingstone.

Shepherd, M. (1990) The "neuroleptics" and the Oedipus effect. *Journal of Psychopharmacology*, **4**, 131–135.

Waugh, E. (1957) *The Ordeal of Gilbert Pinfold*. London: Chapman & Hall.

Whiskey, E., Werneke, U. & Taylor, D. (2001) A systematic review and meta-analysis of Hypericum perforatum in depression: a comprehensive clinical review. *International Clinical Psychopharmacology*, **16**, 239–252.

Zollman, C. & Vickers, A. (1999) What is complementary medicine? *BMJ*, **319**, 693–696.

PSYCHOPHARMACOLOGY

The first use of the word psychopharmacology to describe the study of the effects of drugs upon mental functions and illness was in 1957, when an international society for neuropsychopharmacology was founded, the Collegium Internationale Psychopharmacologicum (CINP). The British Association for Psychopharmacology (BAP) was founded in 1974. Psychopharmacology is an area of research and knowledge rather than a clinical speciality, although many branches of psychiatry draw upon it.

CLASSIFICATION

Drugs with actions in psychiatric conditions are called psychotropic (affecting the mind) drugs. The classification of these drugs has been a somewhat arcane or obscure subject developed more or less historically rather than scientifically; it is now clearer and based first upon their clinical effects and secondly upon their mechanisms of action, if known.

Broadly speaking, psychotropics are classified according to their main therapeutic use into the following groups: antidepressants; antipsychotics (formerly neuroleptics or major tranquillisers); anxiolytics; mood stabilisers; sedatives or hypnotics; antidementia drugs; and stimulants.

There are further drugs, such as those used to treat addictions or reduce craving, that are outside these groups.

For some classes of drugs, the regulatory authorities have defined requirements that must be met before the drug can be allowed an indication and be promoted for clinical use. These groups are further subdivided according to pharmacology, chemistry, or both (see Box 2.1).

Often these subdivisions can be seen to be rather arbitrary and unhelpful. Many, for example 5-HT and noradrenaline reuptake

---

Box 2.1 Factors for classifying psychotropic drugs

Main therapeutic action (e.g. antidepressant)
Clinical feature of action (e.g. sedation)
Overall pharmacological action (e.g. serotonergic)
Molecular mechanism of action (e.g. reuptake inhibitor)
Chemical structure (e.g. phenothiazine)
Source (e.g. original plant – opiates, atropinics)

inhibitors (SNRIs) and noradrenergic and specific serotonergic antidepressants (NaSSAs), have been invented by drug manufacturers largely as a marketing exercise.

The same drug may have several therapeutic uses, for example antidepressants can be used in anxiety states and eating disorders. The molecular mechanism of action may not be known or may seem simple, whereas the pharmacological actions may be complex and affect many systems; but both are related indirectly or obscurely to the therapeutic effect. The molecular target is often a neurotransmitter receptor, a second messenger system, a reuptake mechanism or a membrane ion channel; sometimes it is an enzyme.

Most drugs have known chemical structures, which can be formally described; but these names are too long and complex to be used routinely. However, a chemical group name is often used to describe drugs or compounds that share similar basic chemical structures. Examples are catecholamines, benzodiazepines, butyrophenones, tricyclics, steroids (sharing the C^{17} hydrocarbon ring) and alkaloids (organic molecules containing nitrogen).

Antidepressants

For a new drug to be marketed as an antidepressant, the European Union requires that it be proved superior to placebo in patients with major depression in both the acute phase (6 weeks) and the medium term (relapse prevention in the 6 months after remission). Far fewer studies have looked at the subsequent long-term follow-up (prophylaxis against recurrence). To market a drug for use in the elderly, separate studies are required. Table 2.1 shows the main antidepressants described in this book.

The three main groups are the monoamine reuptake inhibitors (MARIs) that act predominantly by blocking the reuptake of 5-HT and/ or noradrenaline, the monoamine oxidase inhibitors (MAOIs) and a group that potentiate the same transmitters by complex mechanisms. An alternative classification divides the antidepressants into four broad groups – the MAOIs, tricyclic antidepressants (TCAs), selective 5-HT reuptake inhibitors (SSRIs) and a loose group often called atypical antidepressants. MAOIs include 'traditional' or irreversible inhibitors (which can be subdivided according to their structure) and may also incorporate reversible inhibitors of monoamine oxidase-A (RIMAs), such as moclobemide. TCAs include tertiary amines (amitriptyline) and secondary amines (nortriptyline). SSRIs are not usually subdivided, but atypical antidepressants include a wide range of compounds with varied pharmacological activities. They include reboxetine (noradrenaline reuptake inhibitor; NRI), venlafaxine (SNRI), mirtazapine (NaSSA), nefazodone (5-HT antagonist and reuptake inhibitor; SARI) and many others.

Antipsychotics

The occurrence of neurological (Parkinsonian) side-effects indicated that these drugs affected neurons, and the name neuroleptic (seizes

Table 2.1 Classification of antidepressants

Monoamine reuptake inhibitors (MARIs)				Complex		Monoamine oxidase inhibitors (MAOIs)		
TCA	SSRI	NRI	SNRI	NaSSA	SARI	RIMA	Hydrazines	Non-hydrazines
Amitriptyline	Fluvoxamine	Reboxetine	Venlafaxine	Mirtazapine	Nefazodone	Moclobemide	Phenelzine	Tranylcypromine
Imipramine	Fluoxetine		Milnacipran		Trazodone		Iproniazid	
Clomipramine	Paroxetine							
Dothiepin	Sertraline							
Lofepramine	Citalopram							

TCA, tricyclic antidepressant; SSRI, selective serotonin reuptake inhibitor; NRI, noradrenalin reuptake inhibitor; SNRI serotonin and noradrenaline reuptake inhibitor; NaSSA, noradrenergic and specific serotonergic antidepressant; SARI, serotonin antagonist and reuptake inhibitor; RIMA, reversible inhibitor of monoamine oxidase-A.

Table 2.2 Classification of antipsychotics

	Classical (or typical)	Atypical			
Chemical class	Example	Pure D_2/D_3 antagonists	Mixed S_2/D_2 antagonists SDRAs	D_2-sparing pluripotent PRAs	Others
Phenothiazine: a) aliphatic b) piperidine c) piperazine	Chlorpromazine Thioridazine Trifluoperazine Fluphenazine	Benzamides: Sulpiride Amisulpride	Risperidone Ziprasidone (Sertindole)	Clozapine Olanzapine Quetiapine	Zotepine
Butyrophenone	Haloperidol (Droperidol)				
Thioxanthene	Flupentixol Zuclopenthixol				
Diphenylbutylpiperidine	Pimozide				

SDRA, serotonin and dopamine receptor antagonist; PRA, pluripotent receptor antagonist.

neurons) was at first used to describe them; the term antipsychotic is now preferred. Subsequently, newer drugs have been developed to avoid these side-effects. Antipsychotics are usually termed typical (or classical, i.e. causing acute extrapyramidal effects) or atypical (avoiding them), although the distinction is arguable in many instances.

Typical or classical antipsychotics are usually subdivided by chemistry: phenothiazines, butyrophenones, thioxanthenes, benzamides, etc. To some extent, pharmacological activity is usefully indicated by chemistry. For example, butyrophenones have little anticholinergic activity, aliphatic phenothiazines (e.g. chlorpromazine) are potently hypotensive and benzamides are selective antagonists of D_2-like receptors.

Atypical drugs are occasionally classified according to breadth of pharmacological activity. The term 5-HT and dopamine receptor antagonist (SDRA) is used to describe risperidone and ziprasidone. Clozapine, olanzapine and quetiapine have broader actions (pluripotent receptor antagonists; PRAs, according to some manufacturers); amisulpride has many fewer. Chemical distinctions are unhelpful but of academic interest; for example olanzapine, loxapine and quetiapine have structural similarities to clozapine. The structure may help to predict side-effects; for example those like clozapine in structure tend to be sedative and hypotensive.

Table 2.2 shows the main antipsychotics described in this book, classified according to their clinical effects (classical or atypical) and their structure (in the case of the classical drugs), or their pharmacology (in the case of the atypical ones).

ANXIOLYTIC DRUGS

Anxiolytic drugs include benzodiazepines, barbiturates and other sedatives such as hydroxyzine. Buspirone, an azaspirodecanedione, is also anxiolytic, but is relatively slow acting. Many anxiolytics are also used as hypnotics (sleep-inducers), but not all hypnotics are proven anxiolytics – zolpidem (an imidazopyridine), zopiclone (a cyclopyrrolone) and zaleplon (a pyrazolopyrimidine) are chemically distinct and are used only as hypnotics.

ANTIMANICS AND MOOD STABILISERS

For a drug to be officially labelled and promoted as an antimanic, it should improve the acute manic state and not worsen the bipolar condition over the subsequent 6 months. One definition of a mood stabiliser is a drug that improves either depression or mania and does not worsen or precipitate either state.

The mood stabiliser class usually include only lithium and the anticonvulsants carbamazepine and valproate. Other drugs with fairly clear mood stabilising activity are the antipsychotics, especially clozapine, risperidone and olanzapine. The novel anticonvulsant lamotrigine has narrower mood-stabilising actions (see chapter 32).

Stimulants

Stimulants include any drug known to increase activity and alertness. Examples range from methylxanthines (caffeine, theobromine) to amphetamine-like compounds, including methylphenidate.

The amphetamines can produce secondary psychosis and are therefore among the drugs described as psychotomimetic. Others include phencyclidine. Drugs that produce bizarre visual hallucinations are called psychedelic and include LSD.

Drug names

New patented drugs have generally one generic name and a brand name that may vary between countries. Brand names are chosen to be catchy, easy to remember and inoffensive in the languages of the world; their creation is a skill in itself. Generic names tend to have common endings that give a clue to their actions, for example: -ide is used for benzamide structures, mostly antipsychotics, but also moclobemide; - am is for benzodiazepine anxiolytics; and - olol is for beta-blockers.

However, these rules are not absolute. Other features of the generic name may relate to their structure, source or discoverer.

In an attempt to improve communication about drugs, the World Health Organization (WHO) has decided that certain older drugs with more than one generic name should be described consistently in different countries. For example noradrenaline (or levarterenol) will be known as norepinephrine.

When writing prescriptions, using the generic name reduces the risk of error and gives the pharmacist the right to dispense the cheapest form of the drug.

References and further information

British Association for Psychopharmacology (BAP), 6 Regent Terrace, Cambridge CB2 1AA, UK; tel: 01223 358 395; fax: 01223 321 268; e-mail: susan@bap.org.uk; website: http://www.bap.org.uk.

British Medical Association and Royal Pharmaceutical Society of Great Britain (revised 6-monthly) *British National Formulary*. London & Wallingford: BMJ Books and Pharmaceutical Press.

The United Kingdom Drug Information Pharmacists Group, website: http://www.ukdipg.org.uk

The Association of the British Pharmaceutical Industry (2002) *Compendium of Summaries of Product Characteristics 2002*. London: Datapharm Ltd.

Martindale, W. (1999) *The Complete Drug Reference* (32nd edn). London: Pharmaceutical Press. (First published in 1883.)

3. PRESCRIBING IN PSYCHIATRY: INSIGHT, COMPLIANCE AND PSYCHOEDUCATION

The use of drugs in psychiatry differs from their use in other branches of medicine in a number of important ways.

In general, the exact pathological processes, which underlie mental illness, are not clearly known. Moreover, the drugs used to treat mental illness have until recently, in the main, been based to some extent on chance discoveries. We know that chlorpromazine can effectively treat symptoms of schizophrenia, but we do not know exactly how it does this, nor do we know precisely how schizophrenia arises. Compare this situation with, say, the use of propranolol in angina, and the differences are clear; in the latter case there is an understanding of the aetiology in terms of restricted blood flow, and of the mechanism of drug action in reducing the work of the heart.

Of equal importance are the notions of insight and personal belief systems. In many mental illnesses, patients are partly or completely bereft of insight: they do not understand that they are ill. It is not surprising therefore to find that compliance with antipsychotic medication is poor. Why take a tablet for an illness you do not recognise? Perhaps surprisingly, compliance is in fact poor for most conditions and medications, psychiatric or otherwise. There are many reasons for this, but personal belief systems certainly play a part. The medical model dictates that an illness has a biochemical or pathological cause that can be rectified by the administration of some exogenous compound – a drug. Not all people agree with this view. In particular, many do not recognise that biochemical changes might underlie mental illness, object to taking unnatural chemicals as remedies or believe in self-healing, faith healing, homeopathy or natural detoxification.

The explosion of information in this computer age means that people may be well informed, or more often misinformed rather than uninformed. Remember also that patients are likely to be presented with often complex and inadequately explained data in package inserts. The prescriber can no longer simply write a prescription and pass it over to the patient without a word. Indeed, such practice is probably the best way to ensure poor compliance. Today, prescribers are rightly expected to reach a mutual accord with those being treated about which medication is to be prescribed and to be taken.

COMPLIANCE, ADHERENCE AND CONCORDANCE

Compliance may be defined as the degree of conformity between the standard set for treatment and the treatment accepted by the patient. Non-compliance may be partial or complete. Over-compliance suggests that tolerance, dependence or abuse are occurring. Targets of compliance (in the sense of obeying the doctor's instructions) and adherence (sticking to a written order) are now seen in some situations as inferior to concordance, in which the patient, the person who is to take the medication, should, wherever possible, be involved and feel involved in the process of choosing a treatment or indeed in choosing whether or not to be treated. It should also be remembered that patients expect to be treated with honesty and with candour. Furthermore, poor compliance is a common cause for failure to respond to treatment. The topic of psychoeducation is therefore of great importance in successful prescribing.

It is customary to attribute non-compliance to factors in the illness (lack of motivation as part of depression or schizophrenia, poor concentration, or hopelessness; or the time between stopping medication and relapsing may be long), factors in the patient (lack of insight, lack of knowledge, distrust), factors in the drug (low efficacy, delayed action on symptoms, side-effects) and factors in the doctor (failure to explain the drug and to recognise non-compliance). More recently attention has shifted to the quality of the doctor–patient relationship itself, and to concordance in the views of both partners of it, as important determinants of adherence and outcome.

Do not be afraid to tell patients the whole truth, good and bad, about a drug treatment. What little research there is indicates that concordance is not adversely affected by provision of comprehensive information. If a patient tells you that he or she will not take a medication, then this can none the less be considered a successful interaction. It is better to know that someone will not be taking a drug than to assume wrongly that they will and then base a further decision on this assumption. Note also that not to give a patient enough information to allow him or her informed choice, while seemingly the easiest option, is also the one that pays least respect to basic human rights. Decisions about whether or not to take a drug are in essence based on the balance of benefits and disadvantages. Decisions in medicine (for doctor and patient alike) are often made by balancing conflicting evidence. They are best made after discussion with the patient and the patient's relatives or others who have a legitimate interest. Ultimately, however, the doctor, must be prepared to give well-informed advice, acting in the best interests of the patient. In prescribing a drug, the prescriber is tacitly indicating the relatively greater weight of the benefits. For therapy to be accepted, the patient must come to the same conclusion.

Insight

Insight into mental illness has three components:
  (1) awareness that one is suffering from an illness and that this is a mental as opposed to a physical condition;
  (2) awareness that particular experiences (that may include beliefs, impulses and feelings) may be part of an illness; and
  (3) recognition that treatment (that may include drugs) is needed and may help to relieve the illness or some of its symptoms.

Factors affecting insight include: the nature of the illness; the severity of illness; intellectual ability; cultural influences; and family attitudes.

Insight is generally impaired more severely in mania than in schizophrenia and less in depression. Greater severity of the condition is usually associated with more impairment of insight, but surprisingly, within the spectrum of milder (and non-psychotic) depressive conditions insight actually increases with severity. Both general intellectual ability and abstract thinking, which may involve frontal lobe function, are important. As each acute episode settles there is an opportunity for the patient to review his or her condition, and to gain in understanding of how it changes him-/herself and how medication may help. Unwillingness to acknowledge mental illness may arise from alternative explanatory systems, including religious beliefs, or may be denial motivated by the fear of the stigma attached to a medical diagnosis or label. Ethnic variations in relation to medication involve both genetic differences in metabolism and response (pharmacogenetics) and cultural differences in attitudes and beliefs. Families have their own distinct values and experiences that shape their attitudes towards mental illness. Nevertheless, it is usually to the patient's advantage to share the medical model when a treatment is available and especially one in which he/she and his/her family may be expected to take part in monitoring its benefits and risks. Recognition of the early signs of deterioration (prodrome) is a very important part of insight as it enables earlier interventions such as an increase in medication, which may prevent further worsening. Not surprisingly, insight is closely linked to compliance with treatment (see Box 3.1).

REASONS FOR DISCONTINUING TREATMENT, AND TIMING

In general, compliance is particularly poor with antidepressants, antipsychotics and lithium. In clinical trials it is usual to report the proportion of patients discontinuing because of lack of efficacy, and because of side-effects. Newer drugs with fewer side-effects tend to be associated with fewer drop-outs for the latter reason.

In routine practice up to 50% of patients discontinue antidepressants within 3 months, which is too soon. The reasons for stopping in the first few weeks are perceived lack of efficacy, and side-effects. Later, the common reasons for stopping are that the patient feels better, or that he/she fears dependence and does not recognise the importance of continuing, or that long-term side-effects such as weight gain develop, or previously irrelevant side-effects, such as reduced sexual function, assume more significance as depression improves. Some patients stop medication and refuse to restart, seemingly deliberately opting for illness.

In out-patients with schizophrenia, non-compliance with oral medication is as high as 50%. Even in patients on depot injections, a proportion does not accept treatment as regularly as advised, and this is reflected in relapse rates (see Table 3.1).

In the case of lithium, compliance rates tend to be very low. This has important consequences because of the possibility of withdrawal rebound into mania (see chapter 12).

Box 3.1 Factors affecting adherence to medication

Health beliefs	Complex interactions but lay beliefs usually have a negative effect on compliance. Consider, for example, the trend towards natural remedies and the widely held belief that antidepressants are addictive.
Adverse effects	They usually reduce adherence, especially if the patient is not forewarned. Some people equate severity of adverse effects with a 'strong medicine'.
Effectiveness	Rapidly effective drugs may be taken for a short time only. Many people discontinue antidepressants simply because they feel better. Apparent lack of efficacy also reduces rates of adherence.
Relationships	Trust and respect for prescriber are likely to improve adherence. Subterfuge and dismissiveness of patients inquiries are very likely to reduce adherence. Professionals must act to establish a productive therapeutic alliance.
Ease of obtaining medication	Travel to dispensaries, community centres and other inconvenient locations may reduce adherence. Payment for prescriptions can militate against good adherence.
Insight	Complex effects: many patients adhere well while lacking insight. Steps should be taken to establish insight, but prescribers should be aware of the possibility of so-called intelligent non-compliance, a refusal to take medication despite possession of relevant information. In general, however, insight makes adherence to medication more likely.
The setting	Adherence is higher among in-patients than day hospital or out-patients. Supervision by relatives or hostel staff can help, and the attitudes of these people are important. With depot injections the role of the community psychiatric nurse is crucial.

IMPROVING COMPLIANCE

Steps that may be taken to improve compliance are shown in Box 3.2.

It is useful to enquire at the start "Who has sent this patient to the clinic?" or "Why is this patient in hospital?", meaning "Who has urged or insisted that the patient seek medical help?", because very often relations or workmates, social workers or lawyers or other outside professionals have prompted referral and are expecting some change in the patient. Treatment has therefore to be directed towards them, too.

The patient's personality and lifestyle, as well as his/her illness may affect his/her attitude to treatment. Certain side-effects have greater significance for particular individuals. These include weight gain, drowsiness and reduced sexual function. Sometimes the fear of having a side-effect is more important than the actual side-effect. A side-effect that exacerbates a pre-existing physical disorder is also very

Table 3.1 Adherence to depot medication and associated relapse rates in 1 year (Data from an East London clinic, $n=298$)

Depot medication received (%)	Proportion of patients (%)	Relapse rate (%)
More than 90%	60	13
70–90%	21	29
Less than 70%	15	42
Not known	4	–
Total	100	19

undesirable; such side-effects would include urinary hesitancy, cardiovascular and gastrointestinal problems.

Simpler oral regimes, taking medication once a day in the morning or evening, achieve better adherence than more frequent doses or doses at inconvenient times. When enquiring about compliance the patient may be asked "Do you have any difficulty taking all your prescribed medication?" or "How do you remember to take your medication?" For complex regimes, when several drugs are to be taken, a dosette box (containing a week's supply of tablets in separate compartments for each day and each time of administration) is a useful aid.

If drugs are started one at a time, it will be easier to identify the cause of side-effects. The use of low initial doses allows compensatory bodily mechanisms to occur while the dose is increased and this reduces some side-effects and is more acceptable to patients.

Psychiatric illness may impair a person's self-awareness and knowledge of the impression he/she makes on others, and may also diminish the care he/she takes of him-/herself and his/her appreciation of his/her own interests. The doctor must therefore take on a greater responsibility for the person, a quasi-parental role, in order to serve him/her well, and serve the community in which they live. GPs in particular quite commonly leave it to patients to come back to them if they are dissatisfied or not doing well. This level of supervision may be insufficient for some psychiatric patients; the doctor should give them a definite follow-up appointment (and if it is not kept, check up why not, and make another) for a day or two hence, or a week or two, to see whether the prescription has resulted in any changes in terms

---

Box 3.2 Steps taken to improve compliance

Explore patients' attitudes to illness and treatment
Distinguish between illness and personality
Provide clear advice
Take side-effects seriously
Use easy dose regimes
Introduce drugs gradually
Arrange supervision and follow-up
Psychoeducation
Compulsory treatment
Compliance therapy

of side-effects or of symptomatic improvement. It may be important to ask a relative to come to the appointment too (or to phone in with a report). The patient may not have taken the medicine, or may say it has done no good, whereas the relative may have noted a striking improvement; or it may have produced new symptoms, in which case the doctor should learn of this. The telephone can also be useful for the follow-up of patients who have difficulty travelling or are staying at a distance.

An important part of the art of practice is knowing when to follow up, how often, for how long and in what ways. Psychiatric illness in particular is often chronic even though fluctuating in severity or punctuated by long remissions. It is especially important to have some rational plan of when and how to follow it through, and to ask members of the family or community, particularly those close to the patient, from time to time to give their impressions of progress. This may be to a keyworker whose contact number they have, and who collates information for other members of the multi-disciplinary team.

PSYCHOEDUCATION

Psychoeducation is the provision of information about the illness and its treatment in the context of a medical model based on vulnerability, stress and coping. It can help patients and their families to take full advantage of the increasing range of treatments available by providing the right balance of support, encouragement and expectation. There is widespread misunderstanding in the general public about even as common a condition as depressive illness, with attributions to emotional weakness, moral failings and bad parenting, and a lack of recognition that it has a biological basis involving the brain; it is also widely assumed that antidepressants are addictive. After the first episode of illness the patient him-/herself is usually most in need of a psychoeducational approach, but the family also may be usefully involved. Later it may be helpful for groups of patients or a group of families to take part together; sessions might include the use of videotapes or other material to stimulate discussion.

It is usually helpful (and always correct in respect of human rights) to explain to the patient in appropriately simple language what each drug is supposed to do for him/her and the logic of its use, and to add something about the more common side-effects and what they mean. How this is done must be tailored to the previous knowledge and level of understanding of the individual patient, and take into account any obsessional or hypochondriacal tendencies as well as language difficulties. Most pharmacy departments provide comprehensive information on medication that may be particularly useful for those patients who find discussion with a doctor quite daunting. For some drugs, lithium in particular, the pharmacist gives a leaflet with advice on side-effects, interactions and signs of toxicity. Particularly thorough education is useful for patients undergoing long-term treatment for a severe illness, and their relatives. The outcome of treatment depends very much on creating the right psychological conditions as well as prescribing the right drug in the right dose.

RECOGNISING EARLY SYMPTOMS OF RELAPSE

Patients and relatives should be helped to recognise early features of relapse of the illness (sometimes a unique relapse signature) and to know what action to take in order to alert the relevant professionals. By this means it has been found possible to reduce the frequency of full relapse of mania, although not of depression in bipolar patients. Symptoms of relapse of depression can be difficult to distinguish from less sinister symptoms or symptoms due to other causes such as alcohol.

COMPLIANCE THERAPY

A special type of cognitive therapy called compliance therapy has been developed, aimed at improving the patient's insight, attitude to treatment and compliance, and this has been shown to prolong periods of remission from illness and to delay the need for admission to hospital in patients with psychotic disorders. Attitudes can be more important than the illness or treatment in determining the prognosis, and therapy may be able to change these. The therapy includes discussion of the patient's experiences (including the most recent psychotic episode) and the doctor's understanding of them; the experiences of other patient's; ambivalent attitude towards treatment; fears about dependence, loss of autonomy and side-effects; the value of long-term treatment as protection or insurance; and recognising the early signs of relapse and how to respond to them. Some of the ingredients of these cognitive approaches are those of psychoeducation, which is now seen of a routine part of general clinical care by the psychiatrist and the community psychiatric nurse (CPN). Training courses can improve the effectiveness of the therapist or doctor. When psychological means of coping with stress are also included, the approach has further benefits as well as improving compliance.

OTHER FACTORS TO CONSIDER BEFORE PRESCRIBING

Patient–doctor concordance is only the first step in successful prescribing. Some other major considerations are listed below and are discussed in later parts of the book.

- Evidence for the choice of drug, dose and schedule
- Age, physical health and weight
- Drugs recently or currently being taken
- The effectiveness or otherwise of previous drugs
- The target symptoms both short and long term
- Arrangements for continuation of prescribing and monitoring – the role of GP and CPN.

CONCLUSION

Prescribing in psychiatry has changed markedly over the past 10 years or so. While once good prescribing owed more to art and experience than to science, now an evidence-based scientific approach is essential. Drug choice may ultimately also include personal and social factors, but the single most important component is a knowledge of the scientific basis supporting the use of drugs that might potentially be prescribed. By prescribing better medications in conjunction with psychoeducation and other compliance-enhancing measures, we can hope to have a greater positive impact on the lives of people with mental illness. The rest of this book is devoted to a pragmatic evaluation of the scientific basis of drug use in psychiatry.

FURTHER READING

Anderson, I. M. & Tomerson, B. M. (1995) Treatment discontinuation with selective serotonin reuptake inhibitors compared with tricyclic antidepressants: a meta-analysis. *BMJ*, **310**, 1433–1438.

Bhugra, D. & Bhui, K. (1999) Ethnic and cultural factors in psychopharmacology. *Advances in Psychiatric Treatment*, **5**, 89–95.

Demyttenaere, K. (1998) Non-compliance with antidepressants: who's to blame? *International Clinical Psychopharmacology*, **13**(Suppl 2), 19–26.

Fava, G. (1999) Subclinical symptoms in mood disorders:pathophysiological and therapeutic implications. *Psychological Medicine*, **29**, 47–61.

Johnson, D. A. W. (1984) Observations on the use of long-acting depot neuroleptic injections in the maintenance therapy of schizophrenia. *Journal of Clinical Psychiatry*, **45**, 13–21.

Kemp, R., Kirov, G., Everitt, B., *et al* (1998) Randomised controlled trial of compliance therapy. 18-month follow-up. *British Journal of Psychiatry*, **172**, 413–419.

Paykel, E. S., Hart, D. & Priest, R. G. (1998) Changes in public attitudes to depression during the Defeat Depression Campaign. *British Journal of Psychiatry*, **173**, 519–522.

Perry, A., Tarrier, N., Morriss, R., *et al* (1999) Randomised controlled trial of efficacy of teaching patients with bipolar disorder to identify early symptoms of relapse and obtain treatment. *BMJ*, **318**, 149–153.

Surguladze, S. & David, A. (1999) Insight and major mental illness: an update for clinicians. *Advances in Psychiatric Treatment*, **5**, 163–170.

4. CLINICAL TRIALS AND THE DEVELOPMENT OF NEW DRUGS

The development of new drugs involves many different skills. In a pharmaceutical company chemists, guided by a concept of a new treatment, synthesise new compounds by modifying existing molecules. The new compound is quickly screened for the target activity, by biochemists using test-tube techniques and by pharmacologists using *in vitro* methods and animal models. If it is found to be active, it is screened for acute toxic effects. Having passed these tests it will be studied more extensively in animals to establish its pharmacology. Toxicologists will define its safe limits prior to use in people and will study its distribution, metabolism and excretion. Studies of reproduction, teratology and mutagenicity will be carried out. Only after evaluation of the data for several other species and of experience with similar compounds, is the drug studied in people.

Clinical trials are the bedrock of developing medicine, but are fraught with problematic ethical issues. In dealing with issues such as placebo-controlled trials, the liberalisation of patient information and the compassionate use of unapproved drugs, companies need to strike a balance between the necessity of safeguarding patients, maintaining the pursuit of good science and commercial considerations.

The clinical development of a new drug is divided into four phases. Each phase should be conducted by investigators with relevant expertise and facilities. Every study is based upon a detailed protocol approved by a national regulatory body and a local ethics committee (EC), and requires informed consent by the participating individuals.

Phase 1

In Phase 1 the basic pharmacokinetics, tolerability (side-effects), toxicity and mechanism of action are studied. Safety is the most important consideration and extreme caution is the byword. Healthy young male volunteers free from all other drugs are generally used, because there is no risk of pregnancy and consequent teratogenic effects, and their bodies have intact homoeostatic mechanisms and are the most resilient to trauma. Single and multiple doses are studied and responses monitored. Radioactive labelling is sometimes used to assist in studying metabolism and disposition, if these are complex and other assays cannot be used. These studies should reveal a safe starting dose for use in patients. Further Phase 1 studies can be conducted later, in other groups such as the elderly or people with physical illnesses.

Although there is as yet no legislation in Europe or the US demanding separate drug evaluation in older populations, it is now customary for drug companies to provide data examining the clinical pharmacokinetics, safety, efficacy and dose requirements of new drugs in older people.

The International Conference on Harmonisation Guidelines for drug development research in older people (see Swift, 1998) provides a framework for the planning and execution of such studies. Trials of depression in the elderly must be placebo-controlled if a licence is to be granted for treatment of the elderly; this is increasingly difficult to justify ethically, as more safe and effective drugs become available.

Phase II

In Phase II, patients at whom the drug is targeted receive the drug for the first time, taking a range of doses in open studies. These cannot prove efficacy but will give pointers, and are very important for checking tolerability, and determining doses to be used in later studies. Fewer than a hundred patients may be involved.

The later pivotal studies to prove whether the drug is effective usually require double-blind controlled trials against placebo involving 100 or more patients (late Phase II trials). This is the main way in which the original concept of treatment is proved.

Phase III

Phase III contains the main therapeutic studies, to gain information about efficacy and safety in larger groups and more varied settings. A few thousand patients are likely to participate, and these trials provide information about the characteristics of those who do or do not respond.

The results of Phase I–III studies are submitted to the national regulatory agency to seek approval for a licence to market the drug. The time between synthesis and marketing of a new psychotropic compound is about 8–12 years and incurs enormous costs, but offers the potential for substantial profits. As an example, the cost of developing a new antidepressant launched in 1990 was about US$300 million; in the year 2000, the estimate for worldwide sales was US$2.5bn. This was a particularly successful drug. Costs today are much higher.

Phase IV

Phase IV, the post-marketing phase, involves monitoring of the wider and more prolonged use of the drug. Different groups of patients (especially the elderly) are the subject of further controlled trials and the drug is studied in a wider range of conditions and combinations. Data about safety in pregnancy and breastfeeding will gradually become available.

This phase continues while the drug is on the market and determines its efficacy and safety in routine use. The occurrence of adverse drug reactions (ADRs) and the utilisation (marketing, distribution, prescribing and use of drugs in society) are monitored. Spontaneous, voluntary reporting (the Yellow Card System in Britain) and hospital-based intensive monitoring are the most widely used systems for ADR assessment in this phase. ADRs should be reported if they relate to a new drug, represent previously unknown effects, or result in severe impairment, death, or foetal malformation.

At this stage, rarer side-effects should be detected. For instance, if a side-effect occurs in one patient in a thousand, then 3 000 patients (three times the number) will need to receive the drug in order to have a 95% probability that one patient suffers the side-effect. The problem is confounded by the fact that by no means all adverse events will be reported. The Yellow Card system is the most powerful means of detecting new risks and has lead to new psychotropic compounds being withdrawn from the market, for example because of haemolytic anaemia or Guillain-Barré Syndrome. Its usefulness depends upon the regular participation of sufficient numbers of prescribers.

Intensive monitoring includes case control studies in which patients taking the drug are compared with others who are not, but who are matched for relevant factors such as age, gender and diagnosis. Drug utilisation is studied by market research companies who persuade random samples of prescribing doctors to provide copies of their prescriptions.

CLINICAL TRIAL DESIGN

The design of a clinical trial involves a balance between ethical, scientific, clinical and regulatory requirements. The protocol for a trial will be submitted for approval by the Regulatory Authority (Department of Health) who must issue a certificate if it is to proceed. Large multi-centre trials may be submitted to a multi-centre research ethics committee (MREC), but all protocols also need to be submitted by the investigator to the local (hospital level) EC, so that local factors may be considered.

Many studies are based on the randomly assigned double-blind parallel group comparative design, using a placebo and/or active control. This powerful design was conceived by Bradford Hill during the Second World War and strongly advocated by him from 1946. Sometimes, especially for rarer conditions, within-patient designs are used, in which the same patient is studied on different treatments, as in the placebo cross-over study or Latin Square design. Cessation studies are important for studying rebound phenomena and withdrawal syndromes and can help in assessing prophylactic efficacy.

ETHICS

Ethical principles provide guidance as to what ought to be done and what can be done, and are particularly complex in psychiatry, where the ability of the person to make decisions (autonomy) is affected by mental illness. Respect for the individual's rights and his/her desire to contribute to research is balanced by the collective need to develop optimal treatments, and by common sense. Development of better treatment, and knowledge of which treatment is best, can only be achieved by systematic medical experimentation involving patients.

The Declarations of Helsinki (1964 and 1975) provide a framework for ethical clinical research, adopted by the WHO. These, together with local laws and codes, govern the planning of clinical trials. Their application to a specific project is best ensured by a review by a group of people knowledgeable about local, ethical, cultural, medical and legal issues (ECs). The committee should review the research protocol for the questions of informed consent of the subject, the balance of risks and expected benefits, and confidentiality. They should also ensure that proper insurance exists in the event of damage to the individual, arising either from adherence to the protocol (which is the responsibility of the sponsor), or from negligence of the staff.

One important principle is that participation in the study should not deprive the patient of the best available level of care. Patients in a clinical trial generally receive a high degree of attention to their physical and mental condition.

Participation in a trial is voluntary. Consent is given and witnessed after the patient has received adequate and accurate information including a standard form of words, written in a clear way that he/she can understand. The patients should be free to withdraw from the study at any time, and it must be made clear to them that if they do not wish to participate this will not compromise their entitlement to the usual treatment for their condition.

Payments to healthy volunteers who give up their time to participate are considered ethical, but are usually regarded as unethical inducements for patients; the exception may be when the trial entails inconvenience such as frequent blood sampling for pharmacokinetic studies that cannot be done in healthy volunteers.

RANDOMISATION

To prove efficacy in psychiatric conditions it is necessary to design studies that take account of spontaneous improvement, and of bias in the observer or patient, as well as non-specific factors such as the special attention received by the patient. This can be achieved by: having a control group (receiving a comparator); assigning patients at random to receive either the new treatment or the comparator; and conducting the trial double-blind (neither the doctor nor the patient knowing which treatment is received until all the data from the whole trial are gathered and complete). This is the randomised double-blind controlled trial.

Randomisation is particularly important because it can remove bias arising from any demographic or other unpredictable factors in the patient that may affect his/her response to one of the treatments.

PLACEBO

If the new treatment is much better than the standard treatment, then only these two groups are needed. If, however, the new drug is thought to be about as effective as standard treatment, and if the condition is liable to spontaneous improvement, then efficacy can only be proved by comparison with placebo (see chapter 5). Regulatory authorities in many countries require two 'pivotal studies' in separate and independent centres to demonstrate superiority to placebo before a drug can be licensed for use in a psychiatric condition. It is best (ideally) to include both placebo and standard treatment as comparators because this will show whether the standard treatment is effective under the circumstances of the trial. Otherwise the trial fails as a test of efficacy – a 'failed trial'.

The inclusion of placebo in a study will mean that patients cannot be included if they require immediate active treatment, for example because they are severely disturbed.

In deciding whether to ask an individual patient to participate in a study, the investigator and the patient's own physician must balance the needs of the study with those of the patient.

TRIAL PROTOCOL

This should describe the rationale for the study, and set out the hypotheses to be tested. The selection of patients should be based on inclusion and exclusion criteria; the relevant diagnosis is reached according to standard criteria (such as ICD–10 or DSM–IV) and a particular level of severity on a standard rating scale. The age range, sex and race of the patients may be specified. Exclusion criteria will normally include women who are at risk of pregnancy, patients with somatic illnesses and those who are taking certain other medication or have a history of alcohol or drug misuse.

The number of patients to be recruited to the study should be determined in advance, based upon advice from a statistician. In particular, the number should be sufficient to avoid the possibility of a type II statistical error (false negative result, failing to show a difference between two treatments when one does exist). The power of a study is a measure of its ability to demonstrate a difference that exists in response to two treatments. It is determined by the actual size of that difference, known as the effect size (for definitions see chapter 5), the number of patients included in the study and the spread of results between different patients (standard deviation, for example). Thus, the number to be included should be defined by a power calculation, based on specified and justifiable assumptions about the effect size and on an explicit primary hypothesis about the outcome of the study. Negative results, or results indicating equivalence in effect, are invalid if no power calculation is used.

In some study designs, patients are subdivided or stratified, for instance according to the number and pattern of previous episodes (in order to reduce the risk of chance differences between groups affecting study outcome), and assigned randomly to receive one of the study treatments. Stratification is recommended when clinicians are able to identify clearly the patients likely to respond in a particular way.

The dosage may be variable, fixed or variable within pre-set limits. The use of more than one dose range of active treatment allows dose–response relations to be explored, and compared with the incidence of side-effects.

There should be a wash-out period before entry to the study, to avoid interactions between the new drug and previous medication, and to identify patients who improve spontaneously and are therefore best not included. During the trial, additional medication should be avoided as far as possible. The use of night sedation or anti-cholinergic drugs should be disallowed or standardised, by specifying which drug may be used and under what circumstances.

The patient should be assessed regularly, using validated clinical rating scales for his/her condition. The scales chosen should be comprehensive, sensitive to change and easy to apply in the circumstances of the trial. A scale of global clinical state and improvement, such as the Clinical Global Impression Scale (CGI; Guy, 1976) provides a categorical measure of outcome, useful in calculating absolute risk reduction and number needed to treat (see chapter 5) and for making comparisons between effects in different clinical disorders. Self-reports of improvement should also be recorded. In multi-centre studies it is important to hold training sessions to improve interrater reliability, as variability between raters reduces the power of the study.

Side-effects can be measured by standard checklists and by open enquiry. Known side-effects of the class of drug should be included in the checklist, for example sexual side-effects of antidepressants.

Laboratory tests are monitored at relevant intervals for safety checks. Blood levels of the drug are measured both to confirm adherence to treatment and to explore the relationship between blood level and efficacy.

ANALYSIS OF DATA

All the data should be collected before the trial code is revealed (which patient received which treatment). The results are analysed using appropriate statistical methods, preferably by a statistician independent of the investigators and according to a predetermined analytical plan. Analyses that are suggested after the study is conducted are called *post hoc* analyses, and their findings require replication in a further study.

Patients who drop out or are withdrawn because of side-effects, non-response or recovery pose difficulties for the analysis. When studying the results of a trial it is important to know whether the scores from these drop-outs have been included in the graphs and subsequent analyses. For studies testing efficacy, it is preferable to include the data from all patients who entered the trial and received at least one dose of medication. This is called the 'intent to treat' population. To analyse the results, the scores of patients who drop out early may be carried forward to later time points. This is known as intent to treat analysis with last observation carried forward (LOCF). Sometimes graphs are presented only to the time of drop-out, and this has the effect of exaggerating the improvement shown in the rest of the graph. Alternatively, only those completing the full duration of the study are considered (completer analysis). Analysis of the intent to treat population helps to avoid bias that could arise from allowing individuals to be excluded for special reasons.

For example, if the active comparator (the established drug with proven efficacy in the condition) leads to more early drop-outs through side-effects, the new drug with fewer side-effects may appear spuriously to have greater therapeutic efficacy on intent to treat analysis with LOCF. Similarly, if there are many early drop-outs through lack of improvement in the placebo group, then the advantage of the new and effective drug may appear somewhat exaggerated on intent to treat analysis with LOCF, because patients will have remained on it longer and have greater time for improvement. However, this method of analysis is clearly fairer than analysing only completers because they will include all the placebo-responders.

The information gathered during the trial must respect the patients' confidentiality and must be preserved for several years. Pharmaceutical companies are expected to monitor trials to ensure that they are conducted according to international requirements for good practice in clinical research. This includes the external audit of case notes and of the trial record books on behalf of the regulatory bodies.

The results of well-conducted clinical trials should be published even if the results are not favourable to the new drug.

Today, regulatory authorities demand that manufacturers conduct well-constructed trials before a product licence is issued. Most published comparisons of drug treatments will now be robust and carefully conducted. However, statistical analysis tends to be performed by the company's own statiticians.

Nevertheless, some caution is required in interpreting the results of published trials sponsored by manufacturers. The impression of a larger effect may, for example, be given by presenting graphs in which the lower part of the y-axis is omitted, the so-called 'gee-whizz' graph. The pharmaceutical industry exists, in essence, to make money. All companies are therefore keen to have their products seen in a positive light. This is manifested in two important ways. First, the discussion sections of papers will contain the manufacturer's interpretation of the results obtained, and often give a more positive slant than is appropriate. Second, companies may decline to submit for publication the report of any study that does not show their product in a good light. This leads to publication bias, where the literature includes only positive results – equivocal or negative results are suppressed. Systematic reviews are time-consuming, and some of the most comprehensive reviews are published in journal supplements sponsored by a company. All company-sponsored trial reports and reviews should thus be judged with a 'cold and fishy' sceptic's eye and examined carefully for evidence of bias.

CONSORT STATEMENT AND INTERPRETING TRIAL REPORTS

The "CONSORT statement", published in 1996 (Altman, 1996), lists 17 items that should be included in a report of a clinical trial for it to be thorough. The trials of efficacy described above are conducted under relatively ideal conditions, and the findings may not be generalisable to other more natural clinical situations. This is discussed further in chapter 5.

FURTHER READING

Altman, D. (1996) Better reporting of randomised controlled trials: the CONSORT statement. *BMJ*, **313**, 570–571.

Doll, R. (1990) The development of controlled trials in preventative and therapeutic medicine. *Journal of Biosocial Science*, **23**, 365–378.

—— (1998) Controlled trials: the 1948 watershed. *BMJ*, **317**, 1217–1220.

Guy, W. (1976) *ECDEU Assessment Manual for Psychopharmacology*. Rockville, MD: National Institute for Mental Health.

Johnson, T. (1999) Statistical methods and clinical trials. In *Research Methods in Psychiatry: A Beginner's Guide* (eds C. Freeman & P. Tyrer) (2nd edn), pp. 24–61. London: Gaskell.

Peto, R. & Baigent, C. (1998) Trials: the next fifty years. *BMJ*, **317**, 1170–1171.

Royal College of Psychiatrists' Working Party (2000) *Guideline for Researchs and for Research Ethics Committees on Psychiatric Research Involving Human Participants*. Council Report CR82. London: Gaskell.

Swift C. G. (1998) Drug safety and effectiveness in the elderly. In *Textbook on Geriatric Medicine and Gerontology* (eds R. C. Tallis, H. M. Fillit & J. C. Brocklehurst), pp. 1309–1317. Edinburgh: Churchill Livingstone.

5. PLACEBO EFFECTS, EVALUATING EVIDENCE AND COMBINING PSYCHOTHERAPY

PLACEBO EFFECTS

Patients may get better when treated with tablets without any active drug within them. This is called the placebo effect (Latin, 'I shall please'). It was exploited in former times when inert substances (placebos) were given by apparently successful physicians to treat patients. Today placebos are used in orthodox medicine only as research tools, in clinical trials (see chapter 4). By contrast, the placebo effect may add on to the pharmacological effect where an active drug is used and can thereby be an important part of clinical practice.

On the other hand, patients may complain of side-effects when given placebo treatments. This has been called the nocebo effect (Latin, 'I shall harm'); it would have its most extreme form in voodoo death.

On the positive side, factors contributing to the placebo effect include the patient's confidence in the treatment, his/her suggestibility, his/her belief in the potency of a remedy, which may depend in part on its striking colour or bitter taste, his/her acceptance of the doctor's 'gift' of tablets as symbolic or magical, involving concern or care, and the prestige of medical knowledge. These factors may therefore be as important as an individual drug's pharmacological action in determining the benefits and acceptability of treatment. On the other hand, distrust, together with preconceived notions about side-effects, toxicity or dependence may detract from the beneficial actions of the drug.

In psychiatry a medication is seldom prescribed without a dialogue between the doctor and patient. The patient's decision to seek help can herald some improvement. Often the first contact will have entailed the doctor taking a detailed account of the patient's symptoms and background, and providing some explanation in terms of medical diagnosis or formulation of the psychological problem. Reassurance and encouragement may have been given, and the offer of further help. These in themselves are powerful interventions in some cases, and affect the trust and expectation of the patient.

Placebo responses in clinical trials

We have seen in chapter 4 that in order to prove the efficacy of a new treatment, it is necessary to control for the coincidental action of non-specific factors. This is achieved by the use of a double-blind randomised placebo-controlled design, first used in clinical research in the 1940s. In such a design, the improvement that is seen to occur in the group of patients receiving placebo may arise from any of the above factors.

Box 5.1 Factors contributing to improvement on pacebo

Patient	Illness	Doctor	Previous drugs
Trust	Spontaneous recovery	First interview	Side-effects
Expectation	Fluctuating severity	Explanation	Withdrawal/ rebound
Suggestibility	Engagement with doctor	Reassurance	Delayed effects e.g. of depot injection
Decision to seek treatment	Psychotherapy	Physical examination Investigations	Rescue medication
Change of environment, e.g. hospital admission		Bias	

Box 5.1 lists these factors together with other processes that are controlled for by inclusion of a placebo group. The latter include spontaneous improvement as part of the natural history of the illness, the decline in side-effects resulting from previous medication that was stopped, and the course of any symptoms arising from discontinuation, such as rebound exacerbation of the treated condition. During the early stages of the trial it may be permitted to administer limited amounts of additional medication to calm the patient or to help them sleep; this rescue medication is often a benzodiazepine, and is assumed not to have profound enduring beneficial effects. With both depression and the negative symptoms of schizophrenia improvement arises from the social stimulation of repeated contacts with the investigator. The continuing contacts between the doctor and patient may amount to psychotherapeutic interventions, unless this is deliberately and perhaps unethically avoided within the design of the trial. The beneficial effect of simply giving attention to people is known as the Hawthorne effect, after an electricity plant where it was found to improve productivity. Finally, the enthusiasm or other feelings of the doctor for the treatment under investigation may bias the assessment of improvement.

Placebo response rates

The proportion of patients improving on placebo varies between diagnoses and even among groups with the same diagnosis (see Table 5.1). For instance, in depressive illness the rate varies from 25% to 60%. In schizophrenia it may vary from 20% to 50%, depending upon the criterion of improvement that is used and other factors. More chronically ill patients show lower placebo response rates.

Time course of drug and placebo differences

In studies of depression the difference in improvement in the group of patients on active treatment compared with the group on placebo increases gradually, with little difference until about 2 weeks of treatment and the full difference developing by 6 weeks. In schizophrenia too, the advantage of the active treatment develops slowly, with much of the difference becoming apparent between 2 and 6 weeks, but it increases progressively for several months. In panic disorder, placebo response rates of up to 70% are seen. The use of placebo in studies of mania is especially difficult because of the need for rescue medication in more severe cases. The placebo response in mania is commonly thought to be small, but in clinical trials placebo response rates as high as 25% are found, reflecting factors such as additional rescue medication.

Pattern of responses

The time course of improvement in depression differs in patients improving on placebo from those improving on active treatment. The main difference is that improvement on the drug tends to be delayed until the third week and then to be persistent; by contrast patients who improve on placebo are more likely to show earlier improvement that then has a fluctuating course. Patients who show an early improvement during a placebo run-in have been found to show greater subsequent improvement whether they are assigned to receive placebo or drug during the double-blind phase of the trial. For this reason, a placebo run-in is used in some studies to identify and exclude from the study a group of patients whose inclusion would weaken the power of the study. This tends to increase the potential effect size. The pattern of placebo responses in other conditions has been less studied.

Active placebos

The occurrence of characteristic side-effects during treatment with drugs, such as tricyclic antidepressants or classical antipsychotics, has the potential to un-blind the investigator as to which treatment an individual patient is receiving in a clinical trial. Patients too may recognise a drug they have had before. It has been argued that an active placebo should be employed, for example a drug with atropinic effects rather than a totally inactive tablet. However, atropinic anticholinergic drugs, such as hyoscine, were used extensively to calm psychiatric patients (see chapter 1) and may not be entirely devoid of antidepressant properties. Studies using active placebos do not generally show a lower placebo response rate than studies using inert placebos. The problem can be overcome by making videotaped interviews for blinded raters to assess.

EVALUATING THE EVIDENCE

The fact that a variety of non-pharmacological factors may bring about apparent improvement in psychiatric conditions means that in order to prove the efficacy of any new treatment, it must be shown to be superior to placebo. This demonstration should preferably be in the context of a double-blind comparison, to reduce bias. For drug treatments, this requirement is relatively easy to arrange by producing placebo tablets of identical appearance to the drug. But for

Table 5.1 Drug and placebo response rates in clinical trials, drop-out rates and numbers needed to treat (NNTs)

Diagnosis	Treatment (n patients)	Duration	Criterion of improvement	Drop-outs due to inefficacy (%)	Drop-outs due to adverse events (%)	Response (%)	Absolute risk reduction (%)	NNTs (95% CI)
Major depression Bremner, 1995	Mirtazapine n=50 Placebo n=50	6 weeks	50% less HAM–D 17	6 14	6 4	61 25	36	3 (2–6)
Acute schizophrenia Cole et al, 1964	Phenothiazine n=338 Placebo n=125	6 weeks	Much or very much improved CGI	2 29	3 0	75 23	52	2 (2–3)
Mania Tohen et al, 1999	Olanzapine n=70 Placebo n=64	3 weeks	50% less Y-MRS	29 48	0 3	49 24	25	4 (3–10)
Mania Bowden et al, 1994	Valproate n=68 Placebo n=73	3 weeks	50% less SADS–M	30 51	6 3	48 25	23 24	5 (3–14) 5 (3–22)

	Lithium *n*=35			33	11	49		
Panic disorder Oehrberg *et al*, 1995	Paroxetine *n*=60	12 weeks	50% less panic attacks	2	5	82	32	4 (3–7)
	Placebo *n*=60			5	0	50		
Bipolar maintenance Prien *et al*, 1973	Lithium *n*=101	2 years	No relapse	11	1	57	38	3 (3–4)
	Placebo *n*=104			40	0	19		
Schizophrenia maintenance Hirsch *et al*, 1973	Depot fluphenazine injection *n*=40	9 months	No relapse		9	92	58	2 (2–3)
	Placebo *n*=41					34		
Alzheimers dementia Rosler *et al*, 1999	Rivastigmine 6–12 mg *n*=243	26 weeks	CIBIC – plus improvement	2	27	37	17	6 (4–11)
	Placebo *n*=239			2	9	20		

HAM-D, Hamilton rating scale for depression – 17 items; CGI, Clinical Global Impression scale; Y-MRS, Young mania rating scale; SADS-M, schizophrenia and affective disorders scale mania component; CIBIC, Clinician's Interview Based Impression of Change.

Box 5.2 Hierarchy of quality of evidence

(1)   Clear advantage over placebo in at least one randomised controlled trial, preferably replicated at a different centre.

(2)   Series of cases compared to a non-randomised control series.

(3)   Consecutive series of cases described by a respected authority.

(4)   Dramatic results in an uncontrolled series of cases.

(5)   Single case report.

---

psychological treatments it is difficult or impossible to ensure that the patient and assessor are blind to which treatment is being or has been given, or to separate the specific element of the treatment from non-specific elements. Nevertheless, it is imperative that placebo treatment groups should be included if the therapy is to have credibility.

Apart from the parallel group randomly assigned double-blind placebo-controlled trial, other lesser standards of evidence may provide the earliest indications that a treatment is effective. Box 5.2 lists the forms of evidence that may support the use of a treatment, in order of declining conclusiveness.

Systematic reviews and meta-analysis

When several RCTs have been reported with similar designs, these can be analysed together using the method of meta-analysis. This allows the consistency of the findings to be examined, and an overall conclusion to be drawn about the effect size, using the pooled data. The technique of a funnel plot can identify whether there is a gap, suggesting that there may be missing data, such as might arise from a bias to publish positive findings.

The methods of systematic review are intended to identify all available data relevant to the subject being studied. As well as searching a variety of computerised databases, it is important to attempt to include unpublished findings; these may be more negative than those that are readily accessed. They may be obtained by personal communication with investigators, or by approaching pharmaceutical companies and seeking internal reports on studies that were not published.

Size of effect and NNT

Beyond establishing that a treatment is more efficacious than placebo in a condition, it is important to be able to describe the magnitude of the benefit it has (the size of effect). This enables the doctor to tell the patient how likely it is that the treatment will help them; it also enables comparisons to be made with other treatments for the same condition, or indeed for different conditions. One of the simplest measures of size of effect is the difference in the percentage of people improving on the treatment from the percentage who improve on placebo (also known as the absolute risk reduction). To make this comparison, improvement must be defined at the start of the trial using a criterion that can be readily recognised. As an example, the change in the overall clinical state might be used, and the percentage of patients counted who are much improved or very much improved according to the Clinical Global Impression (CGI) scale. Alternatively, if a well-known and validated rating scale is used, then a patient might be defined as improved if his/her score falls below a defined threshold, or if his/her score decreases by the average amount (for instance 20% or 50%) by the end of the trial.

This measure of size of effect can be converted to the NNT, by dividing the difference into 100. For example, in the treatment of depression there is commonly a difference of about 33% between the proportion of patients improved on antidepressant drug and the proportion who improved on placebo. The NNT is then 100/33 or about 3. This means that in order for the drug to bring about improvement in one patient, three patients must be treated, one of whom would have improved on placebo; the third patient will remain unwell. For a drug that is always effective in an otherwise untreatable chronic condition the NNT is 1. A treatment with a large NNT might be considered useful if no other treatments are available, or if it is used as an adjunct to other treatments that are only partially effective and it has few side-effects. At present many research reports do not provide sufficient information about size of effect. Table 5.1 summarises the results of influential clinical trials in different conditions, showing the drop-out rates, absolute risk reduction and NNT. Similarly the frequency of adverse effects can be described in terms of a number needed to harm (NNH).

Table 5.1 follows the convention that NNT is expressed as the next highest integer; for example, a NNT of 3.3 would be tabulated as 4.

Other measures of size of effect

The difference in effect between two treatments can also be described using the scores on rating scales as the difference between the mean scores on drug and placebo divided by the standard deviation of the scores, and this is what is usually called the 'effect size'. Another way of comparing a treatment with placebo is to calculate the ratio of the event occurring, for example the relapse rates; this is called the relative risk reduction. In comparing two different drugs, the risk ratio or the closely related odds ratio may also be used.

Efficacy v. effectiveness

We have seen that the efficacy of a treatment is established by means of double-blind RCTs with placebo control groups, carried out in carefully selected patients under relatively ideal circumstances. The disadvantage of such exploratory trials is that their results may not be generalisable. This is because they tend to have strict entry criteria that exclude many patients, they are conducted at specialised research centres and the outcome measures are often subtle, based on sensitive rating scales. Both the patients and the investigating doctors may be atypical. In clinical practice it is important to know what advantage accrues for everyday patients who are started on a treatment compared with those who are not, and when other interventions are allowed as their doctor judges necessary. This is called effectiveness. In general, treatments that are inconvenient or are associated with unwanted side-effects are less effective, because patients discontinue them before deriving the full benefit.

Explanatory *v.* pragmatic trials

Effectiveness too is measured in RCTs, by including as many patients as possible and continuing to monitor the condition of patients who stop treatment, rather than carrying forward the last value before they discontinued treatment (the pragmatic trial, as opposed to the explanatory trial used to prove efficacy). In this way a treatment of proven efficacy may appear much less effective in the routine clinic.

Pragmatic trials are conducted on treatments of proven efficacy, but explore a practical question and aim to exclude as few relevant patients as possible. The outcomes are then compared after a set interval, for example 1 year, using a range of outcome measures.

Large scale randomised pragmatic trials are needed to detect small but meaningful advantages of treatments, for example with adjunctive drug combinations. Patients are suitable to enter such a study only when the clinician is substantially uncertain which of the trial treatments would be most appropriate for that individual (the 'uncertainty principle') and when the patient is willing to accept any one of the options to which he/she may be randomly assigned.

Consensus statements and clinical guidelines

The complexities and cost of modern medicine have forced a sea change in therapeutic decision-making. In the past, clinicians prescribed drugs, observed their effects and developed an individual view of effectiveness and tolerability. Some would be influenced by clinical trials. Today, clinicians are more often expected to be influenced by published guidelines and consensus statements. Indeed, in some countries managed care arrangements effectively remove from clinicians any individualised choice of therapy by stipulating exactly the sequence of treatment options in a given illness. However, in an age of litigation, guidelines can become a constraint on clinicians, and consensus statements may simply repeat what the guidelines have enshrined as correct.

Ideally, both consensus statements and clinical guidelines should be predominantly evidence-based. That is, the guidance they provide should essentially be a pragmatic summary of a systematic review of published data, which may include meta-analyses of published trials. There is some room to accommodate individual views of clinicians, but perhaps only where there are gaps in the evidence base. Where individual views are allowed to dominate, guidelines merely represent the ideas of the most forceful contributors and may be wildly at odds with published data.

Guidelines should also closely match what is already done in clinical practice. Clinicians are, by nature, likely to change habits only by gradual increments and tend to reject wholesale change. Sadly, many published guidelines are rather too dependent on individual views and recommend practices some way different from that which is current. Even when they are well constructed, guidelines and consensus statements are, for one reason or another, widely ignored. There are, for example, numerous guidelines on the treatment of depression in the community, but prescription surveys repeatedly show that adherence to these guidelines occurs in less than one-fifth of cases.

Nevertheless, prescribing in psychiatry is likely to be increasingly influenced by guidelines and consensus statements. In the UK, for example, the National Institute for Clinical Excellence (NICE) will be publishing guidance on a number of treatments. The role of the individual clinician will evolve into that of assessing the cogency of any guidelines and then of being guided but not governed by them.

COMBINING DRUG TREATMENT AND PSYCHOTHERAPY

Introduction

The value of combining psychological treatment with drug therapy is more difficult to evaluate than the efficacy of a single treatment, because larger numbers of patients must be studied to detect what are likely to be small differences between combined as opposed to single treatments. When combining two treatments, there are several possible outcomes.

A treatment that was not very effective alone may become effective in the presence of the other treatment. This is called potentiation or augmentation. An example would be the need for a patient with schizophrenia to be receiving effective antipsychotic medication in order for progress to be made with problem-solving or psychosocial interventions. Similarly, psychoeducation or compliance therapy may potentiate drug treatment, but add nothing for patients on placebo.

The combined action of two effective treatments may be greater than either alone (addition). However, two effective treatments given together may produce no greater effect than one given alone (reciprocation); this is likely when both share the same mechanism of action.

Complications of combining therapies

Both drugs and psychotherapy are capable of producing adverse effects either alone or in combination. The combined effect may then be less than the greater of the two separately (inhibition).

The use of combined drug and psychological treatments should not distract from giving adequate doses of medication, or from emphasising to the patient the importance of the medicine in his/her treatment or his/her progress. The patient may start with or develop negative views about either drug or psychological treatment; these may benefit from exploration and explanation. If separate therapists give the two treatments, each should be aware of the dangers of splitting, and should usually advise the patient to express any misgivings directly to the other therapist. The prescriber should avoid being drawn in as a second psychotherapist.

For the more difficult personality disorder it is important to be consistent and not be easily persuaded to change from one drug to

Table 5.2 Depressive illness treated with drugs or psychotherapy

Diagnosis	Treatment (n patients)	Duration	Criterion of improvement	Drop-outs due to inefficacy or adverse events (%)	Response (%)	ARR (%)	NNT (95% CI)
Depression Elkin et al, 1989	Imipramine (n=57)	16 weeks	Recovery: HAM-D < 6	33	42	21	5 (3–20)
	IPT (n=61)			23	43	22	5
	CBT (n=59)			32	36	15 (NSD)	
	Placebo (n=62)			40	21		

ARR, absolute risk reduction; NNT, numbers needed to treat; HAM-D, Hamilton rating scale for depression; IPT, interpersonal psychotherapy; CBT, cognitive–behavioural therapy.

Table 5.3 Drug treatment, IPT or the combination in preventing recurrences of depressive illness in older patients

Diagnosis	Treatment (n patients)	Duration	Criterion of improvement	Dropouts due to inefficacy or adverse events (%)	Response (%)	ARR (%)	NNT (95% CI)
Recurrent unipolar depression (Age over 59) Reynolds et al,1999	Nortriptyline plus IPT (n=25)	3 years	No recurrence	12	80	70	2 (2)
	Nortriptyline (n=28)				57	47	2 (2–4)
	IPT (n=25)			7	36	26	4 (3–24)
	Placebo (n=29)				10		

ARR, absolute risk reduction; NNT, numbers needed to treat; IPT, interpersonal psychotherapy.

another without rationale. Also, beware of sudden dramatic improvements apparently as a result of your new treatment; these will often lead to disappointment and to further challenges for additional help.

DEPRESSION AS AN EXAMPLE FOR COMBINED TREATMENT

Table 5.2 shows findings in a study of out-patients with depression treated separately with antidepressant medication, cognitive–behavioural therapy (CBT), interpersonal psychotherapy (IPT) or placebo. A stringent criterion for improvement was applied. The groups treated with imipramine or IPT showed significant benefit, but for CBT the benefit was not significant. It is widely believed that the results of this single trial may underestimate the value of CBT in depression.

CBT

For out-patients with depression most studies of CBT show a slight positive effect, but little or no additive effect. Adjunctive CBT is of most value when the patient is less severely ill or has intractable personal problems. For the prevention of recurrences, inconsistent additive effects have been seen and compliance may be improved.

IPT

IPT is widely practised, and is of most value for more complex clinical conditions, when there are comorbid disorders or when the illness affects broad aspects of the persons life. Its focus is on interpersonal and familial factors. It is effective in milder cases of depressive illness. In combination, there are additive effects on social adaptation but less so on acute symptoms, supporting the notion that drugs help symptoms and IPT helps with the problems.

For recurrences, no benefit was found from adding IPT to amitriptyline in younger patients. However, in older patients, as shown in Table 5.3, the combination of IPT with drug treatment was more effective than IPT alone; the superiority over drug treatment alone was a trend but not statistically significant. No advantage has been found from adding IPT to drug treatment in the prophylaxis of bipolar disorder.

Specific psychological approaches in other conditions

The rationale for the combination differs between conditions. For example, in schizophrenia psychotherapy may help by improving compliance but is unlikely otherwise to help much unless the patient is already benefiting from medication; then CBT may help to reduce the intrusiveness of hallucinations.

In panic disorder drug treatment confers additional benefit to CBT, but CBT is an important addition when phobic avoidances persist (see p. 168). In obsessive–compulsive disorder (OCD) drug treatments are of limited value unless combined with CBT for compulsive behaviour (see p. 173). In bulimia nervosa drug treatment alone can provide short-term and limited relief but CBT is of greater and more enduring benefit, and the addition of drug treatment confers little further advantage (see p. 231).

FURTHER READING

Assessing evidence

Altman, D. G. (1998) Confidence intervals for the number needed to treat. *BMJ*, **317**, 1309–1312.

Brown, T. & Wilkinson, G. (eds) (1998) *Critical Reviews in Psychiatry*. London: Gaskell.

Centre for Evidence Based Mental Health: http://www.psychiatry.ox.ac.uk/cebmh.

Crombie, I. K. (1996) *The Pocket Guide to Critical Appraisal*. London: BMJ Publishing.

Greenhalgh, T. (1997) *How to Read a Paper: The Basics of Evidence-Based Medicine*. London: BMJ Publishing.

Laupacis, A., Sackett, D. L. & Roberts, R. S. (1988) An assessment of clinically useful measures of the consequences of treatment. *New England Journal of Medicine*, **318**, 1728–1733.

Sackett, D. & Cook, R. (1995) The number needed to treat: a clinically useful measure of treatment effect. *BMJ*, **310**, 452–454.

——, Strauss, S. E., Richardson, W. S., *et al* (2000) *Evidence-based Medicine. How to practise and teach EBM* (2nd edn). Edinburgh: Churchill Livingstone.

Tables of NNTs: http://www.jr2.ox.ac.uk/bandolier/band50/b50-8.html.

Placebo

De Craen, A. J. M., Kaptchuk, T. J., Tijsson, T. J. P., *et al* (1999) Placebos and placebo effects in medicine: historical overview. *Journal of the Royal Society of Medicine*, **92**, 511–515.

Harrington, A. (ed.) (1999) *The Placebo Effect: An Interdisciplinary Exploration*. Cambridge, MA: Harvard University Press.

Quitkin, F. M. (1999) Placebos, drug effects, and study design: a clinician's guide. *American Journal of Psychiatry*, **156**, 829–836.

Combination with psychotherapy

Paykel, E. (1999) Prevention of relapse in residual depression by cognitive therapy. *Archives of General Psychiatry*, **56**, 829–835.

Reynolds, C. F., Frank, E., Perel, J. M., *et al* (1999) Nortriptyline and interpersonal psychotherapy as maintenance therapies for recurrent major depression: a randomised, controlled trial in patients older than 59. *Journal of the American Medical Association*, **281**, 39–45.

Rush, A. J. & Thase, M. E. (1999) Psychotherapies for depressive disorders. In *Depressive Disorders* (eds M. Maj & N. Sartorius), pp. 161–206. WPA Series: *Evidence and Experience in Psychiatry*. Volume 1. Chichester: John Wiley & Sons.

DeRubeis, R. J., Gelfand, L. A., Tang, T. Z., *et al* (1999) Medication versus cognitive behavior therapy for severely depressed outpatients: mega-analysis of four randomised comparisons. *American Journal of Psychiatry*, **156**, 1007–1013.

Pragmatic trials

Hotopf, M., Churchill, R. & Lewis, G. (1999) Pragmatic randomised controlled trials in psychiatry. *British Journal of Psychiatry*, **175**, 217–223.

Roland, M. & Torgerson, D. J. (1998) What are pragmatic trials? *BMJ*, **316**, 285.

Doctor–patient relationship

Downes-Grainger, E., Morriss, R. K., Gask, L., *et al* (1998) Clinical factors associated with short-term change in outcome of patients with somatized mental disorder in primary care. *Psychological Medicine*, **28**, 703–711.

Hughes, P. & Kerr, I. (2000) Transference and countertransference in communication between doctor and patient. *Advances in Psychiatric Treatment*, **6**, 57–64.

Tasman, A., Riba, M. B. & Silk, K. R. (2000) *The Doctor–patient Relationship in Pharmacotherapy: Improving Treatment Effectiveness*. New York & London: Guilford Press.

Clinical trials

Bowden, C., Brugger, A. M., Swann, A. C., *et al* (1994) Efficacy of divalproex vs lithium and placebo in the treatment of mania. *JAMA*, **271**, 918–924.

Bremner, J. D. (1995) A double-blind comparison of Org 3770, amitriptyline, and placebo in major depression. *Journal of Clinical Psychiatry*, **56**, 519–525.

Cole, J. O., Goldberg, S. C. & Klerman, G. L. (1964) Phenothiazine treatment in acute schizophrenia. *Archives of General Psychiatry*, **10**, 246–261.

Hirsch, S. R., Gaind, R., Rohde, P., *et al* (1973) Outpatient maintenance of chronic schizophrenic patients with long-acting fluphenazine: double-blind placebo trial. *BMJ*, **1**, 633–637.

Oehrberg, S., Christiansen, P. E., Behnke, K., *et al* (1995) Paroxetine in the treatment of panic disorder. A randomised, double-blind, placebo-controlled study. *British Journal of Psychiatry*, **167**, 374–379.

Prien, R. F., Caffey, E. M. Jr & Klett, C. J. (1973) Prophylactic efficacy of lithium carbonate in manic-depressive illness. Report of the Veterans Administration and National Institute of Mental Health collaborative study group. *Archives of General Psychiatry*, **28**, 337–341.

Rosler, M., Anand, R., Cicin-Sain, A., *et al* (1999) Efficacy and safety of rivastigmine in patients with Alzheimer's disease: international randomised controlled trial. *BMJ*, **318**, 633–638.

Tohen, M., Sanger, T. M., McElroy, S. L., *et al* (1999) Olanzapine versus placebo in the treatment of acute mania. *American Journal of Psychiatry*, **156**, 702–709.

Guidelines

Elkin, I., Shea, T. M., Watkins, J. T., *et al* (1989) National Institute of Mental Health Treatment of Depression, Collaborative Research Programme. General effectiveness of treatments. *Archives of General Psychiatry*, **46**, 971–982.

Hurwitz, B. (1999) Legal and political considerations of clinical practice guidelines. *BMJ*, **318**, 661–664.

In this chapter we are concerned with the physical factors that determine the way in which the drug in a medicine enters the body and travels in the circulation, reaching a well-protected brain. The safe and effective use of modern psychotropic drugs must be informed by the pharmaceutical and metabolic considerations described briefly below.

TERMINOLOGY

It is useful to explain a number of terms used in clinical pharmacology. 'Pharmacokinetics' is the study of all the factors that determine the concentration of the drug at its site of action – what the body does to the drug. 'Pharmacodynamics', on the other hand, is the study of the mechanisms by which a drug exerts its actions – what the drug does to the body. It is the former we are concerned with in this chapter.

Pharmacokinetics uses a range of well-defined terms. 'Bioavailability' is the extent to which the drug reaches the systemic circulation when taken by a patient orally or parenterally, compared with the same quantity of drug given intravenously. In trying to understand the relation between size of dose, concentration in the blood and duration of clinical effect, a simple model is often used (see Figure 6.1). The body is assumed to be a single vessel of fluid in which the drug will rapidly disperse. The 'volume of distribution' of a drug is the volume of the imaginary vessel necessary to account for the amount of drug given at the diluted plasma concentration to which the drug falls shortly after its administration and rapid absorption. For example, say we give 100 mg of drug (A) by the intravenous route (100% bioavailability). A very short time later the concentration of drug (A) in the plasma is found to be 1 mg/l. The volume required to account for all the drug given at the plasma level measured is $100 \div 1$ litres. Thus the apparent volume of distribution is 100/litre.

The volume of distribution of a drug gives some idea of the whereabouts of the drug in the body. A low value (say 5–10 litres) indicates that the drug is concentrated in blood itself. A very high value (say, 1000 litres or more) indicates that the drug is concentrated in the cells or fatty tissues and not the blood.

Elimination of most drugs follows exponential or 'first-order kinetics'. That is, a constant fraction of the whole in the body is eliminated per unit of time, independent of the actual concentration of the drug. This corresponds to an exponential decline in concentration. A few (e.g. phenytoin, alcohol) are eliminated by relatively inefficient processes, by enzymes present in such small amounts that the concentration of drug quickly saturates them. When the enzymes are working thus at maximum pitch, a constant steady quantity of drug is eliminated per unit of time, whatever the body load. This slower process is one of 'zero-order kinetics' and the concentration in the blood declines linearly.

The 'plasma half-life' indicates how long it takes for the concentration of drug in the plasma to decline to half its previous level. It is a convenient measure of persistence in the body, which will affect the

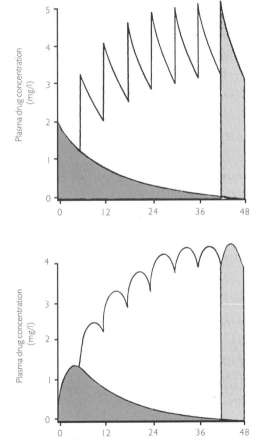

Figure 6.1 Graphical representation of multiple dosing and steady state

The gradual rise in plasma concentration during regular doses of a drug given intravenously or orally. The dosing interval is 6 hours and the half-life is 12 hours. Steady state is approached after 48 hours. The fluctuation of level is greater with the intravenous than the oral route.

frequency of dosing. It is only useful for describing first-order kinetics, as the half-life remains the same whatever the concentration. Another measure is the 'clearance', the fraction of the total volume of distribution emptied, theoretically, of all drug in unit time.

Measurement of plasma concentrations of a drug at various times after a single intravenous dose can show the elimination kinetics, the volume of distribution and plasma half-life, and thereby indicate what dose, repeated in what frequency, should be used to achieve any concentration of drug in the body fluids at a particular time. From a knowledge of a drug's half-life one can predict how long it will take for a steady state to be reached after regular dosing commences (at 'steady state' the rate of removal equals the rate of input). Thus, after the passage of one half-life, the concentration of drug in the blood will have risen to within 50% of the eventual steady state level; after 2 half-lives to within 25%, 3 half-lives 12.5% and so on. After 5 half-lives it will have risen to within 3.125%, or almost 97% of the steady state. Thus, for a drug such as haloperidol, with a half-life of 18 hours, the steady state will have been effectively reached after about 90 hours (5×18) or 4 days. A depot drug such as haloperidol decanoate has an average half-life of about 3 weeks and so during regular dosing the steady state will not be approached until 15 weeks have passed. Depots are unusual in that their apparent half-life is dependent upon rate of drug release, not drug removal.

Under circumstances where the half-life is very long, it is sometimes desirable to give a loading dose (that is a large first dose) or more frequent initial doses to reach the desired steady state level more quickly, and then to reduce the frequency of dosing in order to maintain it. In psychiatry, however, it is rare for high plasma levels to be associated with a more rapid effect.

'Tolerance' is said to have occurred when the same drug effect can be obtained only by increasing the dose (seen with opiates, alcohol and benzodiazepines). This is sometimes for pharmacokinetic reasons – the drug is metabolised more quickly when the body has been exposed to it for longer. Alternatively, tolerance may represent an adaptation to the action of the drug, so a high concentration is needed to bring about the same effect. 'Tachyphylaxis' is the very rapid development of tolerance after only two to three doses; this is most often due to desensitisation of the drug receptors (a process of the receptors becoming less sensitive to a stimulus). Benzodiazepines are a good example here. Tolerance can also arise from slower adaptive changes, including up-regulation of receptors with antagonists, and down-regulation with agonists (see p. 66). 'Dependence' occurs where there are physical or psychological symptoms on attempted discontinuation of the drug, which drive reinstatement of the drug. Drug addiction is characterised by craving, much time spent on drug-seeking and drug-taking behaviour, and both physical and psychological symptoms developing on withdrawal.

Pharmaceutics

A tablet is not all active drug, but contains excipients that bind the ingredients and add bulk to the tablet. It may be covered with a coating, often coloured. An injection has a vehicle; a syrup may have a solvent, a stabiliser and a preservative. Occasionally these supposedly inert substances have unwanted effects, producing, for example, an allergic reaction. (Changing to another brand of the same drug, made up differently, may avoid these adverse effects.) Differences in bioavailability between different brands may sometimes, although rarely, explain the failure of a drug to produce the intended response.

ABSORPTION

Some (a very few) drugs are absorbed from the stomach, others only from a part of the intestine. Delayed gastric emptying may slow the absorption of intestinally absorbed drugs if taken before a meal, when the pylorus is shut. Some drugs, lithium carbonate for instance, are gastric irritants and best taken with some food. The pH of gastric and intestinal contents, the occurrence of intestinal hurry or delay, the nature of the diet and its digestion may all influence the rate of absorption and so the speed of onset of drug action. A partial gastrectomy, malabsorption syndromes and diarrhoea may alter the speed and completeness with which a drug enters the portal circulation from the gut.

With oral preparations of drugs, the rate, and sometimes the extent, of absorption is largely determined by disintegration and dissolution of the dosage form, both processes being a prerequisite for absorption. Tablets and capsules must disintegrate into smaller pieces to expose a greater surface area for dissolution. This process is aided by bursting agents such as starch. Disintegration is often deliberately prolonged (by hard compaction or by incorporating drug in a wax matrix) to provide a reservoir of drug in the gut. Such modified release preparations prolong drug effect and reduce peak plasma concentrations and so may reduce adverse effects (for example, with lithium, venlafaxine and carbamazepine). They may also need less frequent administration (e.g. sodium valproate, venlafaxine).

Dissolution rate is dependent on the size of drug particle, the drug's solubility and the properties (e.g. pH) of intestinal fluid.

Drugs absorbed from the gastrointestinal tract must pass through the intestinal mucosa into the portal circulation and through the liver; some are at once partly destroyed in the mucosa and liver (first-pass metabolism, which may be substantial) before distribution to the rest of the body. Some drugs – diazepam, some antidepressants and antipsychotics, for instance – have therapeutically active metabolites produced in the liver. In contrast, drugs given intravenously, intramuscularly, rectally, sublingually or by nasal spray are distributed first to the lungs and then to the general circulation, brain and body, with a smaller fraction to the liver. By these routes the brain gets a bigger share of the given drug dose than from the same oral dose because of greater bioavailability. The overall effect of the same dose given by different routes may therefore differ markedly.

Liquids or syrups are more quickly absorbed than the contents of tablets because disintegration and dissolution are not required. Diazepam taken as a liquid by mouth, for example, is effective more quickly than the same dose given by intramuscular injection (diazepam is slowly and erratically absorbed from muscle). In psychiatry, liquids are generally used to ensure adherence, rather than to speed the onset of drug action.

METABOLISM

The liver is the chief site of drug metabolism, but gut wall, kidney, lung and placenta may also break down drugs (Figure 6.2), as do the microflora of the gut. Hepatic, oxidative metabolism of drugs is largely controlled by the cytochrome P450 series of enzymes. The activity of this system is at its highest in childhood and declines with age from the early teens. Some liver enzymes that metabolise drugs are reliably increased in quantity, or induced, over a week or more by many substances. These include tobacco smoke, alcohol, phenytoin and some psychotropic drugs (barbiturates, carbamazepine, phenothiazines, orphenadrine). Heavy drinkers, and smokers, people with epilepsy

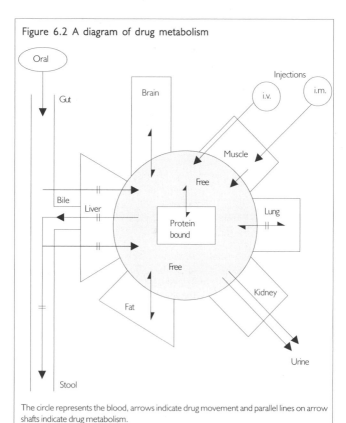

Figure 6.2 A diagram of drug metabolism

The circle represents the blood, arrows indicate drug movement and parallel lines on arrow shafts indicate drug metabolism.
i.v., intravenous; i.m., intramuscular.

and other chronic drug users may therefore need bigger doses of some psychotropic drugs than usual. Carbamazepine induces the liver enzymes that destroy it, and other drugs. Its psychotropic effects may wear off after about 2 weeks of use because additional enzymes become active and the drug is destroyed more quickly. A higher dose is then needed.

In contrast, patients with congestive cardiac failure or other causes of impaired hepatic perfusions arising from liver damage, babies with underdeveloped liver function and the elderly (whose hepatic performance is somewhat diminished) require smaller doses of many psychotropic drugs than the norm for their body weight.

Certain steroids, particularly progestogens and oestrogens, which are used in oral contraceptives, inhibit drug metabolism. A woman taken off 'the pill' may then require more psychotropic drugs as her metabolism increases. Pregnant women, with their raised progesterone levels, metabolise drugs less effectively. Drugs to be continued through pregnancy may need to be reduced in dose if they are subject to metabolic destruction, but should be increased again after delivery.

The outcome of hepatic metabolism is that drugs are made more soluble in water, so that they are less protein-bound and can be filtered and excreted in the kidneys. Drug metabolism is sometimes considered in two phases. Phase 1 involves enzymatic oxidation or reduction, hydroxylation, demethylation and hydrolysis; all produce metabolites that are more water soluble, so a greater proportion of them can be excreted by the kidney. Sometimes these metabolites are pharmacologically as active as the parent compound: for example risperidone (hydroxyrisperidone), lofepramine (desmethylimipramine) and amitriptyline (nortriptyline), but more often they are inert. Phase 2 is the conversion of phase 1 metabolites to conjugates by acetylation, sulphation or conjugation with glucuronic acid; the resultant compounds are very water soluble and are excreted by the kidney. Active metabolites are rarely produced by phase 2 reactions. One of the few important active glucuronides is morphine-6-glucuronide, a metabolite produced from morphine and diamorphine.

Phase 1 metabolism is reduced with ageing, but phase 2 tends to be maintained even in the elderly. Thus, drugs that are metabolised mainly by phase 2, such as oxazepam, do not accumulate to a much greater extent in the elderly. In addition to the decline in liver enzymes including the P450 system (see below) in the elderly, their liver metabolism is more likely to be diminished because of concurrent physical illnesses and their use of medication of other kinds.

CYTOCHROME P450

The cytochrome P450 mono-oxygenase system (CYP) of liver microsomal enzymes is classified using a numerical system. These are enzymes with a haem group containing an iron atom and hence are pink (P) in colour. Certain enzymes are particularly important in relation to psychotropic drugs. For example, the hepatic hydroxylase CYP IID6 plays an important part in the metabolism of tricyclic antidepressants and antipsychotics. About 7–10% of Caucasians have low levels of this enzyme and are slow metabolisers of these drugs. These people can be detected by their slow metabolism of debrisoquine or dextromethorphan. Similarly, a proportion of individuals have low levels of acetylase; this results in them being slow acetylators of drugs including phenelzine. These are autosomal recessive traits. Some drugs inhibit the hydroxylase enzymes – for instance phenothiazines, fluoxetine and paroxetine – leading to increases in the level of tricyclic antidepressants by up to four times.

Over the past 10 years, much has been learned about the various hepatic cytochrome enzymes and their functions. Table 6.1 provides a useful summary. Note that drugs may be metabolised by a number of enzymes and may also inhibit or induce a range of different cytochromes.

Table 6.1 Cytochrome enzymes and psychotropic drugs

CYP	Genetic influence?	Inducible?	Examples of substrates	Inhibitors[1]	Inducers
IID6	Yes (7–10%) slow metabolisers	No	Phenothiazine Butyrophenones Sertindole Risperidone Tricyclics SSRIs Venlafaxine Mirtazapine Propranolol Pindolol	Phenothiazines Tricyclics Haloperidol Fluoxetine Paroxetine Pindolol	None
IA2	No	Yes	Caffeine Clozapine Fluvoxamine Mirtazapine Olanzapine Tricyclics	Fluvoxamine Moclobemide Cimetidine	Smoking[2] Barbecued food[2]
IIC includes IIC9/ 10/19	Yes (2–20%) slow metabolisers (race-dependent)	Yes	Tricyclics Diazepam Moclobemide Phenytoin Warfarin Propranolol	Fluoxetine Fluvoxamine Sertraline Moclobemide Cimetidine	Rifampicin
IIIA3/4	No	Yes	Carbamazepine Nefazodone Quetiapine Tricyclics Olanzapine	Fluoxetine Grapefruit juice[3] Nefazodone Fluvoxamine	Barbituates Carbamazepine Phenyton Rifampicin

CYP, cytochrome P450 mono-oxygenase system; SSRIs, selective serotonin reuptake inhibitors.

1. Inhibitors vary in their potency of effect. Some drugs may be principally metabolised by a particular enzyme and in the process may prevent the enzyme from metabolising another drug. This is competitive inhibition. Other drugs are direct inhibitors of various enzymes. Direct inhibition is usually more profound.

2. Tobacco smoke and barbecued food contain aromatic hydrocarbons that induce CYP IA2 enzymes.

3. Grapefruit juice appears to inhibit CYP3A4 activity in the gut mucosa. Its effect can be an important cause of drug toxicity, for example when it is used to give medicines to children.

ENTERO-HEPATIC CIRCULATION

Drugs of larger molecular size and their metabolites are secreted by the liver into the bile and periodically emptied into the gut from the gall bladder, some to be reabsorbed into the blood. This entero-hepatic circulation of drugs results in a reservoir of drug and metabolites remaining in the bile and gut contents, only some passing out in the faeces. Further, metabolites inactivated by hepatic oxidation may be reactivated by chemical reduction through the activity of intestinal flora. Reactivated drugs then reappear in the circulation and prolong the pharmacological action. Drugs excreted mainly in the bile and faeces therefore take longer to clear from the body than those excreted in the urine. The normality or health of a patient's microflora may influence what happens. Entero-hepatic circulation does not, however, have many clinical consequences in psychiatric practice.

FAT SOLUBILITY

Many drugs are highly soluble in body fat. The brain, being composed largely of lipids, takes up a lot of such drugs. When a drug is first circulating, it rapidly enters the brain because of its high blood supply, but then if it is lipid-soluble it is taken up extensively by the adipose tissue of the body, resulting in it being rapidly withdrawn from the brain again. Thus, the drug is shared unequally between the body and the brain, the body getting most of it. A fat body gets an even larger share, so the brain gets less. A child of 4 years has a brain of almost adult size, which results in the brain getting a larger share of a dose than an adult brain would. Thus, a lipid-soluble drug may have a short activity half-life (in the brain) but a long elimination half-life. The short-acting barbiturates are such drugs, as are some benzodiazepines such as lorazepam. Short-acting barbiturates may show two peaks of effect: one after administration and a second after redistribution from body fat.

RENAL EXCRETION

Some drugs are excreted almost entirely in the urine; lithium and sulpiride are examples. For the most part, however, psychotropic drugs (which are lipid-soluble) need to be metabolised before being excreted (e.g. phenothiazines, tricyclics, benzodiazepines). Good renal function is therefore essential for clearing many drugs and their metabolites from the body. Poor blood flow through the kidney as in cardiac failure or in renal disease such as chronic nephritis, or normally in the infant under 1 year old, may result in partial or complete failure to clear a drug. Normal doses then have the effect of an overdose. The extreme case is prescribing during renal failure treated by dialysis; the drug is only removed periodically in the dialysate and has to be prescribed accordingly. The glomerular filtration rate declines slowly from the age of 30 and the renal clearance of drugs usually declines markedly after the age of 60.

Urinary excretion of drugs that are weak bases or weak acids depends on the urine pH, which may vary with diet and exercise. Conditions that favour salt formation also favour drug excretion. A weak base such as amphetamine is excreted more rapidly if the urine is strongly acid, since it then forms salts that are not reabsorbed; but if the urine is markedly alkaline, the free un-ionized base diffuses out of the renal tubules back into the blood, and drug action on the brain is prolonged. Conversely, the excretion of weak acids such as barbiturates or salicylates can be increased by making the urine alkaline. The urine can be made acid with doses of ammonium chloride or alkaline with sodium bicarbonate or potassium citrate. However, this technique is not often used in clinical practice.

MEASUREMENT OF DRUG PLASMA LEVELS

Since samples of circulating blood are easily drawn, measurement of the amount of a drug in the blood is a simple approach to the question of how much drug is reaching the sensitive areas of the brain – provided a sensitive and specific method exists for analysis of that drug. It is then possible to correlate the therapeutic and side-effects of the drug with its plasma concentration, provided: (a) the clinical effect follows soon after the drug reaches the brain; (b) it is due directly to the drug and not to some metabolite; and (c) the drug–brain receptor interaction is reversible (for most monoamine oxidase inhibitors it is not).

For phenytoin and lithium it is possible to find plasma concentrations associated with beneficial effects, and higher concentrations associated with adverse or toxic effects. These concentrations are similar but not identical in different individuals, which gives rise to the idea of a therapeutic range of values for a given population of patients. Low lithium concentrations have had little effect in treating groups of patients with mania. As the lithium concentrations are raised above 0.7 mmol/l different patients respond as higher concentrations are achieved, but raising the level above 1.4 mmol/l has not produced any further benefits and toxic signs appear. Under these circumstances the therapeutic range of lithium for the treatment of mania is said to be 0.6–1.2 mmol/l (note that estimates vary), which means that the vast majority of patients who respond will be expected to do so on doses producing a plasma level in this range. But one particular individual may do well only at the top of the range, while a second recovers on 0.8 mmol/l and a third may require 1.0 mmol/l. Adverse effects may occur with plasma levels within the therapeutic range, but they usually become dangerous only at levels above the upper limit.

For some antidepressants plasma levels of the drug and its active metabolites can be measured and very approximate therapeutic (target) ranges are known. This is done most commonly for amitriptyline and its metabolite nortriptyline. Nortriptyline itself is unusual in that blood concentrations above a certain level, about 150 ng/ml, are associated with a poor response or side-effects. There is said to be a therapeutic window between 50 and 150 ng/ml.

Phenothiazines are metabolised extensively and some metabolites are active. No clear relationships have been found between the drug levels for individual phenothiazines and clinical response. Haloperidol on the other hand is metabolised more simply. Although its main metabolite, reduced haloperidol, may be active, a relationship has been claimed between haloperidol level and therapeutic response in schizophrenia, with blood levels between 5 and 30 ng/ml. Blood levels greater than this are associated with a poorer clinical response, probably because of side-effects.

In practice blood levels are used clinically only for monitoring lithium, anticonvulsants (including carbamazepine and valproate), clozapine and occasionally amitriptyline and imipramine. One difficulty is that the clinical response (e.g. relief of depression) follows 10 days or more after the establishment of the drug level. What is happening in this time, and how is it related to the quantities of drug arriving over 10 days? (See chapter 7.)

INDIVIDUAL VARIATION

Individual patients differ very considerably in how they absorb and metabolise the same dose of a single drug. For instance, in a group all given 100 mg amitriptyline daily on the same schedule, there is at least a 10-fold difference between the lowest and the highest individual plasma level obtained. For drugs such as carbamazepine and chlorpromazine, which induce liver enzymes, the variability between individuals is even greater. These differences are partly genetic but also reflect age, previous and concurrent drug therapy, physical health and perhaps covert non-compliance. It was therefore hoped that drug level measurements would be a guide in deciding clinical doses for the individual, but this has not on the whole proved possible. Plasma measurements, of course, reveal whether a patient has taken the prescribed drug (though not necessarily in the doses proposed), but they are an expensive way of testing adherence. They have been useful in studying drug toxicity (when linked to abnormally high plasma concentrations of the drug), and they are valuable in the discovery of drug interactions. For example, when fluvoxamine is added to a steady treatment with clozapine, the plasma concentration of clozapine rises 10-fold. This is due to the inhibition in the liver of clozapine metabolism by the cytochrome CYP IA2, an interaction first discovered by plasma measurements. Many examples are now known where one drug inhibits the metabolism of another, or alternatively speeds up its destruction – for instance carbamazepine lowering haloperidol levels by as much as 60% – and blood measurements have been important in the discovery. Other examples include the elevation of tricyclic levels by fluoxetine (inhibition of CYP IID6) and the lowering of clozapine, haloperidol or olanzapine levels by carbamazepine. Assays are therefore valuable in the analysis of unusual or unexpected drug responses.

INTERPRETING PLASMA LEVELS

There are two very important points to remember when interpreting measurements of plasma concentration of drugs. The first is that a blood sample is taken at a moment in time, and the measurement, therefore, applies only to that moment, like a snapshot. Other times of day might yield other values. Therefore, when taking a blood sample always mark the exact time it was drawn and when comparing samples on different days try always to take them at the same time of day, and always avoid times soon after the actual taking of drugs. With lithium this is particularly important because lithium is rapidly absorbed, with the plasma level rising rapidly in the next 4 hours and then falling away exponentially. Blood for clinically useful lithium measurements should be drawn between 8 and 16 hours, preferably 12 hours, after the previous dose. With many other drugs, samples should be drawn when the plasma level is at its lowest (trough level), usually just before the next dose. By always checking through a sequence of plasma level results for a given patient, it is usually quite easy to detect spurious levels produced by a change in sampling time.

The second point is that with most drugs (but not lithium) the plasma proteins modify the values the laboratory returns. Most drugs circulate only partly dissolved freely in the plasma water, and pharmacologically active; but are largely (80–95%) bound reversibly to plasma proteins, especially albumin, and this fraction is pharmacologically inactive. The laboratory reports the total drug in the plasma, free plus protein bound, and unfortunately the latter is subject to hidden changes. If the plasma albumin is low, as in liver disease, the protein-bound drug will be low and the total concentration will be low, but the pharmacological action will be the same because the free drug concentration is the same. Alternatively, the albumin may be normal but its binding capacity for the drug being measured may be low, either because of competitive interference from another drug (very important when using two or more anticonvulsants, for instance carbamazepine with valproate or phenytoin) or because of metabolic interference – the binding is altered in uraemia, diabetes, ketosis and starvation. Or the binding process itself can be increased in some chronic inflammatory conditions (Crohn's disease) or after trauma or surgery, and then bound drug will be high, total drug level high, yet free drug perhaps only just adequate. So total plasma drug concentrations offer many pitfalls, and are not quite the excellent guide to drug therapy that was first hoped. Nevertheless, few drugs are so highly bound to plasma proteins and have such a low therapeutic index that measurements of free plasma levels are necessary.

BABIES AND DRUGS

Many drugs cross the placenta. The baby of a mother taking lithium may be born with hypothyroidism caused by the lithium; a morphine-dependent woman may produce an opiate-dependent infant. With other drugs the chief risk may be to cause an anomaly of development. The greatest risk is in the first 3 months of foetal life, when anatomy is decided, and not thereafter. In deciding whether or not to give such drugs during pregnancy the stage of pregnancy is clearly important, but it is necessary to weigh the pros and cons of treatment for both mother and foetus and not just for one of them.

Drugs also appear in breast milk, in proportion to their free concentration (not bound to protein, or total) in the maternal circulating plasma. Therefore, drugs like phenothiazines and tricyclics, which are mostly protein-bound, are of little import, but lithium, which is free, can matter. These considerations may contraindicate breastfeeding, unless the maternal drug can reasonably be stopped. Infants in the first year of life have poor renal and hepatic function, so clearance of drugs such as diazepam is slow at this time. In practice, however, many psychotropics are given to breastfeeding mothers by necessity. Adverse effects in the infant are rare, though an effect on development cannot be discounted.

If a woman has to take drugs during pregnancy, remember that renal blood flow (and hence urinary excretion) increases at this time, but that the increased progesterone secretion suppresses hepatic metabolism of drugs. Drug dosage may need to be adjusted in the light of those facts, and readjusted after delivery.

DRUG INTERACTIONS

The simultaneous prescription of more than one drug is often necessary. However, drugs may interfere with each other's absorption from the gut, binding in the plasma, excretion in the urine, metabolism in the liver and effects in the brain (see Table 6.1).

Carbamazepine, like barbiturates, stimulates liver enzymes that destroy imipramine, haloperidol, phenytoin and other drugs, and may reduce the clinical effects of these drugs. Monoamine oxidase inhibitors block phenytoin metabolism and may cause phenytoin toxicity. Orphenadrine stimulates the liver enzymes that destroy chlorpromazine, diminishing the levels of chlorpromazine, as well as interacting in the brain to diminish its effects on the extrapyramidal system. In contrast, chlorpromazine, fluvoxamine, fluoxetine and paroxetine prevent the liver metabolism of imipramine. Fluvoxamine slows the elimination of drugs metabolised by oxidation in the liver, including warfarin, phenytoin, theophylline and propranolol. The doses of these drugs should be lowered when prescribing fluvoxamine.

Since the discovery of different cytochrome enzymes, adverse drug interaction can be explained and predicted. The subject has now become extremely complex. Some useful references are listed below.

FURTHER READING

If in any doubt about the interactions between drugs that may be prescribed, consult the *BNF*, which has an appendix of interactions, or the local drug information service.

Cohen, L. J. & DeVane, C. L. (1996) Clinical implications of antidepressant pharmacokinetics and pharmacogenetics. *Annals of Pharmacotherapy*, **30**, 1471–1479.

Ereshefsky, L. (1996) Pharmacokinetics and drug interactions: update for new antipsychotics. *Journal of Clinical Psychiatry*, **57**(Suppl. 11), 12–25.

Glue, P. & Banfield, C. (1996) Psychiatry, psycho-pharmacology and P-450s. *Human Psychopharmacology*, **11**, 97–114.

Meyer, U. A., Balant, L. P., Bertilsson, L. *et al* (1996) Anti-depressants and drug-metabolizing enzymes – expert group report. *Acta Psychiatrica Scandinavica*, **93**, 71–79.

Taylor, D. (1997) Pharmacokinetic interactions involving clozapine. *British Journal of Psychiatry*, **171**, 109–112.

7. PHARMACODYNAMICS: HOW DRUGS AFFECT THE BRAIN

The brain consists of a complex array of neurons, grouped into nuclei that are separated by axonal tracts supported by glial cells, and protected from the circulation by the blood–brain barrier, which is freely permeable to fat-soluble compounds but only selectively permeable to larger or highly charged molecules. The past 50 years has seen an enormous increase in knowledge of cellular function in the brain. But this has led to only a modest increase, mostly speculative, in understanding the pathophysiology of mental illness. There is, however, a clearer understanding of the mechanisms of actions of psychotropic drugs. Unfortunately this does not extend far beyond the primary site of action. We still know little about the more delayed changes that result from drug action, though these are probably more relevant to the slow changes seen in clinical conditions.

Much of our knowledge springs from the discovery of individual neurotransmitters, their synthesis, pathways and receptors. Much remains to be learned about how each neurotransmitter and its neurons interact with others. The more recently discovered neuropeptides are less amenable to pharmacological interventions, but are nevertheless probably very important clinically. More neurotransmitters remain undiscovered, and many receptors unclassified.

In this chapter we will consider individual transmitters that are known to be relevant to understanding drug action. Their synthesis, neuronal pathways and receptors will be summarised.

RECEPTORS

Receptors are the peptide structures to which neurotransmitters and some drugs attach, and which initiate their effects. They consist of a recognition site and an effector. The effector undergoes a change in structure that leads to, for instance, the activation of an enzyme or the opening of an ionic channel. A drug that attaches to the receptor and activates the effector is called an agonist; these are usually related structurally to the natural transmitter. A drug that attaches to the receptor and produces no activation is called an antagonist, because its occupancy of the receptor prevents the agonist or the transmitter from working. The interaction of most drugs with receptors is reversible: a competitive antagonism occurs, in which a higher concentration of the agonist can displace the antagonist and produce an effect.

Occasionally a drug binds irreversibly to the receptor or enzyme (for example some cholinesterase inhibitors and older MAOIs); there is then non-competitive antagonism, and the body must synthesis new enzyme to restore full function. Generally an agonist needs only to occupy a small fraction of the total number of receptors to produce a large neuronal effect, because there are spare receptors. However, an antagonist may need to occupy a certain proportion of receptors before it can have a blocking effect on the transmitters' neuronal action; this is clear in neuromuscular transmission but can also apply in psychiatry (see below).

Partial agonists have to occupy a larger proportion of receptors to achieve an effect. They have a blocking effect upon a full agonist and may not be able to produce the maximum agonist effect. An example is buprenorphine, which can substitute for heroin in opiate addiction, and tends to diminish the effect of any additional heroin that is taken (see chapters 21 and 35).

Inverse agonists are drugs that produce the opposite effect to that of an agonist. This is a complex situation, but one mechanism arises when the receptor is already active in the absence of an agonist. For example, the ionic channel may be partly open. The inverse agonist acts to close it.

As the dose of the drug increases, the quantity bound to the receptor increases in a hyperbolic manner, towards a saturation level. When the relationship between the concentration of an agonist and the response is plotted on a logarithmic scale an S-shaped log dose response curve is observed. In the presence of a competitive antagonist this curve is shifted to the right in a parallel manner (see Figure 7.1).

The dose ratio between the new concentration and the original concentration required to produce a given response is related to the proportion of receptors occupied by the antagonist – the occupancy – by a simple formula Dose Ratio $= 100/(100 - P)$, where P is the percentage of receptors occupied. Thus, when 75% of receptors are occupied, the dose ratio is 4; if 95% are occupied, the ratio is 20. This method has been used to determine receptor occupancy by antipsychotic drugs using positron emission tomography (PET) scanning (see p. 285). At some peripheral synapses, such as the neuromuscular junction, there is a safety factor – a large proportion of receptors has

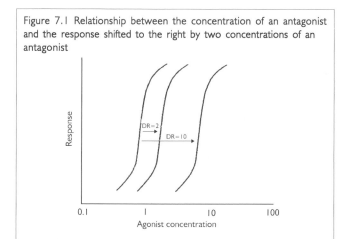

Figure 7.1 Relationship between the concentration of an antagonist and the response shifted to the right by two concentrations of an antagonist

to be occupied, perhaps 80%, before transmission fails. However, if there is no safety factor, and the log dose-response curve is steep, then a small occupancy will produce a large reduction in response.

Up-regulation and desensitisation

Transmitter pathways in the brain are resilient and during exposure to drugs compensatory changes occur. For instance, in the presence of an antagonist the presynaptic neuron may – because of feedback inhibition – synthesise and release an increased amount of transmitter. The metabolites are then detected in increased quantities in the cerebrospinal fluid (CSF). Over the course of a week or more the post-synaptic neurons whose receptors are blocked will respond by synthesising more receptors – up-regulation – akin to the phenomenon of denervation hypersensitivity, which follows transection of a peripheral nerve. Interestingly, the new receptors that appear may have different subunit composition (see below) from the original receptors, and this may endow them with subtle differences in their reactions to agonists and antagonists. For example, an antagonist at the original receptor may be a partial agonist at the new receptors, or an inverse agonist.

On the other hand, exposure to agonist causes two processes of reduced sensitivity. First, there is a rapid desensitisation resulting from a change in the structure of the activated receptor to one that is quiescent. Secondly, there is a reduced synthesis or down-regulation of the number of receptors.

This resilience means there is also a safety factor in brain pathways. Thus, symptoms of Parkinsonism do not develop in young adults until some 70% of dopaminergic neurons in the substantia nigra have degenerated, or until 70% of the dopamine receptors in the basal ganglia are occupied by antipsychotic drugs (see below).

Receptors can be identified by labelling them with antagonists containing a radioactive atom. If these 'ligands' are specific for a particular type of receptor, they can be used to measure the quantity of that receptor and its distribution in the brain. Receptors can then be classified according to the transmitter or agonist, the antagonist, and the type of effect. More recently, receptors have been identified from the RNA that synthesises them. Since the RNA can be cloned, it is easier to study than the receptor itself and can provide the amino acid sequence of the receptor. Most receptors are localised on the surface of the cell in the membrane; but steroid and thyroid hormones interact with receptors that are intracellular.

Receptor classes and structures

Class I receptors

Cell surface receptors on neurons are of two main classes. Class I or ionotropic receptors are ligand-gated ionic channels. Their activation leads to a rapid transient increase in membrane permeability to either (positive) cations (especially sodium or calcium) or (negative) anions (mainly chloride). This causes excitation or inhibition of the postsynaptic membrane. Examples are acetylcholine nicotinic receptors (excitatory)

Figure 7.2 Subunit structure of class I receptor (nicotinic acetyl choline receptor: high-affinity nicotine type)

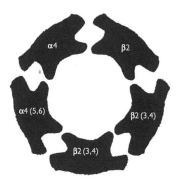

α4   β2

α4 (5,6)   β2 (3,4)

β2 (3,4)

Each subtype of nicotinic receptor is composed of obligatory subunits (in this case α4 β2) and there is variability in the other subunits.

and gamma-aminobutyric acid-A (GABA-A) receptors (inhibitory). These receptors consist of five subunits surrounding a channel in the membrane. For instance, the nicotinic receptor has α, β, γ and δ subunits. (see Figure 7.2). Each subunit has four highly lipophilic stretches in its amino acid sequence and these are thought to be the transmembrane domains. Usually the receptor has two α subunits and three of other types (β, γ or δ), and these five are arranged in a circle. In each subunit one of the transmembrane domains has a series of amino acids with hydroxyl groups; these amino acids may form the lining of the cental pore that enables the conduction of cations through the cell membrane. Binding of the agonist occurs on the α subunits and opens the channel. The subunit structure offers potential for very great multiplicity in structure of the receptor; for example nine varieties of the alpha subunit are known to exist. There are at least three types of nicotinic receptor in the brain, including one with five α subunits . Brain and muscle nicotinic receptors have different subunit composition, and there may be differences in diseases such as Alzheimer's.

Class II receptors

Class II receptors produce slower responses, involving so called G-proteins, which bind to the intracellular portion of the receptor and activate a second messenger. These metabotropic receptors consist of a single long peptide chain with seven subunits within the membrane and a long intracellular loop, which binds the G-protein. Agonist binding causes a change in the structure of the receptor, activating the G-protein that hydrolyses guanosine triphosphate (GTP). The G-protein then dissociates from the receptor and activates an effector protein, which may be an ion channel, or an enzyme. The enzyme then alters the level of an intracellular second messenger. Various second messenger systems may thus be activated or inhibited, including:

- adenylate cyclase (producing cyclic-AMP), which then leads to the phosphorylation (and activation) of other enzymes
- activation of phosphoinositide turnover, controlling inositol triphosphate (IP-3) and calcium release
- the conversion of arachidonic acid to prostaglandins, leukotrienes and other active compounds, and indirect activation of ion channels.

CATECHOLAMINES

Dopamine, noradrenalin and adrenalin are catecholamines and are synthesised from the precursor amino acids tyrosine and phenylalanine, in steps beginning with the action of tyrosine hydroxylase.

Dihydroxy-phenylalanine (DOPA) is then decarboxylated to dopamine. The enzyme dopamine beta-hydroxylase, present in noradrenergic neurons, then converts dopamine to noradrenalin. In the adrenal medulla and adrenergic neurons, noradrenalin is converted to adrenalin by N-methyl transferase (see Figure 7.3).

Dopamine

Tyrosine hydroxylase is the rate-limiting enzyme and synthesis of dopamine can be increased by giving L-DOPA. Dopamine is stored in vesicles and released by nerve impulses. Released dopamine is taken back into the nerve ending by an active reuptake process (the dopamine transporter or DAT). A small portion is also metabolised by intracellular monoamine oxidase (MAO) and by catechol-O-methyl transferase (COMT), the main metabolite being homovanillic acid (HVA).

There are three main dopamine pathways in the brain:

(1) The nigrostriatal pathway, which runs from the substantia nigra to the caudate-putamen in the corpus striatum. This pathway is important in involuntary motor control, including stereotypies. Degeneration of the pathway leads to Parkinson's disease.

(2) The mesolimbic pathway, which extends from the A10 region of the tegmentum, an area of the midbrain close to the substantia nigra, to the limbic areas of the brain. The limbic system is a collection of structures that lie along the medial surface of the brain, especially the temporal lobe. The essential components are the hippocampal complex, amygdala, cingulate gyrus, entorhinal cortex, septal nuclei and nucleus accumbens. There is a mesocortical pathway to the limbic cortex – the medio-frontal, cingulate and entorhinal cortex. The pathway to the nucleus accumbens is important in drive-orientated behaviour and locomotor activation; this tract will support self-stimulation by implanted electrodes, and dopamine injected to the nucleus accumbens causes increased locomotor activity. The nucleus accumbens, the central nucleus of the amygdala and the bed nucleus of the stria terminalis form part of the extended amygdala that is

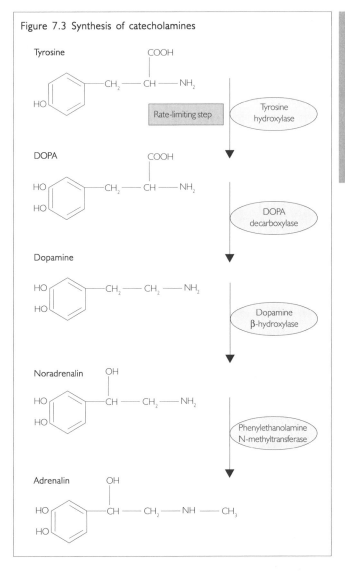

Figure 7.3 Synthesis of catecholamines

thought to be the substrate for the reinforcing actions of all major drugs of misuse. The meso-prefrontal dopamine pathway is part of the mesolimbic system and is activated by stress. It is also postulated to be underdeveloped in schizophrenia, in some theories.

(3) Short dopamine neurons in the hypothalamus secrete dopamine to the pituitary portal blood supply, to inhibit the release of prolactin. Short dopamine neurons exist also in the area postrema in relation to the vomiting centre.

Figure 7.4 The D_1 and D_2 receptor family localisation

D_1 Receptor family		D_2 Receptor family		
D_1	D_5	D_2	D_3	D_4
Caudate-putamen	Hippocampus	Caudate-putamen	N. accumbens	Frontal cortex
N. accumbens	Hypothalamus	N. accumbens	Hypothalamus	Midbrain

Dopamine receptors occur post-synaptically in the terminal areas of these pathways. Also, with the exception of the mesocortical neurons, the other long dopaminergic neurons have inhibitory pre-synaptic autoreceptors; stimulation of autoreceptors inhibits and blockade increases transmitter release. Thus, antipsychotic drugs – by blocking dopamine receptors – lead initially to an increased firing rate of nigro-striatal and mesolimbic but not mesocortical dopaminergic neurons. During long-term treatment the increased firing subsides and the former neurones become quiescent or inactivated.

Dopamine receptors are of two main families: D_1-like and D_2-like (see Figure 7.4). The D_1 type, which includes D_5 receptors, stimulates adenylate cyclase to form cyclic-AMP as a second messenger. The D_2 type is not so linked. Together, D_2, D_3 and D_4 receptors are grouped as D_2-like. The subtypes are differentiated by their antagonists and their location – and more recently by their amino acid sequence, as judged by their m-RNA. The subtypes have become important in understanding the actions of antipsychotic drugs (see chapters 28 and 30). Thus, D_3 and D_4 subtypes of D_2-like receptors are more common in the limbic areas than in the caudate-putamen, where other D_2 receptors predominate. In particular, D_3 receptors are common in the nucleus accumbens as well as D_2 receptors, but not in the pituitary; D_4 receptors are common in the amygdala, hippocampus and frontal cortex. D_5, a subtype of D_1, is present in the hippocampus. The five subtypes of dopamine receptors, so far identified, have different amino acid sequences and are associated with four different chromosomes.

Splice variants

Gene cloning has revealed that some dopaminergic receptors contain one or more repeats of an amino acid sequence in the third loop of the molecule within the cytoplasm; the receptor can occur in short or long forms, which may differ in their second messenger coupling rather than their affinities for drugs. Also there may be amino acid point variations in these segments, which result in further variants of the same receptor. For example, five variants of the human D_2 receptor exist.

Noradrenalin

Noradrenalin is stored in granules in the nerve terminals which, in noradrenalinergic neurons, run very diffusely for several centimetres, each containing several thousand terminal varicosities with granules.

The rate-limiting step in its synthesis is tyrosine hydroxylase, whose action is subject to feedback inhibition. The release of noradrenalin is regulated not only by impulse flow, but also by pre-synaptic receptors, including autoreceptors and opiate receptors. This interaction with opiate receptors means that during opiate withdrawal noradrenalinergic neurons are activated, causing increased release of noradrenalin. In some neurons noradrenalin coexists with neuropeptides, whose release augments the action of noradrenaline.

Released noradrenalin is taken back into the cell by a reuptake mechanism (the noradrenalin transporter, NAT). A small proportion is inactivated by COMT and MAO-A. The main metabolite of brain noradrenalin is methoxy-hydroxy phenylglycol (MHPG), which is measurable in CSF and urine.

Noradrenergic neurons have their cell bodies in the midbrain. The largest group is in the locus coeruleus in the pons (with about 12 000 large cells on each side in humans). Axons from these neurons send extensive branches to the forebrain, including the cerebral cortex, hypothalamus and cerebellar cortex, by pathways including the dorsal and the medial forebrain bundle. A second group is more loosely localised (the lateral tegmental system); their axons running in a ventral bundle with those from the locus coeruleus, supply the amygdala and septum.

Noradrenalin is thought to play an important role in the sleep/wake cycle (including vigilance and REM sleep), reinforcement, learning and affect. Locus coeruleus neurons are activated by unexpected or noxious (painful) sensory events. Severe stress causes an increased turnover of noradrenalin in the brain.

Noradrenalin receptors are subdivided into α and β types. Alpha-1 and β receptors are mainly post-synaptic, α-2 both pre- and post-synaptic. Beta receptors are subdivided into β-1, -2, and -3, all linked to adenylate cyclase but sensitive to different antagonists.

Adrenalin

A smaller group of neurons with adrenalin as the transmitter exists close to the tegmental noradrenalin system. Its function awaits elucidation.

ACETYLCHOLINE

Acetylcholine is synthesised from choline and acetyl coenzyme A by choline acetyl transferase. Choline is the rate-limiting factor in synthesis but not in release. Acetylcholine is stored in vesicles and released by nerve impulses. Within the synaptic cleft it is inactivated by choline esterase. A reuptake process carries choline back into the nerve ending. Choline esterase is inhibited by physostigmine and by organophosphorous compounds, which are used as insecticides (and more recently by drugs such as donepezil).

Cholinergic neurons are widely distributed. There are two major acetylcholine pathways, one from the basal forebrain (including the nucleus basalis of Meinert) projecting to the cerebral cortex and other parts of the forebrain. This pathway includes the septal-hippocampal projection, which is involved in memory. The second is from the midbrain to the thalamus and to the pontine reticular formation.

There are cholinergic inter-neurons in the caudate-putamen that receive an inhibitory input from the nigrostriatal dopamine pathway. This synapse of the nigrostriatal dopamine pathway accounts for the occurrence of Parkinsonism with classical antipsychotics, and the need for anticholinergic drugs to counteract it. Dopamine normally acts on the cholinergic inter-neurons to inhibit their firing. When the D_2 receptors are blocked acetylcholine is released. The anticholinergic drug works by blocking the effect of this released acetylcholine.

Acetylcholine receptors are of two main types, nicotinic and muscarinic. Those in the brain are mainly muscarinic, and at least five subtypes exist (M_{1-5}). They are linked to G-proteins and a variety of second messengers. The M_3 receptor is one of the subtypes in glandular tissue including salivary glands, as is M_4. Atropine is the classical antagonist of M receptors, blocking all subtypes. Many antidepressant and antipsychotic drugs block these receptors, especially in high doses.

Nicotinic acetylcholine receptors in the brain differ from those in skeletal muscle in their subunit composition, and are of at least three types. The three types differ in their localisation, but are found in areas where they may interact with dopamine or with glutamate function, including the neocortex, the striatum, the hippocampus, midbrain and substantia nigra. Nicotine causes dopamine release in the nucleus accumbens. There is also evidence that nicotinic receptors facilitate glutamatergic transmission.

Acetylcholine is thought to play an important part in short-term memory, and in arousal and cortical activation. Degeneration of cholinergic forebrain neurons (and other neurons) occurs in Alzheimer's disease, although the post-synaptic receptors are preserved. The role of glutamate in sensory gating may be modulated by acetylcholine (at nicotinic receptors).

INDOLAMINES

5-Hydroxytryptamine

5-Hydroxytryptamine (serotonin; 5-HT), an indolamine, is synthesised from the amino acid L-tryptophan, converted by tryptophan hydroxylase to 5-hydroxytryptophan, and by a decarboxylase to 5-HT (see Figure 7.5). Synthesis and release can be altered by the availability of L-tryptophan in the diet, which competes with other neutral amino acids for transport into the brain.

Release occurs by nerve impulses and is modulated by the pre-synaptic receptors. After release 5-HT is inactivated by a powerful reuptake mechanism, the serotonin transporter (SERT, see below). A small proportion is broken down by MAO to 5-hydroxy indoleacetic acid (5-HIAA), which appears in the CSF.

The cell bodies of 5-HT neurons are restricted to clusters in the midline (raphé) region of the pons and brain-stem. There are also a small number of cells in the locus coeruleus and in the area postrema.

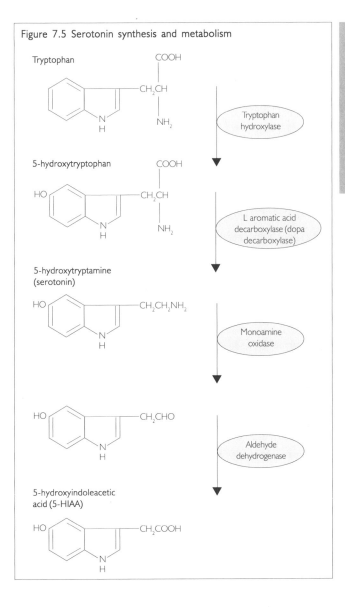

Figure 7.5 Serotonin synthesis and metabolism

In more rostral cell groups, the median raphé sends axons with extensive innervation to the forebrain, including the limbic system and the dorsal raphé, to an extensive diffuse innervation of the cerebral cortex and thalamus. More caudal neurons supply the medulla and spinal cord. 5-HT has both excitatory and inhibitory effects. The neurons discharge rhythmically and they exert a simultaneous modulatory effect in diverse brain regions. The firing frequency is higher during waking arousal and reduced during sleep.

The 5-HT pathways are thought to provide a general behavioural inhibition and seem to be involved in pain suppression, sleep, thermal regulation, sexual and aggressive behaviour, as well as depression and anxiety; but details of these functions are very unclear. Noradrenalin appears to have a stimulating effect on some 5-HT cells.

5-HT receptors

Seven classes of 5-HT receptors are recognised (5-HT-1 to 5-HT-7), with 15 known subtypes (1-A, B, C, etc.). All except 5-HT-3 are metabotrophic (G-protein linked). 5-HT-1A receptors are mainly cell body autoreceptors, which inhibit 5-HT cell firing, but also post-synaptic receptors in the hippocampus. Buspirone is an agonist, the beta-blocker pindolol an antagonist. Functional correlates include anxiety, thermoregulation and the serotonin syndrome. 5-HT-1D receptors are located as nerve terminal autoreceptors; antagonists increase 5-HT release. 5-HT-1D receptors are also found on intracranial blood vessels, where they cause vasoconstriction and are involved in migraine. Sumatriptan is an agonist for both 1B and 1D.

5-HT-2A receptors facilitate excitatory effects on cortical and other neurons. Ritanserin is an antagonist; less specific ones include the atypical antipsychotics clozapine, risperidone, olanzapine, zotepine and ziprasidone. 5-HT-2A antagonists increase slow-wave sleep and decrease paradoxical (REM) sleep; they may also reduce anxiety. However, their most interesting effects are in relation to their ability to restore dopamine cell firing and increase dopamine release; this may lead to less extrapyramidal side-effects (EPS), less cognitive impairment and less reduction of drive as compared with the classical antipsychotics.

The psychotomimetic drug LSD acts on 5-HT receptors. One action is to inhibit cell firing by stimulating autoreceptors, but other actions are thought to be important in its hallucinogenic effects. 5-HT-2A antagonists reduce hallucinations caused by LSD.

5-HT-2C (formerly called 5-HT-1C) receptors are widely distributed in the brain and the choroid plexus. Stimulation causes anxiety, reduces food intake, and stimulates modest prolactin release. Blockade causes weight gain. Strict dieting with low intake of L-tryptophan causes 5-HT-2C receptor supersensitivity. Metachloro phenyl piperazine (m-CPP) is an agonist at 5-HT-2C receptors and can induce anxiety in susceptible individuals. Drugs with strong antagonist actions include ritanserin, mianserin and several atypical antipsychotics – clozapine, olanzapine, zotepine and ziprasidone.

5-HT-3 receptors are pre-synaptic and activate increased release of transmitters in animals. Antagonists include ondansetron, which has anti-emetic effects in man (probably acting in the area postrema), and analgesic effects in animals. There are few 5-HT-3 receptors in the human brain. 5-HT-6 receptors occur in the caudate-putamen and cerebral cortex. Their role is unknown. 5-HT-7 receptors are involved in the control of circadian rhythms, a function of the suprachiasmatic nucleus in the hypothalamus.

Drugs acting on subtypes of 5-HT-1 and 5-HT-2 receptors are being investigated for antidepressant and anxiolytic actions.

SEROTONIN TRANSPORTERS

SERT is a protein with 630 amino acids and 12 transmembrane domains. Both the N- and C- terminals are intracellular, and the transporter exists as tetramers linked by disulphide bridges. Similar transport proteins exist for most other transmitters except acetylcholine (there is a choline transporter instead); they include the transporters for GABA and for noradrenalin, which have very similar amino acid structures, and those for glycine and dopamine.

The SERT has structural similarities to the sodium ion channel. It transports into the cell one sodium ion and one chlorine ion with each positively charged 5-HT, and counter-transports one potassium ion.

TCAs and SSRIs bind to the SERT, preventing 5-HT transport, without being transported themselves. Ecstasy (MDMA) competitively inhibits 5-HT transport and also allows release of intracellular 5-HT from the neuron by reverse transport. It is an amphetamine and is itself transported into the cell by the SERT, probably in exchange for 5-HT.

The TCAs and SSRIs have distinct binding sites on the SERT. These interact with each other and with the transporter site. There are major species differences in the pharmacology of the SERT.

Adaptive changes

Following administration of an SSRI, adaptive changes occur. These include down-regulation of the SERT, with a 50% drop in the number of antidepressant binding sites. The SERT can also be up-regulated by activation of adenosine A_3 receptors. The mechanism of action of SSRIs is discussed in chapter 25.

Other transporters

The noradrenalin transporter (NAT) is one of the sites of action of most tricyclic antidepressants (see chapter 24). The dopamine transporter is one of the main sites of action of cocaine, which increases dopamine release and blocks its reuptake.

HISTAMINE

Histamine-containing neurons exist in the hypothalamus and midbrain reticular formation, and axons are distributed to the hypothalamus and to the forebrain. Histamine is thought to be involved in food intake, hormonal regulation and arousal. Three types of receptors are recognised. H_1 is the site of classical anti-histamines, concerned with allergic reactions; in the brain it is concerned with arousal and possibly with appetite. H_2 receptors are also present in the brain as well as the stomach; their function is unknown but H_2 antagonists, such as cimetidine and ranitidine, may cause hallucinations. H_3 receptors are autoreceptors controlling synthesis and release of histamine.

GABA

GABA is a widespread inhibitory transmitter, mostly in inter-neurons in the brain. It is formed from L-glutamic acid by glutamate decarboxylase. This is a B6-dependent enzyme, and vitamin B6 (pyridoxine, see chapter 38) deficiency leads to low levels of GABA and fits. Released GABA is broken down by a transaminase, but a reuptake mechanism exists to transport it back into the nerve ending. GABA receptors are of two types.

GABA-A receptors

GABA-A receptors are ligand-gated channels for chloride ions. Receptor activation causes hyperpolarisation and reduced excitability of the membrane. The receptor is a five-subunit complex that can be modulated by benzodiazepines, barbiturates and steroids attaching at different sites. It is likely that there are very many different GABA-A receptors subtypes. Benzodiazepines interact with the receptor allosterically (see chapter 34) to potentiate the action of GABA. Benzodiazepine antagonists such as flumazenil block this effect. By contrast inverse agonists decrease the effects of GABA and are anxiogenic. Barbiturates also potentiate GABA but by attaching to a difference site. Picrotoxin blocks the GABA chloride channel and produces seizures. There are thought to be endogenous compounds, which interact at these sites, but they are not yet defined.

GABA-B receptors

GABA-B receptors regulate second messengers and are also inhibitory. Baclofen is an agonist but also releases GABA.

GLUTAMIC ACID

L-glutamate is the principal and ubiquitous excitatory transmitter in the brain. It is formed by transamination of oxoglutarate, a component of Krebs cycle, or from glutamine produced in glial cells. Glutamate has four known roles relevant to psychiatry: it may become excitotoxic; it contributes to epilepsy; it is involved in synaptic plasticity as in learning; and through its interactions with dopamine it may have a role in psychosis (see chapter 13).

Glutamate action is normally ended by active transport back into cells. Under pathological conditions, however, this can operate in reverse, releasing more glutamate. This neurotoxic effect of excitatory amino acids is thought to contribute to damage resulting from ischaemia. Some anticonvulsants such as lamotrigine act largely by reducing glutamate release, through their blockade of presynaptic sodium channels (see chapter 32).

Glutamate receptors are of four main types: NMDA, AMPA, kainate, and metabotropic receptors. NMDA and AMPA types are similar to GABA-A receptors in structure, but contain a cationic channel for sodium and calcium. Both are subject to modulation by other molecules. The NMDA receptor requires glycine (otherwise an inhibitory transmitter in the spinal cord) to occupy a site on the receptor, in order that glutamate may open the channel. D-serine can substitute for glycine.

AMPA receptors operate fast transmission by entry of sodium ions. NMDA receptors permit calcium entry, which activates intracellular changes. The metabotropic receptors are linked to second messengers that result in long-term potentiation (LTP), which gives a basis for synaptic plasticity and learning.

There are major pathways connecting glutamate and dopamine systems. Glutamate projections from the frontal cortex to the caudate-putamen, and to the nucleus accumbens are part of the cortico-striato-pallido-thalamic circuitry that connects back to the cortex. These parallel circuits receive dopamine input at the striatum and accumbens. Phencyclidine (PCP) is thought to bind within the cation channel of the NMDA receptor, blocking glutamate action there but probably increasing glutamate release to act on other receptors. It is psychotomimetic.

NITRIC OXIDE

It was discovered in 1987, in Moncada's laboratory, that nitric oxide (NO) is generated in endothelial cells and mediates vascular relaxation. It is synthesised from the amino acid L-arginine by the enzyme NO synthase (NOS). The synthesis can be inhibited by N-monomethyl arginine (L-NMMA).

There are three distinct forms of NOS, serving different functions. The endothelial form (eNOS) is responsible for vascular tone. The neuronal form (nNOS) is found in the central nervous system in about 2% of neurons (especially the cerebellum and the hippocampus) and in peripheral nerves (e.g. in the gastointestinal and the genitourinary tracts, see chapter 22, p. 225). In both cases NO diffuses from the generator cell to the effector cell, where it complexes the iron of guanylate cyclase and activates this enzyme, leading to the production of cyclic-guanosine monophosphate. This intracellular second messenger phosphorylates enzymes that produce responses, particularly relaxation of smooth muscle. Within the central nervous system (CNS), NO may be involved in adapting blood flow to the metabolic needs of local cells. It is also involved in long-term potentiation, and probably memory. This occurs when glutamate acts on NMDA receptors and activates nNOS; the NO then diffuses to the pre-synaptic terminal and increases the production of glutamate.

An inducible third form (iNOS) occurs in macrophages and is involved in inflammation and cytotoxicity. High levels of NO formed in ischaemic brain tissue may also produce tissue damage.

HORMONES AND RECEPTORS

Hormones have important interactions with neurotransmitters and their receptors. For example, high levels of thyroid hormones lead to the upregulation of noradrenalin β-receptors, contributing to the features of sympathetic overactivity in thyrotoxicosis. High levels of oestrogens, as occur in pregnancy, have antipsychotic-like effects on dopamine receptors, and lead to upregulation of receptor numbers; after delivery the decline in oestrogen levels leaves these receptors exposed. High levels of steroids derived from progesterone also occur in pregnancy; they have actions at GABA-A receptors similar to benzodiazepines.

Given these actions it is not surprising that endocrine conditions and the puerperium are associated with psychiatric disorders.

PEPTIDES

Many peptides have roles as neurotransmitters or modulators; more than 80 have been identified. These include opioid peptides, substance P, cholecystokinin (CCK), corticotrophin releasing factor (CRF), vasointestinal peptide (VIP), neurotensin, somatostatin and angiotensin II. The most studied are the opioids because of the existence of drugs such as morphine and naltrexone, which are agonist and antagonist; at least three types of opioid receptors – μ, δ, and κ – are recognised.

In the brain these peptides are often found co-localised in the same neurons as classical transmitters. Thus, dopamine is found with CCK or neurotensin, acetylcholine with substance P, GABA with somatostatin or CCK, 5-HT with thyrotropin releasing hormone (TRH), and so on. Here they may potentiate transmission under particular circumstances, such as high frequency. Otherwise the peptides have their own roles. CCK analogues can induce panic attacks. Oxytocin and vasopressin affect memory and learning. Somatostatin affects motor activity and sleep. Antipsychotic drugs increase levels of neurotensin. CRF can cause arousal. Cytokines regulate inflammatory responses in the brain. Novel compounds blocking substance P at neurokinin NK-1 receptors are being investigated for antidepressant activity.

FURTHER READING

Cooper, J. R., Bloom, F. E. & Roth, R. H., (1996) *The Biochemical Basis of Neuropharmacology* (7th edn). Oxford: Oxford University Press.

Dalack, G. W., Healy, D. J. & Meador-Woodruff, J. H. (1998) Nicotine dependence in schizophrenia: clinical phenomena and laboratory findings. *American Journal of Psychiatry*, **155**, 1490–1501.

Kramer, M. S., Cutler, N., Feighner, J., *et al* (1998) Distinct mechanism for antidepressant activity by blockade of central substance P receptors. *Science*, **281**, 1640–1645.

Moncada, S. (1999) Nitric oxide: discovery and impact on clinical medicine. *Journal of the Royal Society of Medicine*, **92**, 164–169.

Page, C. P., Curtis, M. J., Sutter, M. C., *et al* (1997) *Integrated Pharmacology*. London: Mosby.

Rang, H. P., Dale, M. M. & Ritter, J. M. (1999) *Pharmacology* (4th edn). Edinburgh: Churchill Livingstone.

Schloss, P. & Williams, D. C. (1998) The serotonin transporter: a primary target for antidepressant drugs. *Journal of Psychopharmacology*, **12**, 115–121.

8. PRINCIPLES OF PRESCRIBING: THE LIFE CYCLES AND ADVERSE DRUG REACTIONS

GENERAL PRINCIPLES IN PRESCRIBING

Prescribing is often based upon a hypothesis about the condition from which the patient is suffering. The outcome of treatment may then support or refute the original hypothesis. We set out here some general principles that underlie a rational approach to prescribing throughout the life cycle. This is followed by discussion of possible reasons for failure of treatment, and for the occurrence of unwanted or unexpected results.

Work with a few established drugs and know them well

Begin by knowing the use of a few drugs thoroughly rather than a large list superficially. Start with drugs whose dose range, side-effects, contraindications and interactions are known from extensive use in clinical practice. Use newly launched drugs, about which there is limited experience, only if they have some clear advantage. Try and ensure that you evaluate the evidence about a new drug as comprehensively and objectively as possible, rather than taking manufacturers' claims at face value. Decide for which patient groups you may recommend the new drug.

Avoid prescribing more than one drug of the same chemical class at the same time

There is usually no clinical advantage in giving two tricyclic antidepressants, say, amitriptyline with imipramine, or two sedative phenothiazines, say chlorpromazine with thioridazine. Treatment is complicated needlessly, and patient and nurse are burdened with extra tablets without point. Acknowledge that the effects of drug treatment may often be limited, and resist the temptation to indulge in very high doses or polypharmacy simply to be seen to be taking action.

Identify appropriate target symptoms

Identify carefully the symptoms that are obvious and likely to improve with treatment, and monitor these. Be sure that the symptoms targeted to monitor improvement are part of the illness, rather than of the patient's personality. Sleep and appetite often improve in depression before other symptoms do. Where possible, use recognised, validated, simple assessment scales to monitor response to treatment, for example the Montgomery-Åsberg rating scale for depression (Montgomery & Åsberg, 1979) or the Young scale for mania (Yound *et al*, 1978).

If a drug fails, change to one with different pharmacological action

When a drug fails, change to a drug from a different group. If an adequate dose of an SSRI doesn't relieve depression, try a drug with a broader spectrum of pharmacological actions, which might include a tricyclic drug or an SNRI or MAOI rather than another SSRI.

Change one thing at a time

Only by doing this can one learn whether a particular treatment is effective or ineffective, and whether new symptoms are side-effects of that drug. It may be best to add the new drug before stopping the previous one, so that the symptoms of discontinuation do not become confused with those of the new drug.

Prescribing as required can be risky

Prescribing 'as required' is potentially dangerous because staff who may not have the appropriate clinical or pharmacological knowledge are authorised to give unlimited extra doses of potentially toxic and interacting drugs. The best practice for discretionary medication is to write instructions limiting the reasons for giving the drug, the number of repetitions and their duration. For example, 'Repeat dose once, if patient unable to sleep, any night in next five', or specify the maximum dose in 24 hours. Do not prescribe on an 'as required' basis any drug that does not have a prompt therapeutic effect.

Avoid prescribing more than three psychotropic drugs at once

Every symptom does not have to be treated. Attempting to do so results in excessive prescribing. A large number of medicines is a burden to the patient and relative or nurse. Errors of dose and timing are more likely to occur and error disrupts the regular timetable of medication. Prescribing more drugs increases the chance of drug interactions, and requires more knowledge.

Hypnotics may not be necessary to control insomnia

Sleep hygiene (see below, p. 83) is often effective and can obviate the need for drugs. The prescription of a hypnotic to control sleeplessness in depression or psychosis can be avoided by giving antidepressants or antipsychotics that are themselves sedative. Where hypnotics are required initially, they may (and where possible should) be tapered and stopped once the primary condition begins to respond to treatment. Improvement in sleep is a useful symptom to monitor during treatment.

Time tablet-taking to suit the patient's lifestyle

Prescribing a drug to be taken three times a day can become an unthinking habit. Perhaps the drug can be given once a day at a convenient and easily remembered time such as 'on going to bed'. Dose related side-effects are more likely with the midday dose because it is so close to the early morning dose. Lunchtime medication also tends to be omitted by people at work, who forget in the press of the day's events or are embarrassed about taking tablets in public. People who work unusual hours may need advice about timing. Those who continue drinking alcohol will need advice on when to take their drugs and on safe limits to drinking.

Do not reject drugs too soon as ineffective

Prescribe a big enough dose for long enough to be sure a drug has had a fair chance to work before concluding that it has failed. The response to a particular dose of a drug cannot always be predicted accurately, but can be deduced from trial and observation. The discovery of an effective drug and its optimal dose is of such tremendous importance to a patient with a lifetime of chronic or recurring illness that months of careful trial of drugs is worthwhile.

Check what medication is being taken

If in any doubt about what is being taken, have patients bring all their medication with them, including unused medication from previous prescriptions. Go through the packets, asking how many they are taking, and checking that they know what each is for.

PRESCRIBING AND THE LIFE CYCLE

Women may become pregnant

Psychotropic drugs may harm the developing foetus. Before prescribing to a woman of childbearing age, enquire about the last menstrual period, contraception and the patient's intentions about getting pregnant.

Prescribing for someone known to be pregnant

A recurrence of a depressive illness or an attack of schizophrenia during pregnancy can be devastating for the mother and potentially a serious threat to the well-being and sometimes life of the unborn child. Where there is a serious risk of such recurrence, the prophylactic use of an antidepressant, or of an antipsychotic, may be necessary. Psychotropic drugs may increase the risk of congenital deformities in the baby. Such abnormalities occur in at least 1–2% of pregnancies anyway, with no known cause. Animal experiments with drugs sometimes suggest teratogenicity, but because the experiments are not on humans, and usually with high doses of drugs, such suggestions have to be regarded with reserve. Human experiences of the drug, with careful collection of statistics over a long period, are a truer guide. However, it is fair to say that although some commonly used and older psychotropic drugs do increase the risk of damage to the foetus, most do not do so to a great extent. The risk must be balanced against the consequences of serious mental illness to the mother and her family. Remember that a drug is likely to be more of a risk for the foetus in higher dosage, and during the first 3 months of foetal life. New drugs or those with known risks (such as carbamazepine) should be avoided. Your local pharmacy department is a good source of information on the use of drugs in pregnancy, and a national information service is available (Newcastle Information Service on drugs in pregnancy, tel: 0191 232 1525).

As drug metabolism may be altered during pregnancy, it may be necessary to adjust dosage in pregnancy, and to readjust soon after childbirth.

Breastfeeding and infancy

Most drugs cross the placental barrier, and also appear in breast milk. The neonate may show withdrawal symptoms if its mother is dependent on opiates or alcohol; or may be limp or even goitrous if she takes lithium. The effects of lithium are, however, transient, with no evidence of lasting harm. Even though the amounts of drug in milk may not be great, the neonate up to about 1 year has less than a child or adult in the way of liver enzymes to destroy active drugs, as well as relatively poor renal function; therefore drugs tend to persist in its body. On present knowledge the doses of phenothiazines, tricyclic antidepressants and anticonvulsants administered to babies in the breast milk of mothers on these drugs appear to be unimportant. Where the mother is taking lithium or diazepam, however, the baby may be affected. New mothers will need to be informed about the risks to the baby of breastfeeding while taking these drugs, and assisted in the choices she makes as to how to feed her baby and whether to continue on the drugs. If in doubt, consult a pharmacist, who will usually have ready access to the most up-to-date information and who may well be able to offer useful advice.

Older people

Growing old is associated with relative metabolic impairment, often aggravated by chronic disease. Kidneys no longer excrete so well; livers no longer metabolise so quickly. Small doses of drugs consequently last longer, accumulate more and exert bigger effects. The ageing brain becomes more sensitive to some drugs: benzodiazepines, classical antipsychotics and anti-Parkinsonian drugs especially. These changes occur at different ages for different people and at different rates for different drugs but are particularly marked in the very old. Older people have more diseases and take more drugs, often from two or more sources. They have therefore a much greater tendency to toxic reactions, accidental overdosing and drug interactions, than the young.

Older people are also more likely to have some degree of cognitive impairment. Impaired memory and concentration cause instructions about drugs to be forgotten or muddled. If patients with memory difficulties are in charge of their own medication, the treatment plan should be as simple as possible: few drugs (preferably no more than three) taken on a regular, easily remembered schedule, linked to the fixed points of the day, such as at meals or when going to bed. Out-patients need written instructions of which medicines to take and when to take them. A relative, friend, community nurse or warden may be able to share responsibility for giving the drugs or for reminding a forgetful patient to take them. A drug wallet or dosette box may help (see p. 27). Complications may arise from self-medication with analgesics, laxatives, drugs left over from a previous illness, or even drugs prescribed for someone else. Psychiatric disorder in the elderly person, especially acute brain syndromes (see chapter 16), often results from or is aggravated by taking too much prescribed and non-prescribed medication.

Insomnia in the elderly

Insomnia with a request for hypnotics is such a common problem in the care of the elderly that a special comment about sleep hygiene is required. First find out if the complaint can be treated by simple measures before prescribing a hypnotic. Some lonely old people go to bed in the early evening and get 5 or 6 hours sleep before their 'insomnia' begins; an after-lunch nap may be prolonged to 6 o'clock. So find out the hours they spend in bed asleep, or trying to sleep, and get independent confirmation. Reading or less time in bed, or taking part in interesting things that require some activity during the day, may give better sleep. Rising at a regular time helps to set circadian rhythms, including the sleep–wake cycle. Improved bedroom comfort such as correct temperature, quiet and pillows at the right height help to promote sleep. Sometimes diet is the culprit. Too much coffee causes excessive arousal by bedtime. Alcohol taken in the early evening may wear off in the night and is a diuretic. Too much fluid during the day can result in repeated waking with a full bladder. Too much food of the wrong kind causes indigestion. Constipation can lead to restlessness. Too much smoking may impair sleep. Medical problems interfere with sleep. Proper attention to pain, breathlessness, coughing, frequency of micturition and the correct timing of diuretic tablets may result in improved sleep. It is also crucial to consider whether the insomnia is the presenting feature of an underlying depressive illness.

An occasional dose of a hypnotic may be used, but look out for unwanted effects. Aim for an early trial without hypnotics again, because the need for them may vary over time and with changing circumstances. Long-term use is generally ineffective and produces dependence. Chloral hydrate preparations, or promazine may be given in doses about half the size for a younger adult. A short-acting benzodiazepine such as temazepam produces less hangover. Zopiclone and zolpidem may also be suitable but are no less addictive. Avoid barbiturates and long periods of benzodiazepines. However, for patients who have taken barbiturates or benzodiazepines for a very long time without increasing doses, the sensible and humane course may be to continue the prescription and perhaps try to wean them from it very slowly. The alternative will be an unhappy patient and possibly withdrawal fits or a psychosis. Excessive night sedation is dangerous. It can cause confusion, incontinence, restlessness, wandering (especially at night but sometimes by day) and impairment of balance with a risk of falling. Chest infections are also more likely in older people who are heavily sedated.

Treatment failure

The fact that a drug has been prescribed is no guarantee that it has been taken correctly (see chapter 3). Mistakes in administration of drugs do occur. Furthermore, some patients may secretly avoid taking their tablets. Then liquid preparations may be more effective than tablets, and injections surer still.

Freedom from common side-effects also suggests non-compliance. Blood level measurements may sometimes help assess the reason for failure. Of course, the prescribed dose may have been too little, or the illness may truly not be responsive to the drug. However, there must be evidence that the drug has been taken before concluding that there is no response.

True allergic or toxic sensitivities to drugs are rare, whereas psychological sensitivities are common. Psychological sensitivities may take the form of anxiety, misattribution of normal somatic sensations to side-effects of the drug, mistrust of doctor or nurse, and exaggerated ideas about 'drugs' and their risks. These include poisoning, addiction and loss of self-control. As discussed in chapter 3, health belief systems vary and misinformation is widespread. The patient who has confidence in his/her doctor will tolerate many side-effects without complaint. Such side-effects may only be elicited on direct enquiry.

Two of the most common reasons for poor results in drug treatment are inadequate dosage and failure to go on long enough. Media criticism of over-prescribing or of turning people into 'addicts' or 'zombies' sometimes persuades doctors to prescribe too little. Some patients try to control their own treatment and demand changes of dose or drug. This may reflect lack of knowledge and insight. The doctor should be the technical expert here, with enough clinical knowledge not to be diverted from assessment of the seriousness of the illness and the pharmacological measures it requires. Nevertheless, remember that the patient is well placed to evaluate the benefits and disadvantages of treatment. If a high dose is given too soon, intolerable side-effects may occur before the drug has time to produce beneficial effects.

ADRs

ADRs may result from predictable pharmacological actions (type A) or may be unusual responses of an individual (type B, idiosyncrasy). New mental or physical symptoms other than usual side-effects may appear early or late in the course of treatment. It is important to recognise when the symptoms result from idiosyncrasy, that is some individual variation of metabolism or unusual immunological response (allergy). In such a case, continuing the drug may be dangerous, and it may be impossible ever to give it again. It can be a serious matter if a patient with recurrent depressions or a schizophrenic illness cannot have the clinical benefits of an antidepressant or an antipsychotic because of the risks of idiosyncratic response. Therefore, it is important to collect satisfactory evidence and to identify the particular drug before condemning it. Establish that the patient means the same as the doctor when saying he/she has an allergy to a drug.

Unexpected results have many possible causes. The symptoms may be those of toxic overdose, taken by mistake or design, or resulting from a dispensing or nursing error. Alternatively, the patient may be intolerant of a usually safe dose of the drug because of an inability to metabolise it normally. That may happen because of an individual metabolic difference, for example confusion on nortriptyline in a poor metaboliser (CYP IID6); agranulocytosis on clozapine is more likely in HLA types B38 and DR4. Alternatively, some other drug (prescribed, illicit or over-the-counter) taken at the same time interferes with normal metabolism. Attention to the dose or to the other drugs may put matters right. There may be a coincidental onset of a physical illness, which makes the patient intolerant of his/her usual dose, or more vulnerable to a side-effect, or produces symptoms such as fever, vomiting or diarrhoea, which are mistaken for a toxic reaction.

Complementary medication may result in adverse effects either through one of the intended ingredients of a herbal remedy, or through contamination with a toxic herb, the inclusion of a heavy metal or the illegal inclusion of a medicine such as a sedative or corticosteroid.

The idiosyncrasy may not be caused by the drug you have prescribed but by some other drug the patient has taken or even food. For example, bronchospasm can result from aspirin sensitivity; urticarial rash and fever can be produced by crabmeat. Remember that an allergic idiosyncrasy is sometimes due to the coating of a tablet (for instance tartrazine in children), or to the excipient or vehicle (for instance the oil of a depot injection) and not to the active drug itself. The idiosyncrasy may be due to a toxic metabolite, for example m-CPP, causing anxiety on trazodone, or agranulocytosis with chlorpromazine; or it may be allergic, such as a rash or cholestatic jaundice (also with chlorpromazine, or clopenthixol). The allergy occurs after drug or metabolite react covalently with protein to form an immunogen, to which antibodies arise.

The symptoms of idiosyncrasy may be:

(a) in the skin – urticaria, maculopapular rash, or exfoliative dermatitis;

(b) in the liver – jaundice;

(c) in the blood – sudden drop in white count (neutropenia or even agranulocytosis). This may present with fever, sore throat or rash. Platelets or red cells may also be depressed with consequent purpura or anaemia;

(d) Stevens-Johnson syndrome – a severe multi-organ inflammatory reaction with skin and mucosal lesions and pneumonia;

(e) Guillain-Barré syndrome – a peripheral neuropathy;

(f) a sudden rise in temperature – with joint pains, swollen lymph glands, and urticaria; 8–10 days after starting may be due to serum sickness.

(g) neuroleptic malignant syndrome (see below);

(h) in the kidney – albuminuria, haemoglobinuria and signs of oliguria and nephritis; and

(i) in the lung – bronchospasm.

What to do in case of suspected idiosyncrasy

Although it is sometimes possible to treat through a mild rash, this carries the risk of a more severe reaction and it is generally advisable to stop the suspected drug, which is especially likely to be one started about 10 days earlier: stop all drugs if a single culprit is not apparent. Take 10 ml blood and deep freeze the serum for possible later immunological study for autoantibodies or viruses. Take a careful drug and chemical history, not only of what a doctor has prescribed, but of what nurses have given or the patient taken of his/her own accord; for instance, proprietary medicines, foods, drinks or industrial chemicals, soaps or washing powders on the ward. Seek information about rare side-effects of the drugs being used; the temporal relationship of the exposure to the drug is more important than the frequency with which the effect has been reported. The GP and hospital records and in-patient prescription sheets should be clearly marked so that the prescriber is aware of previous serious reactions.

The advice and help of physician, dermatologist or clinical pathologist should be sought. Treatment with corticosteroids may be needed to help the patient recover from the damage. Blood and urine tests may be needed. Skin tests (prick and scratch or patch) may be advisable to confirm the existence of hypersensitivity. There may be a possibility of desensitisation.

Idiosyncrasy established to one phenothiazine antipsychotic, for instance, does not necessarily contraindicate all. The idiosyncrasy is related to the chemical structure of the drug rather than its pharmacological action. However, it will be safer to move to a drug of a different chemical class. If the patient's psychiatric state requires drug treatment, start cautiously with another drug, small doses at first, slowly increasing, with daily monitoring of skin (for rash) and temperature, and twice weekly blood cell counts, liver function tests and urine analyses until 4 weeks have passed.

All serious ADRs and all ADRs to new drugs should be reported to the Committee on Safety of Medicines (Freepost, London SW8 5BR), either by Yellow Card or on the same forms provided in every issue of the *BNF*.

If it is safe to do so, the link between the drug and the idiosyncrasy may be proved by re-exposure in a double-blind way, with placebo control. In some instances of hepatic sensitivity the drug can be given again later without the problem recurring, but the advice of a physician must be sought and blood tests monitored.

Look out for these

Besides idiosyncrasy or allergy, many unusual reactions are simply rarely observed side-effects, caused perhaps by a rapid rise to high drug dose in treatment, or by a rapid drug withdrawal, outpacing the CNS's capacity to adapt. Others are the signs of interaction with another drug. But some reports of unusual reactions are mistaken: not due to a psychotropic drug at all but to a missed organic illness, or to some other chemical with which the patient has been in contact, possibly self-prescribed. This is why unusual reactions should be investigated, in the fullest possible way (including a postmortem if the patient has died), instead of jumping to a guessed conclusion. In its early days chlorpromazine was thought to damage the liver frequently: but later study showed there had been coincidental infective hepatitis.

ADRs are an important cause of ill-health and death; in the elderly they can account for around 10% of all admissions. Although many drug reactions are described in their place elsewhere in this book, it may be helpful to list some that are not always considered, but are important.

Rapid rise to high dose

- Dystonia owing to antipsychotics or to SSRIs, especially paroxetine, presents with bizarre postures of tongue, back, or limbs, which may be thought to be attention-seeking (hysterical) or neurological disease.
- Akinetic mutism or stupor owing to very high doses of antipsychotics (beyond those causing Parkinsonian symptoms).
- Ataxia, clumsiness, slurred speech and vomiting owing to toxic lithium levels.
- Rash (lamotrigine).

Rapid withdrawal after long-term treatment

- Delirium tremens, from alcohol.
- Epileptic fit, from benzodiazepine, barbiturate or anticonvulsant.
- Mania, 2–4 weeks after stopping lithium abruptly.
- Headache, nausea, vomiting and insomnia from imipramine or amitriptyline, or a phenothiazine.
- Severe Parkinsonism, with rigidity and salivation, from cessation of an anti-Parkinsonian drug.
- Sudden reduction of high dose of sedatives or opiates may result in confusional state.
- Dizziness and 'flu-like malaise after stopping venlafaxine or SSRIs, e.g. paroxetine.
- Nausea, feeling of unsteadiness, as if on a boat, and visual illusions together with severe anxiety after stopping benzodiazepines.

Some of these reactions may even occur during treatment, or when the patient has missed only 1 or 2 day's tablets (for instance over a weekend), for example with paroxetine or venlafaxine, or panic attacks with short-acting benzodiazepines.

Pharmacodynamic drug interactions

- Lithium toxicity at relative low or therapeutic blood levels, especially in combination with antipsychotics or other drugs.
- Parkinsonism from tricyclic or SSRI plus lithium.
- Serotonin syndrome: high fever, myoclonus, chorea, confusion, fits and coma caused by combination of drugs

increasing serotonin function, e.g. clomipramine, SSRIs or venlafaxine with MAOIs, lithium, L-tryptophan or carbamazepine.

- Severe throbbing headache with hypertension and sometimes fever from MAOI with amine drug such as tricyclic, pethidine or ephedrine (in cold cure)

Pharmacokinetic drug interactions

- Fluvoxamine plus clozapine: clozapine levels may be increased 10-fold by the addition of fluvoxamine. This can induce seizures.
- Naproxen plus lithium: NSAIDs can inhibit renal excretion of lithium and increase plasma levels by up to 50%. These interactions can produce permanent neurological damage and can be fatal.
- Warfarin and antidepressants: most antidepressants inhibit the metabolism of warfarin via a complex mechanism. Bleeding can result.

Neuroleptic malignant syndrome

This consists of generalised muscular rigidity (which can make swallowing and breathing difficult), pyrexia, autonomic instability and lowered consciousness. Rhabdomyolysis occurs with myoglobinuria and acute renal failure; occasionally this is the main manifestation of the condition, rigidity not being apparent. Respiratory failure may result from rigidity of the chest wall and require ventilation. Laboratory findings include raised creatinine phosphokinase (CPK), leucocytosis and low serum iron. It occurs during treatment with antipsychotics and is thought to be due to diminished dopamine function in the basal ganglia and possibly the hypothalamus. Its cause is unclear but antipsychotics must be stopped or the outcome may be fatal, with hyperpyrexia, renal failure, respiratory failure or pneumonia. It is more likely to occur during an intercurrent physical illness, or in a patient with catatonic features. A detailed physical examination and investigations should be made. After full recovery for 2 weeks the patient may be able to tolerate the same drug again without a recurrence, but it is best if possible to use drugs of a different class. All classes of antipsychotics can cause it. For severe cases respiratory paralysis may require urgent ventilation. Treatment may be tried with bromocriptine (5–60 mg daily) or with dantrolene, which acts directly on skeletal muscle; the advice of a physician should be sought.

Unexpected Parkinsonism

Do not forget that haloperidol, even when given for only a short period, can provoke this reaction, which may then continue for weeks after the drug has been stopped. SSRIs too have been known to produce extrapyramidal side-effects that persist for months. Also, a drug-free patient who develops a depressive illness may show some signs of Parkinsonism, which will disappear again as the patient recovers.

Table 8.I Neuroleptic malignant syndrome (NMS), serotonin syndrome and lithium toxicity

	NMS	serotonin syndrome	lithium toxicity
NMS			
Antipsychotic	++	0	+/–
Lead-pipe rigidity	+++	0	0
Catatonia/stupor	+++	0	0
Slow onset	++	0	++
Autonomic instability	++	+/–	0
Raised CPK	+++	+	+/–
Serotonin syndrome			
Serotoninergic drugs	0	+++	0
Chorea/myoclonus	0	+++	+
Shivering	0	+++	0
Agitation	0	++	0
Lithium toxicity			
Lithium	0	0/+	+++
Vomiting	0	0	+++
Cerebellar signs	0	0	+++
Non-specific signs			
Hyperpyrexia	++	++	+
Sweating	+++	++	+/–
Confusion/coma	+++	++	++
Hypertension	++	++	0

CPK, creatinine phosphokinase; 0, absent; +, mild; ++, moderate; +++, marked; ++++, marginal.

Differentiating unusual neuromuscular side-effects

Three conditions, serotonin syndrome, neuromalignant syndrome (NMS) and lithium toxicity have overlapping clinical presentations and Table 8.1 compares their features, grouping together those most characteristic of each.

It is clear that although these conditions share certain non-specific symptoms such as pyrexia, sweating and lowering of level of consciousness, they can usually be distinguished by cerebellar signs and vomiting (lithium toxicity), rigidity (NMS) and agitation, shivering and severe chorea (serotonin syndrome).

Further reading

Buckley, P. F. & Hutchinson, M. (1995) Neuroleptic malignant syndrome. *Journal of Neurology, Neurosurgery and Psychiatry*, **58**, 271–273.

Davis, D. M. (1991) *Textbook of Adverse Drug Reactions* (4th edn). Oxford: Oxford University Press.

Mir, S. & Taylor, D. (1999) Serotonin syndrome. *Psychiatric Bulletin*, **23**, 742–747.

Montgomery, S. A. & Asberg, M. (1979) A new depression scale designed to be sensitive to change. *British Journal of Psychiatry*, **134**, 382–389.

Morin, C. M., Colecchi, C., Stone, J., *et al* (1999) Behavioural and pharmacological therapies for late-life insomnia. *Journal of the American Medical Association*, **281**, 991–999.

Ragheb, M. & Powell, A. L. (1986) Lithium interactions with sulindac and naproxen. *Journal of Clinical Psychopharmacology*, **6**, 150–154.

Sayal, K. S., Duncan-McConnell, D. A., McConnell, H. W., *et al* (2000) Psychotropic interactions with warfarin. *Acta Psychiatrica Scandinavica*, **102**, 250–253.

Taylor, D. (1997) Pharmacokinetic interactions involving clozapine. *British Journal of Psychiatry*, **171**, 109–112.

Young, R. C., Biggs, J. T., Zeigler, V. E., *et al* (1978) A rating scale for mania: reliability, validity and sensitivity. *British Journal of Psychiatry*, **133**, 429–435.

United Kingdom Psychiatric Pharmacists Group website: http://www.ukppg.ppg.uk – this links to other sites, including the FDA.

9. THE COST OF TREATMENT

In former times prescribers could base their practice wholly on their knowledge of clinical pharmacology. Today, a much broader perspective is required. For decades, drugs used in psychiatry have been cheap to purchase and price differences have been small. In addition, the pressure to control healthcare spending has not been so keenly felt as during the past decade. Modern psychotropics are comparatively expensive to buy and differences between them, both pharmacological and financial, relatively large.

Drug choice is now a complex process that takes into account relative efficacy, safety and cost-effectiveness. The last of these is one consideration in the growing discipline of pharmaco-economics, a knowledge of which is essential for effective prescribing.

Drug costs

The pharmaceutical industry is a global business that depends on sales of drugs for its livelihood. The cost of a drug is essentially determined by profit considerations and market forces.

By the time a drug is licensed for use in clinical practice (see chapter 4), it may have only 5 or 10 years of patent remaining. The pharmaceutical manufacturer must therefore set a price for its drug that is likely to recoup its research and marketing costs quickly, and to generate enough profit to allow growth of the business. Increased competition and patent expiry eventually lead to a reduction in price and in profit margins.

On the expiry of a patent, other manufacturers are usually allowed to produce the drug and to market it. Having spent nothing on the drug's development, the manufacturer of the generic product can set a price substantially lower than that of the developer.

Generic preparations must pass stringent tests to ensure uniform content, stability and bioavailability and so may generally be considered to be equivalent to the developer's branded product. Small differences in colour, palatability and storage requirements occasionally make the prescribing of a branded product preferable to a generic one. Examples are, however, rare and the cheaper generic product is usually the one to prescribe. In any case, most hospital pharmacies practice generic substitution, whereby they may supply any preparation of the same drug against a prescription for a branded product. Conversely, community pharmacies are legally obliged to supply the product requested by trade name. Where none is specified, the cheapest available generic will be dispensed. With stiff competition, the cheapest generic version may change from week to week. As a result, patients may receive two or three different generic forms in the same container. This can lead to confusion and perhaps even poor compliance. A few prescribers request branded products to avoid this possibility.

In hospitals, drugs are usually less expensive. This is largely because manufacturers often offer discounts in order, indirectly, to promote the use of their products. The hospital purchase price of a product may, in some cases, be less than half of the cost in the community. Price differences are, however, partly offset by the levying of VAT on hospital purchases (community purchases are exempt). Perhaps more importantly, patients prescribed drugs in hospital usually receive only discounted medication during their stay, but continue to be prescribed non-discounted drugs (from GPs) once discharged. The cost of long-term treatment in the community then quickly offsets any small gains made while in hospital. (This is well known and explains why manufacturers are happy to discount on hospital purchases.) Many hospitals and trusts now disregard the unrealistic discounted price of drugs that they purchase and base their decisions on the cost in the community.

PHARMACO-ECONOMICS

This is a complex subject with a growing importance in all areas of medicine, including psychiatry. The pharmaco-economics of a new drug are now considered in the same light and with the same scrutiny as other more established factors, such as efficacy and safety. An understanding of pharmaco-economic principles is essential to clinicians practising in psychiatry.

Pharmaco-economic evaluations of medical treatments vary in their sophistication and accepted validity.

Cost analysis

The most rudimentary form of evaluation is cost analysis, which simply compares costs of treatments, but ignores the outcomes of these treatments (e.g. a comparison of the costs of using either dothiepin or amitriptyline in depression).

Cost minimisation analysis

A similar method is cost minimisation analysis, which compares costs of treatments and assumes equal outcomes based on literature evaluation. In our dothiepin/amitriptyline example, the cheaper amitriptyline would be favoured in this type of analysis.

Cost-effectiveness analysis

A more sophisticated method is the cost-effectiveness analysis, which compares healthcare costs and therapeutic outcomes. In such an evaluation, dothiepin might be found to be more cost-effective than amitriptyline (despite being more expensive) if it were shown to be better tolerated and produce fewer adverse effects.

Cost-utility analysis and cost–benefit analysis

Still more complex are cost–utility analysis and cost–benefit analysis, both of which aggregate outcomes to a single value for comparison.

These methods are rarely used in psychiatry, partly because of the inherent difficulty in weighting psychiatric outcomes to provide a single numerical value. An example is the calculation of quality-adjusted life-years for patients on a new treatment such as clozapine.

The methods described incorporate different ranges of outcomes in the analysis. Ideally, all potential outcomes and costs should be considered. The box below (Box 9.1) shows some of the factors that might be considered in a pharmaco-economic evaluation of the antipsychotic clozapine.

A full cost-effectiveness analysis or cost–benefit analysis would include all of the outcomes in the box in order to establish the relative cost-effectiveness or cost-benefit of two or more antipsychotics. The same principles apply to analyses of other psychotropic drugs: essentially all direct and indirect costs of treatment should be included. Direct costs are those incurred as a result of treatment and include only those factors directly related to healthcare or social care, for example capital costs, overheads, staff and treatment costs, hospital and social security payments. Indirect costs include those incurred by society, such as absence from work and loss of earnings and productivity (for patients and carers).

The results of pharmaco-economic evaluations are grossly affected by the inclusion or otherwise of direct and indirect costs. Likewise, as with clinical efficacy trials, study design has a profound bearing on results obtained. Indeed, many pharmaco-economic studies are much less scientifically robust than their clinical efficacy counterparts: prospective, randomised, controlled trials are uncommon.

Pharmaco-economics is a rapidly developing subject area that is likely to have an increasing influence on drug choice. At present, pharmaco-economic evaluations have only an indirect influence on prescribing, but, as the scientific validity of studies improves, clinicians can soon be expected to take full account of pharmaco-economic issues when deciding upon drug choice.

THE COST OF TREATMENT AND DRUG CHOICE

Clinicians are now expected to have a wide knowledge of a drug's properties before prescribing it. Factors that need to be considered

---

Box 9.1 Costs and benefits of pharmaco-economic evaluation of clozapine

Potential costs	Potential benefits
Purchase of clozapine	Reduction in symptoms
Monitoring	Reduced length of hospital stay
Clozapine clinic staff	Reduced readmission rates
Admission to hospital to start clozapine	Improvement in quality of life
Burden of adverse effects	Reduction in movement disorders
Community psychiatric nurse visits	Reduction in social security payment
Out-patient appointments	Reduction in care-giver burden
Hostel accommodation	Increased productivity in society

include efficacy, tolerability, safety, frequency of dosing, cost and cost-effectiveness. Two other factors are perhaps of more practical use (see chapter 5). The effectiveness of a drug is a measure of its usefulness in normal clinical practice – a property that may or may not relate to its efficacy, which is what is measured in clinical trials. The number needed to treat (NNT) provides an estimate of the number of patients who needed to receive a drug (or any intervention) for one of those patients to experience a specific benefit or adverse event (see chapter 5). In the past 20 years or so there has been an explosion of information on these issues that few clinicians can assimilate and keep up to date with.

Help is at hand in several forms. The BNF is updated every 6 months and contains brief clinical details alongside general advice on prescribing of individual drugs. Costs are also included, but cost-effectiveness is not covered. *The Extra Pharmacopoeia* (Martindale), updated every 2 years or so, has more detailed information and cites individual clinical studies. Both publications are available on CD-ROM and can be included in hospital networks.

Hospital pharmacists are also useful sources of information. Some hospitals have drug information departments staffed by pharmacists with wide experience of psychotropic drugs. Hospital and drug information pharmacists can provide information on all aspects of drug use (including cost and cost-effectiveness) and can usually provide useful primary references or summary reviews. In many units, pharmacists are the only personnel available to devote enough time to drug treatment issues to keep abreast of the subject. They are thus a useful resource and can make worthwhile contributions to the multi-disciplinary team.

Pharmaceutical price regulation

In the UK the profits of pharmaceutical companies are regulated by the Government through the Pharmaceutical Price Regulation Scheme (PPRS). This controls the maximum (but not the guaranteed) profits companies can make on the capital they have invested in research, development and manufacturing for sale to the NHS. The scheme began in 1957 and is reviewed at intervals of about 5 years. From 1999 there was a 4.5% price reduction on branded medicines, and there is a common allowable return on capital of 21%, which can be increased up to 30% by innovation and productivity, but not by price increases. New products entering the market are priced at the discretion of the company, and not controlled.

In addition the PPRS sets an allowance for expenditure on the promotion of products, which is governed by total NHS sales, and allocated to each company according to a formula. Companies with more products have a larger allowance. The average is 7–8% of income from NHS sales. The level of expenditure on research and development is negotiated with each company, but generally the maximum is 23% of total NHS sales. The PPRS was to be the sole mechanism for ensuring that medicines are available to the NHS at reasonable prices. It was also intended to promote a strong and profitable industry in the UK.

However, the Government has further influenced prescribing by means of an approved list for some classes of drugs, and through the National Institute for Clinical Excellence.

Further information on the PPRS is available from The Association of the British Pharmaceutical Industry, 12 Whitehall, London SW1A 2DY (tel: 020 7930 3477).

FURTHER READING

Aitchison, K. J. & Kerwin, R. W. (1997) Cost-effectiveness of clozapine. A UK clinic-based study. *British Journal of Psychiatry*, **171**, 125–130.

Davies, L. M. & Drummond, M. F. (1993) Assessment of costs and benefits of drug therapy for treatment-resistant schizophrenia in the United Kingdom. *British Journal of Psychiatry*, **162**, 38–42.

Hotopf, M., Lewis, G. & Norman, C. (1996) Are SSRIs a cost-effective alternative to tricyclics? *British Journal of Psychiatry*, **168**, 404–409.

Martindale, W. (1999) *The Complete Drug Reference* (32nd edn). London: Pharmaceutical Press. (First published in 1883.)

Meltzer, H. Y., Cola, P., Way, L., *et al* (1993) Cost effectiveness of clozapine in neuroleptic-resistant schizophrenia. *American Journal of Psychiatry*, **150**, 1630–1638.

Morris, S., Hogan, T. & McGuire A. (1998) The cost-effectiveness of clozapine: a survey of the literature. *Clinical Drug Investigation*, **15**, 137–152.

Rosenheck, R., Cramer, J., Xu, W., *et al* (1997) A comparison of clozapine and haloperidol in hospitalized patients with refractory schizophrenia. *New England Journal of Medicine*, **337**, 809–815.

Sacristán, J. A., Gómez J. C., Martin J., *et al* (1998) Pharmacoeconomic assessment of olanzapine in the treatment of refractory schizophrenia based on a pilot clinical study. *Clinical Drug Investigation*, **15**, 29–35.

Woods, S. W. & Baker, C. B. (1997) Cost-effectiveness of newer antidepressants. *Current Opinion in Psychiatry*, **10**, 95–101.

10. CONSENT TO TREATMENT AND GOOD PRESCRIBING HABITS

In general all patients have the right to have a proposed treatment explained to them and to decide whether or not to accept it. But psychiatric patients can pose three kinds of difficulty here.

Some psychiatric patients may accept a treatment although they have not understood the explanation or what they are agreeing to. Perhaps they agree in an attempt to please the doctor, or are giving way to what they feel is pressure, or they regard the treatment as a punishment that they believe they fully deserve. This is not real consent; it is termed incompetent and is not acceptable.

Others fail to give consent not because they necessarily disagree but because the very nature of their illness makes such consent impossible. They may be mute, in catatonic stupor, suffer from a state of continuous indecision about everything, entertain bodily delusions or have a marked thought disorder that makes it very difficult to be sure what they mean when they speak.

Some refuse in clear consciousness and after discussion. They do not believe they are ill or need treatment, or may fear side-effects of drugs or the way they are given. It may none the less be in the patient's best interests to have the proposed treatment, even a matter of death if they do not have it.

Without 'real' consent, or with refusal, treatment would be an assault and illegal. The Mental Health Act (MHA) 1983 provides a way forward, a procedure allowing treatment of the non-consenting patient by making safeguards for both patient and medical and nursing staff. The patient must be detained under a Section of the MHA. An informal patient in hospital may have to be detained for this purpose. This needs recommendations by a doctor approved under Section 12 of the Act as having special knowledge of psychiatry, and of another doctor who is not on the hospital staff, most often the family doctor, who knows the patient, and an application by an approved social worker or nearest relative. The MHA Section 2, lasting 28 days, or Section 3, lasting 6 months, are thus completed; both can be cancelled at any time before they expire. Mentally disordered offenders detained through a Court under Sections 36, 37, 38 or transferred from prison under Sections 47 or 48 also satisfy the legal requirements.

This procedure can take time, especially at weekends. In dire emergency common law allows doctors to act for the patient on their own initiative alone, avoiding the MHA procedure. For example, medication is given under common law in a life-threatening situation, often at first contact and in a crisis. Alternatively, a seriously dehydrated patient with depression who is refusing all fluids could justifiably be given intravenous diazepam or even electroconvulsive therapy (ECT) forthwith in order to get him/her to drink again. The keeping of full written records of what is being done at all times is an important additional safeguard. The patient's relatives should also be kept fully informed; it is hoped they will concur in the treatment, but their approval is not needed and they cannot bar it.

The treatments controlled by the MHA and discussed here are psychotropic drugs, and the surgical implantation of sex hormones to reduce male sex drive. Leucotomy, a purely surgical procedure, and ECT are also controlled.

DRUG TREATMENT WITHOUT CONSENT

Drugs may be given without the patient's consent if the patient is detained. This includes drugs, such as lithium and clozapine, that require blood tests. After 3 months' treatment under Section 3 the responsible medical officer must sign a certificate that the patient understands the nature, purpose and effects of the drug and agrees to continue. Otherwise a second opinion must be obtained from an independent second opinions approved doctor (SOAD) approved by the Mental Health Act Commission (MHAC) (Sections 58(1) b and (3) b). Long-stay in-patients may agree to treatment without understanding, so it is wise to have a documented second opinion, as above, if there is the slightest doubt.

Surgical implantation of hormones (but not of drugs) to reduce sex drive as a medical treatment for a mental disorder requires for all patients, whether detained or not, the patient's agreement plus a SOAD's approval (Section 57). This affected the use of oestrogen implants but does not affect depo-Provera or goserelin (see chapter 39).

BOURNEWOOD

The 1983 MHA does not fully address the question of patients (particularly those with dementia or learning disabilities but also some with severe schizophrenia or depressive illness) who are unable to give informed consent, but none the less conform with hospitalisation or treatment. This gap in the law was recently tested in the Bournewood judgement (House of Lords, 1998). Despite a contrary prior conclusion in the Court of Appeal, the House of Lords ruled that in such circumstances appropriate care could legally be provided under the "doctrine of necessity". One of the three law Lords giving this (unanimous) judgement commented that such care or treatment contained "none of the safeguards" of the MHA. Subsequent Government guidelines confirmed that informal admission and treatment of compliant incapacitated patients was appropriate but suggested regular assessment of capacity during admission and consultation with relatives or carers.

OUT-PATIENTS

Patients under Section 2 or 3 may be permitted leave from hospital (Section 17) on specified conditions and are said to be liable to be detained. The conditions may include that they continue to take medication. This condition may continue (according to the 1999 Code of Practice of the Mental Health Act) until the Section expires. If the patient then refuses medication, he/she cannot be compelled to take it unless he/she is recalled to hospital, formally and in writing, and this can only be done if his/her condition warrants it (Code of Practice 20.11). A section affecting a patient on leave cannot be renewed when it expires unless the patient requires to be detained in hospital. Grounds for recommending compulsory readmission to hospital, besides the features of acute mental illness, include preventing further serious deterioration in the patient's health as well as dangerousness.

A Guardianship Order (Sections 7 and 8) can require a patient to attend for treatment but does not authorise any treatment, including drugs, against the patient's wishes. Likewise, a Community Supervision Order (Section 25) requires the patient to live at a specified address and to allow access to professionals, but does not permit treatment to be given against the patient's wishes. A Probation Order, with a condition of treatment imposed by a Court, similarly does not compel the acceptance of medication, except that non-compliance with medical advice might warrant recall of the order.

The supervision and treatment orders introduced by the Criminal Procedures (Insanity and Unfitness to Plead) Act 1991, which provides more flexible disposal by courts of offenders found unfit to plead or not guilty by reason of insanity, are based on agreed treatment and supportive programmes on a voluntary basis. Thus, if the client refuses medication at a later date, it cannot be imposed.

Restriction Orders (Section 37/41 of MHA) imposed by the courts when patients, if untreated, are considered a likely serious danger to the public, allow for longer-term treatment when they are on leave in the community. If the patient no longer complies with medication, the Home Office (which controls the patient's whereabouts) usually orders his/her recall to hospital. When restricted patients are conditionally discharged from their detention in hospital by a mental health tribunal, it is now usual to incorporate a long-term plan of management, supervision and, where appropriate, long-term medication as part of the process.

Consent to physical examination and treatment by the mentally disordered is not covered by the MHA, whether patients are detained or informal. The MHA Sections apply to treatment for mental disorder only. But such patients, who may be unwilling or incapable of agreeing to necessary physical procedures, have a Common Law right to be treated appropriately. The medical and surgical treatment must be "in the best interests of the patient" and, by implication, to preserve life, health and well-being. Full consultation (with relatives, multi-disciplinary team and specialists) is required and most hospitals now have clear guidelines with proper documentation to record that the necessary steps have been followed.

The procedures outlined above apply to England and Wales. Very similar practices are followed in other parts of the UK. Scotland has a community treatment order and such legislation in England and Wales is currently proposed in a Government Green Paper.

GOOD PRESCRIBING HABITS

In-patients

The prescription sheet serves five separate but interrelated functions:
- it is the means of ordering drugs from the pharmacy
- it is the instruction sheet for nurses giving patients the drug
- it records the administration
- it is an important part of the patient's record of treatment
- it may also become a legal document in litigation.

Different hospitals have different designs of treatment chart. The following procedures are worth putting into practice:
- the patient's surname, first name, date of birth, hospital number and ward should always be on the prescription sheet; do not leave it to someone else
- date the prescription
- use the proper name of the drug, not its trade name, unless a particular brand is intended. State the form (tablet or liquid) in which the drug is to be given
- write, preferably print, in English when the drug is to be given and avoid medical Latin, or abbreviations such as bd or prn (pro re nata), which can result in error
- in writing 'as required' medication, give maximum dose at a time, indication (e.g. sleeplessness, agitation), its possible frequency and total amount permitted within 24 hours. For use in acute disturbance, limit number of days it is valid, e.g. 7. Do not write 'oral/IM', but write separate prescriptions for each route, or it may later be impossible to tell which route was used. Moreover, for many drugs smaller doses are needed intramuscularly
- sign the prescription legibly with name as well as initials
- at the same time as you prescribe a drug, write in the case notes what you have prescribed and give a reason, assessing the effects of the previous drug if there was one
- when changing a prescription, date the crossing-out of the previous drug when the new drug is written in. Record your decision and the reasoning behind it in the case notes
- in patients receiving long-term care, review medication at least monthly; in acute cases, at least weekly. Check from time to time how the nurses are giving out a prescription; for instance, night sedation may be given routinely needlessly, or too early, or daytime sedation may be over-used
- see that old prescription cards are filed in sequence with a date on the front, so that it is a simple matter to find out what medication the patient had been receiving at an earlier date.

Out-patients

The hospital pharmacy may supply drugs for out-patients, usually on a special hospital card, otherwise drugs for out-patient treatment in the NHS may be prescribed on form FP10 (HP), pads of which are provided by the hospital. A FP10 form is, in effect, an order to a commercial pharmacist to supply the drugs written on it to the patient whose name appears at the top, in return for payment, part of which is met by the patient and the remainder by the NHS. The FP10 form is also a set of instructions to the pharmacist about what to print on the label so that the patient may know what he/she is taking, how often to take it and for how long. The FP10 may become a legal document in cases of litigation. Since the FP10 form cannot be a record of treatment unless carbon copies are kept, a note of the prescription should also be made in the patient's case notes, dated and signed. Remember to observe the following. Write the patient's full name and address at the top, and print the proper name of the drug. Specify the form in which it is to be dispensed, the frequency with which it is to be taken and the number of tablets, capsules and so on that are to be given to the patient. The pharmacist must supply what is written, standard preparation or particular commercial brand except in the case of Government approved listed drugs, mainly benzodiazepines, for which a generic brand may be dispensed even when, for instance 'Valium', a brand is written (see chapter 5).

If you do not wish your patient to know the drug name (a very rare event) delete the letters NP at the top of the prescription form, otherwise the dispenser will write the name of the drug on the container label. Sign and print your name legibly; if there is a mistake the dispenser will be able to contact you.

Explain to the patient why the drug is being given and tell him/her, or a responsible relative, how often to take it, what serious side-effects to expect and how to cope with them. Failure to take drugs results in part from poor education and inadequate discussion.

Since the FP10 is in the patient's charge between leaving the out-patient clinic and reaching the dispensing chemist, opportunity for forgery arises. To avoid forgery print the drug name in bold capitals and the quantity in Arabic numerals and in words. Leave no free space below the prescription and initial alterations.

Prescriptions ordering controlled drugs are covered by certain restrictions (see chapters 21 and 35).

Remember, FP10 pads can be stolen and used to forge prescriptions. Lock them up.

One principle governing the role of the hospital or GP in prescribing is that the doctor who has clinical responsibility for that element of a patient's care should do the prescribing. The high cost of new medicines and the fact that hospital doctors may prescribe drugs to treat conditions with which the GP is less familiar have led to the need for shared-care for some conditions. This is most appropriate for the long-term management of chronic but stabilised illness, such as bipolar affective disorder. For these conditions the hospital doctor and GP agree on a written arrangement – protocol – setting out who does what, for instance the arrangements for prescribing, blood tests and medical review. Other suitable groups might include those with schizophrenia, those with Alzheimer's disease receiving cholinesterase inhibitors, and prescribing for substance misusers. In the modern NHS shared-care arrangements between primary and secondary care are usually decided by committees, including members from hospitals, health authorities and primary care groups (PCGs). In the future, direct negotiations between PCGs and secondary care trusts is likely.

Dependence on prescribed drugs

Usually anxiety, tension, worrying or helplessness first bring these patients to medical attention. They request regular doses of minor tranquillizers, analgesics or appetite suppressants to avert symptoms and maintain a sense of well-being, but they do not become dependent on 'hard' drugs. By the time they reach psychiatric out-patients they may have been provided with drugs for years. Referral may be by GPs no longer agreeable to prescribing such drugs long-term, or patients themselves influenced by the media emphasising the dangers and wish to withdraw.

The psychiatrist may advise continuing the supply of drugs but must take steps to ensure that drug intake does not steadily increase, as it may easily do, by agreeing with the family doctor for only one person to prescribe the drug and to fix what the dose shall be. On the other hand, if it is agreed that the aim is withdrawal, appropriate psychological help is needed. Whichever course is decided, the longer-term management is a matter for the family doctor.

FURTHER READING

House of Lords (1998) *R. v. Bournewood Community Mental Health NHS Trust ex parte L. (by his friend)*. Houes of Lords Judgement, 25 June 1998.

Kearney, N. & Treloar, A. (2000) In the light of Bournewood. Changes in the management of elderly incapacitated patients. *Psychiatric Bulletin*, **24**, 52–54.

Shaw, M. (2001) Competence and consent to treatment in children and adolescents. *Advances in Psychiatric Treatment*, **7**, 150–159.

11. DEPRESSIVE DISORDERS

EPIDEMIOLOGY

Depressive disorders are common both in the community and in people presenting in a primary care setting. One-month prevalence rates in the community (using standardised screening and detection instruments) of about 5–7% have been reported in Europe, Australia and the US. In patients presenting to their GP rates are as high as 10%. Still higher rates (20–30%) are found in people with significant physical illness in the general hospital setting.

Depressive disorders are associated with very considerable loss of general health and work capacity. Susceptibility to physical illness increases and hospitalisations for such illness tends to be prolonged. Patients with depression also consult their GPs more often than those free of depression, often with somatic complaints that mask their depression. Mortality is also increased in the context of depressive disorders (particularly in older people), partly, but not entirely, owing to suicide. People with depressive disorders lose more than five times as many days from work as non-depressed controls. They also have an increased mortality, and a specific association with cardiovascular problems.

CLINICAL FEATURES AND CLASSIFICATION

Low mood is one of the cardinal features of depression – as well as sadness this can encompass loss of interest, loss of the capacity to enjoy, anger and irritability, a sense of emptiness and a loss of motivation. All these feelings can also occur normally but transiently in response to stress, loss or other adverse life circumstances. It is helpful to compare the patient's feeling and behaviour with that of others, and more especially with that of people who resemble the patient in gender, ethnic and social background. Comparison with the individual's past mood states is also helpful. Some patients can recognise in themselves whether their current mood state is inappropriate; indeed, patients with recurrent depression are often the first to notice early signs of depressive relapse – but the last to notice their own emerging recovery.

True depressive disorders are associated with a cluster of symptoms and signs that affect several areas apart from mood. Thought and cognition may be affected in terms of poor concentration, loss of confidence and self-esteem, pessimism about the future, preoccupations with guilt or worthlessness, and thoughts of death or suicide. Motor activity may be altered, in the form of restlessness, agitation or, in contrast, slowing and loss of facial expressiveness. There may be a host of bodily symptoms including sleep disturbance (initial insomnia, early waking or excessive sleep), poor appetite, loss of energy, exhaustion, aches and pains and constipation. These bodily symptoms may be the most prominent feature in the minority of patients with depressive disorders who do not admit to depressed feelings but are preoccupied with their physical health. Only when directly asked do such patients admit to psychological symptoms. These patients may be regarded as having masked depression. Such patients may be first referred by their GPs to physicians and surgeons who must be aware that depressions can masquerade as other illnesses.

Within the broad rubric of depressive disorders, the International Classification of Diseases (ICD–10; WHO, 1992) recognises several subtypes. Major depressive episode is divided into mild (in which most daily living functions are satisfactorily maintained, albeit with difficulty); moderate (with obvious difficulty in maintaining social and work roles) and severe (with, usually, marked agitation or retardation and inability to function in a normal way). Major depressive disorder may occur with or without psychotic symptoms (delusions or hallucinations that are usually mood-congruent). Severe major depressive disorder with prominent biological symptoms is sometimes known as melancholia. Other depressive subtypes include:

- Dysthymia – in which the symptoms are relatively mild but chronic (lasting 2 years or more per episode). Dysthymia and major depressive disorder can coexist as double depression.

- Seasonal depressive disorder – has a clear pattern of autumnal onset and spring relief and is often associated with hypersomnia, lethargy and increased appetite, especially a craving for calorie-rich food such as chocolate.

- Atypical depression – may be characterised by reversed biological symptoms (overeating rather than loss of appetite; hypersomnia; mood worst at the end rather than the beginning of the day) and/or by extreme sensitivity to being rejected in relationships.

- Bipolar depression – in which episodes of mania (see chapter 12) also occur. Bipolar depression may also be rapid cycling, with cycling sometimes accelerated by antidepressants. SSRIs and bupropion are less likely to trigger manic switches in bipolar patients.

- Secondary depression – term used for depressive disorders that develop in the presence of another psychiatric or physical disorder. The link may be psychological, physiological or both. In such cases both the primary condition and the depression itself need to be treated.

- Brief recurrent depression – in which the episodes are very brief (less than 2 weeks) but may be severe and associated with suicidal intent. Patients with borderline personality may present in this way. Response to antidepressant treatments is usually disappointing.

THE AETIOLOGY OF DEPRESSIVE DISORDERS

The predominant biochemical theoretical model about the underlying pathophysiology of depressive disorders, the biogenic amine hypothesis, has been central to depression research for 40 years and is

DRUG TREATMENT

based largely upon the effects of drugs. Drugs such as reserpine, which deplete the biogenic amines noradrenalin, serotonin and dopamine can cause depression-like symptoms (though apparent agitation in such patients may also have been owing to the extrapyramidal side-effect of akathisia); conversely most antidepressants are thought to increase the synaptic availability of biogenic amines. On this basis, it was thought that depression arose from underactivity of certain central pathways for these amines, particularly noradrenalin and serotonin (5-HT). An alternative version of this theory emphasises adrenergic-cholinergic dysregulation and resultant cholinergic dominance as the main biochemical mechanism.

Recent evidence supporting a role for catecholamines in depression comes from studies of the drug alpha-methylparatyrosine. This inhibits the synthesis of noradrenalin and dopamine, causing a transient relapse of depressive symptoms when given to euthymic medication-free subjects with a history of major depression. Likewise, the role of 5-HT is supported by the finding that recently recovered patients with depression relapse quickly in response to a drink containing amino acids without L-tryptophan.

There is evidence that the turnover of 5-HT in the brain is low in some patients with depression, as measured by levels of the metabolite 5-hydroxyindole acetic acid (5-HIAA) in the CSF. This abnormality is also linked to a risk of violent suicide attempts, and in other contexts to violent behaviour. Low levels of 5-HT have also been found at postmortem in suicide victims. For most patients with depressive disorders, however, no differences in the metabolites of 5-HT, noradrenalin (methoxy-hydroxyphenylglycol, MHPG), or dopamine (homovanillic acid, HVA) are found. In recent years interest has focused more on depression-related alterations in the number or sensitivity of pre- or post-synaptic receptors for these transmitters. Findings of 5-HT-2 receptor levels in the brains of suicides postmortem have been interesting but inconsistent. Other neurotransmitters including GABA and several neuropeptides have also been implicated in the pathophysiology of depressive disorders.

Several other biological abnormalities have been described in depressive disorders. These include abnormalities in neuroendocrine function, particularly raised levels of cortisol, and resistance to suppression by dexamethason (the dexamethasone suppression test), and blunting of the thyroid stimulatory hormone (thyrotropin; TSH) response to thyrotropin releasing hormone (TRH). Raised levels of corticosteroids may be relevant as these can alter synaptic connectivity, especially in the hippocampus.

More specific pharmacological probes such as clonidine (α-2 agonist) and D-fenfluramine (releasing 5-HT) have been used to assess central noradrenalin and 5-HT receptor function, by measuring the release of growth hormone, prolactin or cortisol evoked by the drug. Peripheral markers in the form of monoamine receptors or uptake sites on platelet or lymphocyte membranes have also been widely studied. The results suggest some patients with depressive disorders do indeed have abnormalities in receptor function in depression, in some cases reflecting underlying traits (blunted growth hormone response to clonidine) and others (such as the dexamethasone suppression test

(DST)) normalising with recovery from depression and thus indicating depressed state. No biological marker with acceptably high sensitivity and specificity for depressive disorder (or any of its subtypes) to be of clinical use has yet been identified.

Neuroimaging studies (particularly using PET) reveal abnormalities in cerebral blood flow and glucose metabolism in some patients with depression, particularly in the frontal cortex and the limbic system. PET scans show a widespread reduction in brain 5-HT-1A receptor numbers in depression, and no change with treatment.

There is also considerable genetic evidence for depressive disorders having a biological substrate. Family studies demonstrate that rates of depressive disorder are about three times higher than expected in first-degree relatives of probands with unipolar depression and about four times higher in relatives of bipolar subjects. Twin studies show much higher concordance for depressive disorders in identical than in dizygotic twins, and adoption studies show increased frequency of depressive disorders in the biological but not the adoptive relatives of depressed probands.

Psychosocial factors also clearly play an important part in determining vulnerability of depressive disorders and in determining when episodes occur. Specific vulnerability factors include early maternal loss; social isolation; having several children under the age of 14 at home; being widowed, divorced or separated; alcohol or other substance misuse; and physical illness. Women are more vulnerable to unipolar (but not bipolar) depressive disorders than men. This is largely accounted for by increased vulnerability to depression in women in the months after childbirth. Low educational level also seems to increase vulnerability to depression in women but not in men.

Depression often occurs in the context of adverse life situations, especially loss events – loss of loved ones, loss of self-esteem through failures in work, the declining powers of middle-age, sudden misfortunes and sexual disappointments. The psychosocial vulnerability factors outlined above appear particularly important in determining whether an individual develops a depressive disorder in the context of such adverse life events. There is also evidence that the availability of social support, for instance a confiding relationship, may protect against life event induced depressive disorders.

It must be stressed that apparently understandable depressive disorders may be no less disabling than those arising in the absence of clear psychosocial triggers. They may also be associated with risk of suicide. Psychological understandability does not make depressive disorders any less amenable to pharmacological treatments, although psychological therapies should also be considered. CBT and IPT may have similar efficacy to antidepressants in mild to moderate depression, but in severe depression they are useful only as adjuncts (see chapter 5).

Depression can be an important symptom in conditions associated with brain damage – stroke, head injury, epilepsy, Parkinsonism, multiple sclerosis – rheumatoid arthritis and other physical illnesses associated with chronic disability. Cancer, some endocrine (especially thyroid, adrenal and parathyroid) disorders, vitamin deficiencies and viral infections are also associated with high rates of depressive symptomatology. Some drugs (e.g. oral contraceptives, methyldopa, reserpine and tetrabenazine, topiramate, lipid-soluble beta-blockers, mefloquine ('Lariam') and retinoids) predispose to depression; others (such as amphetamines and short half-life SSRIs), if stopped after long use, may result in depression. Alcohol or substance misuse will contribute to the emergence of depressive disorders and also interfere with their treatment.

IMPROVING RECOGNITION AND DIAGNOSIS OF DEPRESSIVE DISORDERS

The majority of people with depressive disorders do not receive appropriate treatment for their depression. There are several obstacles both to the recognition of depressive disorders (by patients and carers as well as by physicians) and to patient acceptance of the need for treatment. Patients may (often rightly) fear the stigmatisation associated with a psychiatric diagnosis. They may also consider their depressive symptoms to be a manifestation of weakness of character or a failure to pull themselves together; these wrong but understandable notions are often fuelled further by the feelings of low self-esteem and worthlessness integral to the depressive disorders themselves. GPs, physicians and psychiatrists alike must also guard against the temptation to dismiss persistent and disabling depressive symptoms as understandable reactions to illness or adversity.

Prominent somatic symptoms, particularly in the context of masked depression (in which the core mood-related symptoms are less prominent), may be further barriers to recognition. The pattern of somatic presentation may vary between ethnic groups and at different ages. Similarly the presence of true somatic pathology may both contribute to the depression itself and obscure its diagnosis. This is particularly problematic in older patients who not only have a greater likelihood of true somatic pathology but also tend when depressed to have less prominent mood symptoms but rather complain of bodily aches and pains and of sleep disturbance. Somatic symptoms most often associated with underlying depressive disorder include pain, sleep disturbance, constipation, exhaustion and loss of appetite.

A further diagnostic trap most often seen in older patients is the overlap in symptoms between depressive disorders and the dementias. Older people may fear dementia – when depressed these fears may reach delusional intensity. Severe depression may present with prominent loss of daily living skills, poor memory and poor concentration in the relative absence of overt low mood. Such depressive pseudodementia is usually characterised by a short history, the absence of dyspraxias or of focal neurological signs, and good insight into performance failure accompanied by an attitude of 'don't care' indifference. It must, however, be remembered that depressive symptoms may be prominent at all stages in true dementia. Though spontaneous remission rates are relatively high, such depressions of dementia have been shown to respond well to antidepressant treatments, particularly SSRIs and moclobemide, which would also be expected to have little if any adverse effects on cognitive function; in general these drugs have little or no anticholinergic properties.

Other important differential diagnoses include primary anxiety disorders and bereavement reactions. Anxiety symptoms are extremely common within depressive disorders and screening for core depressive symptoms and signs (see below) should always be undertaken before initiating symptomatic or behavioural management. As can be seen from chapter 15, many antidepressant drugs are in any case effective treatments for generalised anxiety disorder, panic disorder and phobic disorder. Depressive symptoms are almost invariably present following bereavement. In uncomplicated bereavement reactions, however, preoccupation with loss and grief are very prominent, as is withdrawal from social activities. Second-person auditory hallucinations of the deceased are also common. Persistence of depressive symptoms or hallucinatory experiences beyond 2–3 months (bearing in mind the wide range of cultural conventions concerning appropriate behaviour after bereavement), preoccupation with guilt and with a wish to be dead, and a failure to begin resuming social functioning all suggest that the bereavement has triggered a true depressive disorder.

Within a clinical interview, it is particularly important to use open-ended questions and to allow patients enough time to express their feelings and experiences. Reflective comments 'So you've been feeling sad … tell me more about that' and supportive legitimisations 'I can understand that those feelings are very painful' are helpful. It is also important to explore the range of possible depression-related experiences, including sleep and appetite disturbance, mood fluctuation and reactivity, subjective ability to concentrate, and the ability to enjoy everyday activities. Suicidal thoughts should be explored gently 'Have you ever felt that life was not worth living … tell me more about that'. Such questioning is extremely unlikely to trigger suicidal activity and may provide considerable relief to patients who have felt unable to express their most burdensome preoccupations.

Several self-report screening questionnaires have been developed to aid in the recognition of depressive disorders. These include the Zung scale (Zung, 1965) and Beck Depression Inventory (Beck *et al*, 1961). These are of course no substitute for a clinical diagnosis but are helpful in identifying subjects in whom further assessment is indicated. Clinical diagnosis may be facilitated by semi-structured interview schedules such as the Prime-MD (Spitzer *et al*, 1995), and the present state examination scales (such as the Hamilton Depression Rating Scale (Hamilton, 1960) and the Montgomery-Åsberg Depression Rating Scale (Montgomery & Åsberg, 1979)) are also available for measuring severity of depressive symptoms once a diagnosis is made. These are useful adjuncts to monitoring treatment response.

THE MANAGEMENT OF DEPRESSIVE DISORDERS

Initial assessment of a patient with a depressive disorder should generate a treatment plan that may include both psychosocial and physical treatment elements (which usually work additively rather than in opposition) and should address the main objectives of management. These are to:

- improve signs and symptoms of depression

DRUG TREATMENT

- restore psychosocial and work functioning
- reduce risk of relapse (return of symptoms within 6 months of their resolution)
- reduce risk of recurrence (return of symptoms more than 6 months after their resolution: effectively a new episode).

The first step, having established a likely diagnosis of depression and comorbid conditions, and explored the psychosocial context, is to offer the patient an explanation of his/her symptoms, sympathy and encouragement.

The person with depression often feels alone. Mustering the concern of relatives and friends may be helpful. A temporary change of environment, such as staying with a friend, may bring some relief. Admission to hospital may relieve environmental anxieties and obligations, but should not be rushed into. Admission may well be correct where there is a serious risk of suicide or of danger to others, antisocial behaviour, or a particularly unhelpful environment. On occasion, compulsory admission will be life-saving. However, the person with depression who is still working may not need to stop work, or have everyday social links and responsibilities taken away.

If possible, a patient admitted to hospital should be observed for up to 1 week with as little medication as possible, in order to clarify his/her symptom pattern and any response to non-specific treatment. During this time insomnia or daytime restlessness may need to be treated symptomatically with benzodiazepines or low-dose sedative antipsychotics. It should, however, be remembered that such symptoms usually respond well to antidepressant drugs once these are initiated.

Specific treatments such as antidepressant medication should be seen as part of an overall treatment plan, which usually includes providing support, advice and encouragement, enlisting the help of others, relatives and community psychiatric nurses, guiding the patient regarding prognosis and assessing clinical state and suicide risk until recovery. In the longer term, selected patients may benefit additionally from psychotherapeutic exploration of past and present relationships and roles, with the aim of improving their psychological adjustment.

Specific treatment

The somewhat faster onset of action and very high response rate (in well-selected cases) to ECT makes it preferable to antidepressant drugs (or psychological treatments) in very severe depression or where there is a risk of suicide. Other indications for ECT as treatment of first choice include delusional depression (which is unlikely to respond to antidepressants alone but can be treated with a combination of antidepressant and antipsychotic) and severe depressive retardation (with stupor and/or poor food and fluid intake). It is not clear whether small doses of antipsychotics such as flupentixol or chlorpromazine have a general antideressant effect or reflects improvement in items such as agitation and sleep.

Antidepressant drugs are, however, useful in the majority of patients with major depression or dysthymia and can often restore patients to their premorbid level of functioning within 1–2 months, as well as being useful in preventing relapse and recurrence. Their efficacy (compared with placebo) has been demonstrated in clinical trials in patients with all but the very mildest forms of depressive disorder. There is little evidence for differences between antidepressant classes or between individual antidepressants in overall efficacy in mild to moderate depression. Drugs with a broad spectrum of pharmacological action (such as TCAs, SNRIs and NaSSAs) may, however, be superior to SSRIs in melancholic, psychotic or very severe depressive disorders. Choice of drug should be based mainly on side-effect profile and the possibility of adverse interactions with other drugs. Other factors to consider include the presence of comorbid physical conditions, such as cardiac disease, prostatism and epilepsy, or of comorbid psychiatric disorders such as panic, obsessive–compulsive disorder (OCD) and eating disorder. Further relevant issues in antidepressant selection include vulnerability to specific side-effects (such as the increased risk of postural hypotension and to falls in older patients, weight gain, sexual dysfunction or drug-induced sedation – which may, where agitation is prominent, be desirable), dosing regimen, prior personal or family history of response to a particular antidepressant or antidepressant class, the clinician's experience of particular drugs and the patient's preference.

The drawbacks of antidepressant drugs are their slow onset of action, usually taking at least 10 days for the improvement to be distinguishable from placebo and 4–6 weeks for full effect (up to 12 weeks in older patients); their side-effects; and in some cases their toxicity in overdose. Side-effects range from the minor and irritating (dry mouth, constipation, headache and nausea) through the potentially disabling (postural hypotension, urinary retention, impotence and blurred vision) to the potentially life-threatening (cardiac dysrhythmias). In addition, response rates to antidepressants alone are only 60–70%, which must be set against a placebo response rate of about 30%. These aspects should all be explained to patients starting antidepressant treatment, and the opportunity should be taken to explore the patient's own understanding of his/her illness and its possible treatment. This should increase doctor–patient concordance with an agreed treatment plan as well as increasing drug compliance.

Drugs that are cardiotoxic in overdose should be avoided in patients with a heart disease or who are a suicide risk. In the latter situation steps should also be taken to limit their access by prescribing for only 1 week at a time, or entrusting a relative to supervise the medication.

Individual antidepressant drugs are discussed in more detail in chapters 24–27. Their classification is set out in chapter 2. Here we summarise the classes of antidepressants and their properties:

- TCAs – amitriptyline, imipramine, clomipramine, etc. These inhibit the reuptake (to varying degrees) of both noradrenalin and serotonin and also directly block (again to varying degrees) neurotransmitter receptors (notably a-noradrenergic, muscarinic and histaminergic) (see chapter 24).

- SSRIs – fluoxetine, paroxetine, sertraline, citalopram and fluvoxamine. They selectively block serotonin reuptake and have relatively little receptor-blocking effect (see chapter 25)

- MAOIs – traditional MAOIs including tranylcypromine, phenelzine and isocarboxazid. These require a low tyramine diet and have similar receptor-blocking effects to the TCAs.

More recently a selective reversible inhibitor of MAO-A (a RIMA), moclobemide, has been introduced that does not require dietary restriction and is relatively free of receptor-blocking effects (see chapter 27).

- Other reuptake-blocking antidepressants – including venlafaxine (noradrenalin and serotonin); bupropion (noradrenalin and dopamine); reboxetine (noradrenalin only); trazodone and nefazodone (serotonin) (see chapter 26).

- Miscellaneous – a further group includes mirtazapine and amoxapine, as well as lithium, lamotrigine and L-tryptophan (see chapter 26).

TCAs

Typical TCA side-effects (mainly attributable to their multiple receptor-blocking actions) include dry mouth, constipation, sedation, loss of visual accommodation, urinary retention and postural hypotension. Cardiac dysrhythmias may also occur, particularly in overdose. Within the TCA group, amitriptyline is sedative, imipramine less so, and desipramine and nortriptyline even less. These drugs have the advantage of having been widely used and having proven efficacy in a variety of settings. In general, dosage should be titrated up to the maximum tolerated. Patients metabolise TCAs and their (often) active metabolites at widely varying rates, which is why different people require different doses. In physically frail patients or where compliance is in doubt, plasma level monitoring may be useful.

TCA side-effects are worse in the first days of treatment, or just after each dose increase. The patient who has had the purpose and side-effects of the drug explained is more likely to tolerate a dry mouth and other side-effects without asking for the treatment to be changed. If postural hypotension is a problem, changing to nortriptyline or lofepramine may be helpful.

The whole of a day's dose can be taken as a single daily dose if side-effects do not prevent it: the customary ritual thrice daily has no other advantage because tricyclics have a long half-life. In fact, taking a large dose at night when the patient is lying down minimises the hypotensive and other side-effects and utilises the sedative effect; the patient is asleep when he/she might be experiencing them most. A single dose each day will also aid adherence.

SSRIs

This group of drugs, by virtue of their lack of receptor-blocking activity, carry a low burden of TCA-like side-effects. Side-effects more commonly associated with SSRIs (headache, nausea, nervousness, diarrhoea, insomnia and loss of appetite) are usually mild and transient and the SSRIs are also much safer than TCAs in overdose.

SSRIs are usually given in a single daily dose, in the morning with food. They vary quite widely in plasma half-life however, with fluoxetine (and its major active metabolite norfluoxetine) having the longest half-life and paroxetine the shortest. This is relevant in terms both of the interval necessary between stopping an SSRI and starting an MAOI (5 weeks for fluoxetine) and of the possibility of SSRI discontinuation reactions. These occur more commonly with shorter half-life (paroxetine, sertraline) than longer half-life (fluoxetine) SSRIs.

Despite their relatively alerting profile, SSRIs are often effective in the long-term in relieving anxiety symptoms within depression.

Several SSRIs inhibit CYP450 enzymes and have potential interactions with other drugs.

The good tolerability of SSRIs has resulted in their being used with success in people with very chronic depressive disorders (particularly dysthymias) in which the depressive symptoms have been wrongly thought characterological. This has resulted in popular claims that these drugs may alter personality or make people feel 'better than well'. No objective evidence exists to support the use of SSRIs as lifestyle drugs.

MAOIs

The traditional MAOIs are seldom used in first-line treatment of major depressive disorder despite their well-established efficacy. This is mainly because of the potential for causing hypertensive and hyperthermic reactions to high intake of dietary tyramine (as in cheese, pickled herrings and red wine) or to sympathomimetic agents (such as proprietary cold cures). They are, however, particularly effective for atypical depressive disorders (see above). They may also be useful in refractory depression (see below). The effect of these irreversible MAOI drugs continues for up to 4 weeks after the patient has stopped taking them, the time required to synthesise fresh enzyme to replace that inactivated by the drug. This is important because dietary restrictions and avoidance of sympathomimetic drugs should be maintained for at least 2 weeks after the MAOI is discontinued.

RIMAs

Moclobemide is the first of a new class of drugs, the reversible inhibitors of monoamine oxidase A (RIMA). Clinical trials suggest that it has equivalent antidepressant efficacy to TCAs or SSRIs. There is little evidence to suggest that it has the same preferential action as traditional MAOIs in atypical or refractory depression. Moclobemide carries much less risk than the traditional MAOIs of interaction with foodstuffs and with other drugs and, being reversible, the risk of an interaction with an SSRI lasts only for a few days after it is stopped.

OTHER ANTIDEPRESSANTS (REUPTAKE BLOCKERS AND MISCELLANEOUS)

The drugs listed in these categories are discussed in more detail in chapter 26. Bupropion has a similar side-effect profile to SSRIs but carries a risk of seizures. Like trazodone and nefazodone, it has a short half-life and should be given in divided doses. It may be useful in smoking cessation as well as in depressive disorders. Venlafaxine may, in high doses, be effective in refractory depression. Unlike TCAs and SSRIs, little if any adverse sexual side-effects are associated with nefazodone, mirtazapine and bupropion. Lamotrigine is effective in bipolar and unipolar depression and in prophylaxis of rapid-cycling BP II disorder (see chapter 32).

Refractory depression

If first-line antidepressant treatment fails to alleviate depressive symptoms, it is necessary to review the clinical situation thoroughly (see Box 11.1).

Was the right dose prescribed? Did the patient take the drug as instructed? Did side-effects prevent a high enough dose being achieved? Conversely, lack of side-effects may be a pointer to inadequate dosage, particularly of TCAs. The effects of phenytoin, carbamazepine and other drugs concurrently taken may decrease antidepressant drug levels. Laboratory measurements help to decide if plasma levels are within the therapeutic range – these are usually available for amitriptyline, imipramine and their metabolites. Were benzodiazepines or anticonvulsant drugs being taken while ECT was given, and suppressing a fit?

Failure of treatment should lead to review of the diagnosis. Is there an unrecognised medical illness? Thyroid disease in particular should be excluded. Is there a personality disorder as well as depression? Is there a problem with alcohol or substance misuse? Are there marital difficulties undermining recovery?

If the first treatment is not successful because of side-effects, a change to another drug of the same class may be helpful if the side-effect profile is slightly different, for instance another SSRI or TCA.

Box 11.1 Management of treatment-resistant depression

Check dose and compliance	Blood levels
Adjust dose	
Review diagnosis	
Review physical condition	Blood tests
Consider comorbid problems	Personality disorder
	Alcohol/drug misuse
	Marital problems
Change to different class of antidepressant	Try broader-spectrum drug, amitriptyline or SNRI
Combine antidepressant and antipsychotic	e.g. MARI plus chlorpromazine
Augmentation	Lithium, L-tryptophan
Combined SSRI and atypical antipsychotic	e.g. fluoxetine plus olanzapine
Combination of antidepressants	TCA plus MAOI
Triple drug therapy	TCA, lithium, L-tryptophan
ECT	
Psychosurgery	

SNRI, selective noradrenalin reuptake inhibitor; MARI, monoamine reuptake inhibitor; SSRI, selective serotonin reuptake inhibitor; TCA, tricyclic antidepressant; MAOI, monoamine oxidase inhibitor; ECT, electroconvulsive therapy.

In patients in whom a treatment trial has been adequate, there is only limited (uncontrolled trials) evidence that changing to another antidepressant in the same class is useful, but a change to a different class of antidepressant may induce improvement. In particular a drug with a broader spectrum of pharmacological actions (such as amitriptyline, an SNRI or an NaSSA) may be more effective for severe depression than a SSRI. On the other hand, an SSRI may be more effective if severe anxiety or panic attacks exist, or if side-effects of TCAs have limited the dose that is accepted.

MAOIs are sometimes useful when TCAs have failed. Their use following SSRIs is problematic, because of the risk of serotonin syndrome (see chapter 8).

AUGMENTATION STRATEGIES

Adding lithium carbonate to the antidepressant that has failed alone to relieve the depression has been shown to be successful in 50–60% of cases of refractory depression. Open studies in older people suggest similar efficacy for lithium augmentation to that found in open and controlled studies in younger subjects with refractory depression. There is also some evidence supporting augmentation with tri-iodothyronine, based on short-term studies.

COMBINATION STRATEGIES

Combination antidepressant treatments are widely used and may act by increasing the overall spectrum of antidepressant action. In the case of combined administration of TCAs and SSRIs, resultant increases in plasma levels of the TCA may be important. The combination of an SSRI with an NARI can also be justified, as this avoids some side-effects of TCAs, and also avoids the increased level of side-effects resulting from higher doses of SNRIs.

L-tryptophan has also been extensively used as an adjunct to an MAOI or tricyclic, with the further addition of lithium in triple therapy. Tryptophan is now used much less because of reports of an eosinophilia-myalgia syndrome (probably caused by a contaminant rather than the L-tryptophan itself).

The combination of TCAs and MAOIs has also been advocated. The combination is potentially dangerous because of the risk of the serotonin syndrome, or hypotension. Clomipramine or the SSRIs must not be combined with an MAOI, and tranylcypromine is more hazardous in combination than other traditional MAOIs. Probably the safest combination is amitriptyline or imipramine, to which phenelzine is later added. There is little evidence for the use of moclobemide in this context. If using a TCA/MAOI combination, low blood pressure and other combination side-effects must be looked for. The treatment is therefore best started in hospital, where good observation is possible. Otherwise, the patient should be seen every second or third day as an out-patient. The doses of tricyclic drug and MAOI may be increased, depending on symptom response and side-effects, in small increments to the maximum dose levels of each, as if used on its own.

COMBINING ANTIDEPRESSANT AND ANTIPSYCHOTIC

For psychotic depression the combination of an MARI with an antipsychotic such as chlorpromazine is comparable in efficacy to ECT. Such co-administration is likely to increase the level of TCAs and therefore TCA-related side-effects. However, this is not thought to explain the efficacy of the combination. An atypical antipsychotic such as olanzapine has also been used with some success in combination with an SSRI for refractory non-psychotic depression, although the pharmacological rationale has not been established.

THE USE OF ECT

ECT is an important treatment option in refractory depression; antidepressants can usually be continued during ECT administration but an antidepressant that has failed to induce remission is unlikely to prevent relapse (see below) following ECT-induced remission (see chapter 40).

OTHER STRATEGIES

Other more speculative pharmacological cocktails for refractory depression include the addition of pindolol (see page 254) and the use of drugs (such as glutethimide and ketoconazole) that reduce corticosteroid levels.

Continuation treatment

Antidepressant drugs begin by suppressing symptoms rather than abolishing the underlying malfunction. If the drugs are stopped as soon as the patient has lost all symptoms, relapse is likely. All patients responding to antidepressant treatment should continue on the same dose of drug for 6–9 months after recovery. In primary care, such continued treatment is rare and the majority cease medication within a few months. When a clinical decision is made to stop antidepressant medication, it is advisable to taper the dose over a period of at least 4 weeks. Both TCAs and SSRIs can cause symptoms if discontinued too abruptly.

This continuation phase of treatment is thought to allow time for the episode of illness to resolve. Continuation of combination antidepressant treatment should be used in patients responding acutely to such combination treatment. In patients responding to ECT, subsequent continuation treatment should be either with an antidepressant that has not failed to induce acute response, or with combination treatment (e.g. antidepressant and lithium). Antidepressants are also probably useful in the continuation treatment of patients responding to psychotherapy.

Maintenance treatment

Depression may become progressively more difficult to treat with each successive new episode. In the light of this and of the great burden of distress and poor functioning associated with recurrent depression, consideration should be given to long-term (maintenance) treatment in patients at risk of such recurrence.

Maintenance treatment with TCAs or SSRIs (which should be at full dose for maximal effect) has clearly been shown to reduce risk of recurrence in patients with major (unipolar) depressive disorder at high risk of such recurrence. For patients with bipolar disorder, mood stabilisers such as lithium or carbamazepine are preferable to avoid triggering mania or rapid cycling. Lithium is also a useful option in the maintenance treatment of unipolar depressive disorders, and reduces the high mortality from suicide in recurrent affective disorders.

Selection of patients for maintenance treatment

Maintenance treatment is indicated in patients with three or more past episodes of major depressive disorder. Strong consideration should also be given to maintenance treatment in those with two or more episodes if recurrence has occurred within a year after discontinuation of medication, if there is a strong family history of bipolar or major depression and if the past episodes were life-threatening and/or sudden in onset.

FURTHER READING

Overviews

Checkley, S. A. (ed.)(1998) *The Management of Depression*. Oxford: Blackwell Science.

Pech, P. (1999) Pharmacological treatments of depressive disorders: a review. In *Depressive Disorders* (eds M. Maj & N. Sartorius), pp. 89–127. Chichester: John Wiley & Sons.

Honig, A. & van Praag, H. M. (1997) Depression: Neurobiological, Psychopathological and Therapeutic Advances. Chichester: John Wiley & Sons.

Guidelines

Paykel, E. S. & Priest, R. G. (1992) Recognition and management of depression in general practice: consensus statement. *BMJ,* **305,** 98–102.

Anderson, I. M., Nutt, D. J. & Deakin, J. F. W. (2000) Evidence-based guidelines for treating depressive disorders with antidepressants: a revision of the 1993 British Association for Psychopharmacology guidelines. *Journal of Psychopharmacology*, **14**, 3–20.

American Psychiatric Association (2000) Practice guideline for the treatment of patients with major depressive disorder (revised). *American Journal of Psychiatry*, **157**(Suppl.), 1–45.

Donoghue, J. & Taylor, D. (2000) Suboptimal use of antidepressants in the treatment of depression. *CNS Drugs*, **13**, 365–383.

World Health Organization (1992) *The ICD–10 Classification of Mental and Behavioural Disorders*. Geneva: WHO.

Drug treatment

Elkin, I., Shea, T. M., Watkins, J. T., *et al* (1989) National Institute of Mental Health Treatment of Depression, Collaborative Research Programme. General effectiveness of treatments. *Archives of General Psychiatry*, **46**, 971–982.

Kuhn, R. (1958) The treatment of depressive states with C.22355 (imipramine hydrochloride). *American Journal of Psychiatry*, **115**, 459.

Relapse prevention

Reimherr, F. W., Amsterdam, J. D., Quitkin, F. M., *et al* (1998) Optimal length of continuation therapy in depression: a prospective assessment during long-term fluoxetine treatment. *American Journal of Psychiatry*, **155**, 1247–1253.

Prevention recurrence

Kupfer, D. J., Frank, E., Perel, J. M., *et al* (1992) 5 Year outcome for maintenance therapies in recurrent depression. *Archives of General Psychiatry*, **49**, 769–773.

Hochstrasser, B., Isaksen, P. M., Koponen, H., *et al* (2001) Prophylactic effect of citalopram in unipolar, recurrent depression. Placebo-controlled study of maintenance therapy. *British Journal of Psychiatry*, **178**, 304–310.

Reynolds, C. F., Perel, J. M., Frank, E., *et al* (1999). Three-year outcomes of maintenance nortriptyline treatment in late-life depression: a study of two fixed plasma levels. *American Journal of Psychiatry*, **156**, 1177–1181.

Pathophysiology

Berman, R. M., Narasimhan, M., Anand, A., *et al* (1999) Transient depressive relapse induced by catecholamine depletion. *Archives of General Psychiatry*, **56**, 395–403.

Sargent, P. A., Kjaer, K. H., Bench, C. J., *et al* (2000) Brain serotonin1A receptor binding measured by positron emission tomography with [11C] WAY-100635: effects of depression and antidepressant treatment. *Archives of General Psychiatry*, **57**, 174–180.

Reid, I. C. & Stewart, C. A. (2001) How antidepressants work. New perspectives on the pathophysiology of depressive disorder. *British Journal of Psychiatry*, **178**, 299–303.

Healy, D. & Savage, M. (1998) Reserpine exhumed. *British Journal of Psychiatry*, **172**, 376–378.

Augmentation strategies

Katona, C. L. E., Abou-Saleh, M. T., Harrison, D. A., *et al* (1995). Placebo-controlled trial of lithium augmentation of fluoxetine and lofepramine. *British Journal of Psychiatry*, **166**, 80–86.

Aronson, R., Offman, H. J., Joffe, R. T., *et al* (1996) Tri-iodothyronine augmentation in the treatment of refractory depression. A meta-analysis. *Archives of General Psychiatry*, **53**, 842–848.

Shelton, R. C., Tollefson, G. D., Tohen, M., *et al* (2001) A novel augmentation strategy for treating resistant major depression. *American Journal of Psychiatry*, **158**, 131–134.

Personal accounts

Wolpert, L. (1999) *Malignant Sadness*. London: Faber.

Styron, W. (1991) *Darkness Visible*. London: Jonathon Cape.

Rating scales

Beck, A. T., Ward, C. H., Mendelson, M., *et al* (1961) An inventory for measuring depression. *Archives of General Psychiatry*, **4**, 561–571.

Hamilton, M. (1960) A rating scale for depression. *Journal of Neurology, Neurosurgery and Psychiatry*, **23**, 56–62.

Montgomery, S. A. & Åsberg, M. (1979) A new depression scale designed to be sensitive to change. *British Journal of Psychiatry*, **134**, 382–389.

Spitzer, R. L., Kroenke, K., Linzer, M., *et al* (1995) Health-related quality of life in primary care patients with mental disorders. Results from the PRIME-MD 1000 Study. *JAMA*, **274**, 1511–1517.

Zung, W. W. K. (1965) A self-rating depression scale. *Archives of General Psychiatry*, **12**, 63–70.

12. TREATMENT OF MANIA AND BIPOLAR DISORDER

The manic syndrome is one of the most clearly defined in psychiatry, but the diagnosis is often missed or mistaken for schizophrenia or personality disorder (Box 12.1 shows the inclusion criteria used in research for the diagnosis of mania).

As well as the alteration of mood with either elation or irritability, characteristic features include overtalkativeness, overactivity, flight of ideas and distractibility. A failure of judgement may be obvious too. Grandiosity and decreased need for sleep complete the picture. The majority of patients show all of the listed symptoms, although flight of ideas, distractibility and sexual disinhibition are less frequent, and fewer patients have delusions or hallucinations.

Irritability leads to verbal and even physical aggression, and exasperation with imposed restraints leads to feelings of persecution.

Lack of judgement may cause irresponsible, impetuous acts that may be criminal or socially unacceptable. A previously well-conducted person may start to drink heavily, get involved in fights and become promiscuous.

In the milder forms, racing thoughts and cheerfulness, without outwardly visible overactivity or pressure of speech may be the only abnormalities. Sometimes those who know the patient can see he/she is unwell even though speech, mood and activities seem within the normal range to strangers; the term hypomania should be reserved for these milder conditions that would be recognised as pathological only by those who are familiar with the patient or with psychiatry.

The term dysphoric mania describes those in whom manic symptoms are accompanied by marked anxiety, irritability or depression; these symptoms tend to emerge in more severe stages of mania, but some patients present throughout with a hostile-paranoid pattern rather than the pure elated-grandiose one. Older people often present with irritability rather than elation as the most prominent presenting feature.

Box 12.1 Diagnostic criteria for mania

Distinct period of elation or irritability.
Three of the following:
   overactivity
   increased talkativeness or pressure of speech
   flight of ideas or racing thoughts
   inflated self-esteem or grandiosity (which may be delusional)
   decreased need for sleep
   distractibility
   indiscreet behaviour with poor judgement (sexual, financial, etc.).
Marked impairment in occupational or social function.
Duration of more than 1 week.

Manic episodes may develop slowly over some days, or rapidly over a few hours. They may start from a normal state or follow a depressive illness. They may succeed psychological stress, surgery or infection. In particular they may follow childbirth or the use of antidepressants, ECT or other drugs – especially corticosteroids, psycho-stimulants, dopaminergic drugs (L-dopa, bromocriptine) or anabolic steroids. They may result from discontinuation of drugs – especially lithium, but also baclofen, clonidine or fenfluramine. Sometimes episodes are seasonal, occurring more often in the summer. Some follow organic brain damage, particularly in the right frontal or temporal lobes, from causes such as head injury, stroke, HIV infection, multiple sclerosis, epilepsy or cerebral tumour. These are referred to as secondary mania.

Manic episodes may last only a few days or weeks but usually continue for months, unless treated. Most patients with mania suffer at other times with episodes of depression and are called bipolar-I. Unipolar mania is less common (5–10% of cases) and otherwise resembles bipolar mania. It is included in bipolar-I disorder. Some patients with recurrent depression have hypomanic episodes not requiring hospitalisation and are called bipolar-II.

Mania can affect people of all social and occupational groups. Hypomanic traits and episodes can be associated with successful leadership, productivity and creativity. Manic episodes, however, are very disruptive and can be socially disastrous and there is a high rate of divorce, and of suicide, in bipolar patients. Fortunately effective treatment often improves the quality of the marriage, and lowers the suicide risk.

RAPID CYCLING

If the patient has four or more affective episodes in a year, he/she is said to be in a phase of rapid cycling. This can occur at the onset of illness but is much more common later in its course. It is also more common in females. Antidepressant medication (particularly tricyclic MARIs) can increase the frequency of cycling, and withdrawal of antidepressants can then restore normal cycling. Some cases of rapid cycling are associated with clinical or subclinical hypothyroidism. Ultrarapid cycling describes four or more episodes a month. Rare cases exist of patients who oscillate from mania to depression and back again every 48 hours. Ultradian cycling (within a day) has been described in otherwise typical bipolar patients; mood changes occur in a matter of minutes or hours, resembling the changes in borderline personalities.

MIXED AFFECTIVE STATES

Depression occurs as an integral part of bipolar disorder, and often either precedes or succeeds an episode of mania. The switch between mania and depression may occur suddenly but is usually more gradual, with an intervening mixed state or period of normality. Sometimes the whole affective episode contains a mixture of manic and depressive symptoms. The best-recognised mixed states are manic stupor and depression with flight of ideas. Transient depression of mood is very common in mania and the term mixed state is best reserved for when the syndromes of both mania and depression are consistently present. The term dysphoric mania is used when the depression or anxiety are less pronounced.

NATURAL HISTORY OF BIPOLAR DISORDER

Mania is very rare before puberty and there may be a hormonal interaction with genetic expression and brain development in bipolar disorder. The peak age of first hospitalisation is in the late teens, the median in the mid-20s. There have often been earlier milder affective episodes. First episodes of mania continue to be seen in late life; an onset over the age of 60 is more likely to be associated with organic brain disease.

The great majority of patients with mania have more than one episode because bipolar disorder is a recurrent illness. The onset may become more rapid in later episodes. The average interval from one episode to the next tends to decrease during the first five episodes, for instance from 5 years between the first and second episode to 2 years between the fifth and sixth. However, in an individual there is great variability in the length between episodes and a tendency for clustering at times of particular stress. A long interval between the first and second episode is especially likely if the first episode followed adverse life events.

There is an increased rate of adverse life events in the month before mania, but the proportion of episodes arising in this way is small. The first episode is more likely to be triggered by life events than later episodes. Insomnia or sleep deprivation may trigger a manic episode, for instance when flying overnight from West to East, or in fathers following the birth of their children.

Patients may increase or decrease alcohol or drug misuse when manic or depressed. These drugs can alter the course of bipolar disorder by triggering mania; they diminish impulse control, impair judgement and are serious risk factors for suicide. Cannabis may increase psychotic symptoms in mania and induce mania, as may cocaine and other psychostimulants. Therefore the recognition and treatment of alcohol and drug misuse in bipolar patients is a matter of urgency.

Psycho-dynamically mania is regarded as a defence against depressive feelings and cognitions.

PATHOPHYSIOLOGY

The effects of drug treatment suggest that mania involves overactivity of certain central dopamine (and noradrenalin) pathways and possible underactivity of certain acetylcholine and serotonin pathways. Thus, antipsychotics with antimanic actions block dopamine and in some cases noradrenalin receptors. Also, an amino acid drink lacking tyrosine can deplete brain dopamine function and reduce the severity of mania. Glutamate pathways may also be active. There is limited direct biochemical evidence to support these views. The accelerating course

DRUG TREATMENT

of recurrences, decreasing relationship to life stresses and the increasing speed of onset with subsequent episodes may reflect a process of electrical kindling in limbic brain structures, similar to that occurring in epilepsy. Increased activity of glutamate neurons, perhaps in the excitatory pathway from the frontal cortex to the ventral striatum, has been suggested. Some treatment-resistant patients show evidence of neurological damage such as hyper-intensities on magnetic resonance imaging (MRI) scan, reduced caudate volume, or electroencephalogram (EEG) abnormalities.

Raised intracellular calcium levels have been found in the blood cells in mania, as have raised levels of the intracellular messenger protein kinase C.

TREATMENT

Treatment has three aims:

    (1) managing the patient and the problems created by the manic conduct;

    (2) controlling with drugs the abnormal mental state and behaviour, including any depressive or mixed phase following mania;

    (3) preventing further episodes.

MANAGING THE PATIENT

Do not argue with the patient – humour him/her, attempt to establish rapport by discussing the changes he/she will have noticed, his/her lack of sleep and his/her difficulties with family and friends and at work. Use these as the grounds on which he/she needs your help, possibly with drugs. Maintain gentle, calm, friendly handling, steering him/her away from extravagant behaviour and indiscretion. Explain to the family that mania is an illness that causes a temporary restlessness, loss of judgement and sense of proportion, from which recovery is expected, so it is best if they are tolerant and forgiving, avoiding provocative challenges. In the first episode the family will need much counselling. Mania is the most genetic and often the most insightless form of mental illness. Most manic episodes are best treated in hospital, not only to give family and society relief from a trying responsibility, but also to avoid long-term damage to career and marriage. Much skill is needed in achieving this by persuasion. Compulsory admission under the MHA is often necessary for severe mania, because of refusal to accept treatment or the likelihood of poor adherence to drug treatment out of hospital or, indeed, in it.

In hospital, give as much living space as possible; confinement breeds conflict. Two patients with mania on a ward can cause chaos. It may be necessary to prevent use of the telephone, to remove cheque books and credit cards, warn the bank, stop car driving and ban business engagements. The patient's demands can be seemingly endless. If you remain firm on limits understood and agreed by staff, family and associates, patients usually accept them. They may not understand the restrictions but, provided you remain friendly and calm, they may follow them to please you. The less cooperative patient needs either individual attention or nursing in a locked intensive care ward to prevent him/her from leaving.

ANTIPSYCHOTICS

Mild mania may be treated with antipsychotic drugs such as haloperidol 5–15 mg daily. Lithium treatment is also useful but improvement takes 1–2 weeks. Moderate or severe mania is usually most rapidly controlled by antipsychotic drugs. Phenothiazines (e.g. chlorpromazine) and thioxanthenes (e.g. zuclopenthixol) are effective, but the butyrophenone haloperidol is often particularly useful in a dose of 5–10 mg three times a day. The more disturbed patient may be given haloperidol (5–10 mg) intramuscularly at 2 hourly intervals until he/she is calm (chapter 14, p. 156 and following). Haloperidol (5–10 mg) may also be given intravenously. Larger intramuscular doses (above 10 mg) are discouraged because they are excessive in some patients, and because their effect may last for several days, obscuring the diagnosis and making further management difficult; the patient may no longer appear very disturbed but is likely to deteriorate unless treatment is continued. A better approach is to give smaller doses but more often.

Haloperidol tends to produce initial sedation, which wears off after a day or so during continued treatment. If the patient remains very behaviourally disturbed, chlorpromazine or zuclopenthixol may be more useful because they are more sedative than haloperidol. However, many patients with mania resent being made to feel drowsy and this limits the doses they will accept. Chlorpromazine is hypotensive and should be used cautiously, especially in the elderly.

EPS, particularly dystonia, may be less of a problem with larger doses of haloperidol, but may emerge as the dose is reduced or some days after it is discontinued. Anti-Parkinsonian medication should therefore be continued for at least 7 days after haloperidol is stopped.

Rapid improvement in mania occurs for 1–3 days after starting medication, and more gradually over the next 2 weeks. There is no evidence that increasing the dose of haloperidol above 30 mg per day achieves greater long-term improvement. Generally the more sedative drugs do not produce greater long-term improvement than the less sedative haloperidol.

For patients with mania whose failure to improve is owing to poor compliance, depot antipsychotic medication including haloperidol decanoate can be used. The acetate of zuclopenthixol in a depot formulation ('Acuphase') has a duration of action of up to 3 days and a more rapid onset than the decanoates; still it requires 2–8 hours for its effects to develop. It is useful in very disturbed patients who persistently refuse oral medication, during the first few days of treatment, and who would otherwise need repeated intramuscular injections.

Tardive dyskinesia

The use of intermittent courses of antipsychotic drugs in schizophrenia is particularly prone to induce tardive dyskinesia. For this reason some authorities urge that antipsychotic drugs should be avoided as far as possible in the management of bipolar patients. However, in practice antipsychotic drugs are widely used, even in conjunction with mood stabilisers.

ATYPICAL ANTIPSYCHOTICS IN MANIA

Of the new atypical antipsychotics, olanzapine (in doses of up to 30 mg/day) is effective in acute mania, but it is not yet fully clear how it compares with haloperidol. Risperidone in doses of up to 6 mg/day is also effective, including in combination with lithium or valproate. A transition from mania to depression may be less likely with these drugs than with haloperidol. Clozapine is sometimes effective in treatment-resistant mania, including rapid cycling.

OTHER SEDATIVE DRUGS

For those who are not adequately sedated by antipsychotic drugs, or to avoid such drugs, sedation may be achieved by a benzodiazepine such as diazepam (5–20 mg intravenously or 30 mg orally). For intramuscular use lorazepam is absorbed faster and causes less local pain. Lorazepam (up to 8 mg a day or more) can be used alone or as an adjunct to other antimanic drugs for short-term treatment. (The *BNF* upper limit is 4 mg per day, equivalent to 40 mg of diazepam). Depersonalisation, dissociation and disinhibition are potential problems with benzodiazepines, and in the longer term dependence and withdrawal symptoms. Respiratory depression can occur, so flumazenil must always be on hand.

ANTIPSYCHOTIC-RESISTANT MANIA

A proportion of patients (about 50%) show only partial improvement, or initial improvement followed by partial relapse, with antipsychotic drugs. The main alternatives or adjuncts to the antipsychotics are lithium and anticonvulsants, particularly valproate or carbamazepine.

Lithium

About 50% of patients with mania show a good response to lithium, which usually requires 3 weeks to approach its full effect on mania. Used alone it is more useful in mild than in severe cases. Patients who respond tend to be those with classical mania rather than mixed, dysphoric or schizoaffective, and those with a family history of bipolar disorder. Patients who have benefited previously from lithium are more likely to do so again (lithium-responders). Those in a rapid cycling phase and those with mania secondary to organic brain disease tend not to respond to lithium.

Doses in acute mania

The narrow gap or overlap between therapeutic and toxic blood levels of lithium necessitates careful monitoring of blood levels, usually based on samples taken 12 hours after the last dose. Increasing plasma levels of lithium above 0.8 up to 1.4 mmol/l are associated with higher rates of response in mania, but levels above 1.2 require special care in monitoring to avoid toxicity. When a suitable patient does not respond at a lower dose it is necessary to increase the level to the top of the therapeutic range before concluding that the individual is non-responsive. Many of the features of toxicity may reflect high intracellular and brain, rather than extracellular, levels; hence, in assessing toxicity and efficacy, clinical judgement rather than blood levels should be paramount.

Lithium–antipsychotic combinations

Combinations of high levels of lithium with high doses of antipsychotics including haloperidol have been associated with severe neurological symptoms resembling lithium toxicity (see p. 334), perhaps because antipsychotic drugs can increase intracellular lithium levels. This reaction is uncommon and it is generally safe to combine haloperidol (up to 30 mg per day) with lithium at levels of up to 1 mmol/l. Thus, when combining these treatments the blood levels should generally be maintained below 1 mmol/l; staff should be advised to observe and report the development of neurological symptoms, and lithium should be temporarily discontinued if signs of toxicity such as vomiting, cerebellar signs or clouded consciousness develop.

The combination of antipsychotics and lithium can occasionally lead to troublesome sleepwalking requiring reduction of doses.

Valproate in acute mania

Valproate (p. 343) is effective in a proportion of patients with mania, including non-responders to the antipsychotic drugs lithium and carbamazepine. Most of the improvement occurs within days of achieving therapeutic levels (50–100 mg/l). The drug is generally well tolerated but side-effects include vomiting, tremor, weight gain, rash, transient hair loss and, potentially, acute liver damage, which is a rare complication occurring mainly in children. Liver function tests should be monitored every 3–6 months. For sodium valproate the starting dose is 600 mg daily or 500 mg modified release, rising to 2000 mg according to clinical response. A rapid titration of dose may be used from the start, such as up to 1500 mg (20 mg/kg). Semisodium valproate ('Depakote') is licenced for the treatment of mania. The starting dose is 750 mg daily.

Carbamazepine

Carbamazepine is effective almost as often as lithium in mania. There is some delay in its action but less so than with lithium. More severely ill patients with mania, including those with mixed or dysphoric mania, can benefit from carbamazepine, and a history of non-response to lithium does not reduce the chances of responding to carbamazepine. Patients with no family history of mania may have a greater chance of responding, and mania secondary to brain damage can also benefit.

The dose of carbamazepine used in acute mania is similar to that used for epilepsy, except that the starting dose has to be less gradual to avoid delay. Starting with 400 mg daily, the dose can be increased according to response and side-effects to a maximum of 1600 mg daily. Blood tests should be monitored (p. 347).

Combination treatment

Less than half of patients with mania respond adequately to monotherapy with a single drug, antipsychotic, lithium or valproate. Judicious combinations are often required. It is common to combine an antipsychotic with lithium or valproate. Table 5.1 (p. 42) summarises the evidence for these drugs as monotherapy in mania and Table 12.1 shows the evidence for their combined use.

Combining mood stabilisers

The view that polypharmacy may be justified in order to gain control of resistant bipolar disorder has gained ground in recent years. Carbamazepine is difficult to combine because it induces liver enzymes that metabolise other drugs. However, lithium is not metabolised and many patients who fail to improve when taking carbamazepine alone do so when lithium is added. This combination – as with antipsychotics – increases the risk of lithium neurotoxicity. The combination of lithium and valproate is the safest and often most efficacious. Carbamazepine can also be combined with valproate but pharmacokinetic interactions occur and more careful monitoring of dose is needed.

OTHER DRUGS

Topiramate is another anticonvulsant that has been used in bipolar disorder; controlled trials are awaited. Lamotrigine can improve bipolar depression but probably not mania (see p. 246). Gabapentin has been widely prescribed, is well tolerated and has minimal pharmacokinetic interactions, but controlled trials have proved negative. Calcium antagonists including verapamil and nimodipine have also been used, but, again, controlled trials have not confirmed their efficacy.

USE OF ECT IN MANIA

Many clinicians reserve ECT for only the most severe and drug-resistant patients with mania, and it is possible that more widespread use would be justified. In early reports about two-thirds of patients given ECT in mania showed marked improvement. In a double-blind trial ECT was superior to lithium during the first 8 weeks, especially for severe mania and for mixed states.

FOLLOW-UP AFTER A MANIC EPISODE

The return of a patient's mental state to apparent normality does not allow lessening of clinical vigilance. Within hours or days a swing into a dangerous (suicidal) depressive state may occur. Also, the picture

Table 12.1 Numbers needed to treat (NNTs) in placebo-controlled trials of antipsychotics in combination with lithium or anticonvulsants in mania

Treatment group (combination with)	Treatments (n=patients)	Duration (weeks)	Criterion of response	Drop-outs due to inefficacy (%)	Drop-outs due to adverse events (%)	Response (%)	ARR (%)	NNT (95% C.I.)
Mood stabiliser[1]	Risperidone (n=75)	3	50% less Y-MRS	39	39	59	17	6 (4-82)
	Placebo (n=75)			55	55	42		
Mood stabiliser[2]	Olanzapine (n=229)	6	50% less Y-MRS	4	28	68	23	5 (3-9)
	Placebo (n=115)			13	18	45		
Antipsychotics[3]	Valproate (n=69)	3	50% less Y-MRS	1	9	70	24	5 (3-13)
	Placebo (n=67)			3	13	46		

1. Yatham, 2000.
2. Tohen et al, 2000.
3. Muller-Oerlinghausen et al, 2000.
ARR, absolute risk reduction; Y-MRS, young mania rating scale.

may change subtly with irritability and a mixed affective state, heralding the development of depression. These call for a reduction or even cessation of antipsychotic drugs, while continuing a mood stabiliser, and considering an antidepressant. Equally, severe extrapyramidal side-effects may suddenly develop, requiring a reduction of dose of antipsychotic and adjustment of dose of anticholinergic. Many patients are still on antipsychotics when discharged from hospital. As their condition stabilises, over the subsequent 6–12 months, attempts should be made to withdraw antipsychotic medication.

PROPHYLAXIS OF BIPOLAR DISORDER

Selection of patients

Maintenance treatment should be considered after a second episode of bipolar disorder, especially if the interval between episodes has been less than 5 years. Because the interval between the first and second episodes tends to be longer than the intervals between subsequent episodes, maintenance treatment should be used after a first episode only if the dangers of a subsequent episode are thought to justify it – for instance if the episode was severe and disruptive, had a relatively sudden onset and was not precipitated by external factors, or if the person's job is very sensitive or there is a risk of suicide. Because of the risk of withdrawal mania on sudden discontinuation of lithium, prolonged maintenance treatment should not be started in patients who are likely to comply poorly.

Lithium maintenance

Patients who are more likely to benefit are those with typical bipolar disorder having complete recovery between episodes, or a family history of bipolar disorder. Patients with a rapid cycling phase of illness are less responsive to lithium. Other factors militating against prophylactic efficacy are poor adherence to treatment and drug misuse. A large proportion of patients at risk do not seek treatment, and many who do none the less adhere poorly to lithium. There is also the risk of withdrawal mania in those who stop treatment too abruptly, for instance when feeling no need for it during a mild upswing of mood. However, where steps are taken to encourage and check adherence, low relapse rates and affective morbidity on lithium can be achieved. This is part of the rationale for specialist lithium or affective disorder clinics, or for shared-care protocols.

Patients are less likely to adhere if they are younger, male and have had fewer previous episodes. The reasons they give for stopping are its ineffectiveness, drug side-effects, feeling well and in no need of treatment, finding it inconvenient and not wanting to depend on medication, and feeling less energy or drive. The side-effects most often given as reasons are excessive thirst and polyuria, tremor, memory impairment and weight gain.

In order to increase adherence, the doctor should take side-effects seriously, keep lithium levels as low as possible, educate the patients and their families about their illness and the use of lithium and discuss adherence with the patient. Pharmacists should be able to provide information sheets about lithium for the patient, and cards on which doctors can record blood test results and doses. Sometimes manipulation of dose schedules can be helpful, for instance switching from once daily to twice daily doses, and patients have individual preferences. Regular contact and counselling can be useful. It may be helpful to plot a life chart with the patient, to improve his/her understanding of the impact of his/her condition. It may also be helpful to give him/her a daily mood chart or diary to complete and bring for review at his/her next appointment, if his/her mood has been unstable.

In spite of these measures many bipolar patients tend to drop out of lithium treatment. Cognitive therapy may be helpful by altering the patients understanding and attitude towards their illness and treatment, and therefore improving compliance.

Lithium lessens both the severity and the frequency of episodes. Usually it also stabilises the mood between major episodes. But only 50% of those started benefit in terms of reduced hospitalisation over 5 years. The mortality rate (high because of suicides and cardiovascular deaths) can be reduced on lithium to that of the general population.

Blood levels and monitoring

Blood levels lower than those for acute mania are sufficient in prophylaxis (0.5–1.0 mmol/l). For some patients lower levels than this would suffice. In the elderly a level of 0.5 mmol/l is recommended. During less stable phases lithium levels should be monitored frequently, and even in the most stable the tests of lithium level, renal function and thyroid function should be done at least once a year.

Antidepressants and lithium

Depression occurring during lithium treatment can be treated with MARIs. In patients with bipolar-I disorder the course of antidepressant treatment should be gradually discontinued as the depression improves, in order to reduce the risk of triggering a manic episode and to avoid the induction of rapid cycling. For patients with a predominantly depressive pattern of bipolar disorder (bipolar-II) the combination of lithium and an MARI may be more effective in preventing depression than either drug alone. SSRIs such as paroxetine are less liable to induce mania than the TCAs. However, some bipolar patients are readily switched into mania on particular SSRIs.

Discontinuation of lithium

Symptoms of anxiety, irritability and emotional lability can occur following sudden discontinuation. Abrupt cessation of lithium in bipolar patients leads to the development of mania 2–3 weeks later in up to 50% of patients. Discontinuation should therefore be gradual. Patients whose mood has been stable are less likely to relapse on stopping than those who have continued to show mild mood swings (meta-stable). Lithium may be reduced at the rate of a quarter to an eighth of the original dose every 2 months. The high risk of occurrence of mania on abrupt discontinuation of lithium should be part of the

DRUG TREATMENT

information given to patients. Patients should be advised not to taper off lithium in less than 2 weeks.

Alternatives to lithium in maintenance

Even in favourable clinical trials lithium maintenance was unsuccessful in over 30% of patients and more recent studies that include a broader range of manic patients (see p. 8) put the failure rate much higher. For non-responders an alternative is carbamazepine. Rapid cycling patients are more likely to benefit from carbamazepine than from lithium. In longer-term use there may be partial loss of efficacy by the third year, though it is not clear to what extent poor adherence to medication is responsible.

Side-effects of carbamazepine can be minimised by using slow-release formulations or by commencing treatment with low doses (100–200 mg at night) and increasing every few days to the maximum dose that is well tolerated (usually 400–600 mg, maximum 1600 mg daily). Patients should be informed of the risk of side-effects, including blood disorders (see p. 346), and told to report to the doctor possible symptoms such as sore throat, rash or fever.

Some patients benefit more from the combination of lithium and carbamazepine than from either drug alone. There have been reports of reversible neurological side-effects characterised mainly by confusional states and cerebellar signs similar to those of lithium toxicity.

Valproate has been studied less but may be useful in those who are resistant to lithium or carbamazepine. The combination of lithium with valproate produces less neurological problems than the combination of lithium and carbamazepine.

Other anticonvulsants used in maintenance treatment include lamotrigine for rapid-cycling bipolar-II disorder.

Antipsychotic drugs should be avoided if possible for long-term use in bipolar patients because of sedative effects and tardive dyskinesia. Brief intermittent therapy is possible in which the patient commences an antipsychotic, particularly at night, when he/she senses a period of lability of mood or insomnia.

However, for those who have frequently recurring episodes and either do not benefit from or do not adhere to oral medication, depot antipsychotic medication can provide long periods of stability.

Resistant bipolar disorders attract polypharmacy, which may be necessary but can lead to the creation of a drug fog. Fear of relapse prevents attempts to reduce overmedication. A sensible course is to remove at least some medicines by stages, and to review the value of others. If possible in such cases, try to limit medication to mood-stabilising drugs and an antipsychotic or an antidepressant. Daily mood charting is helpful to document changes associated with the introduction or removal of individual drugs. A combination of drugs may thereby be found that provides the best control.

Pregnancy and childbirth in bipolar disorder

In the first trimester lithium carries a risk of cardiac malformations, such as Ebstein's anomaly, in the foetus. Recent cohort studies suggest the risk of major congenital abnormalities may be 4–12%, compared to 2–4% in women taking other drugs not known to be teratogenic. The anticonvulsants carbamazepine and valproate in early pregnancy are associated with brain and neural tube developmental defects in about 1% of births. Because of the possible developmental effects upon the child, pregnancy in bipolar patients should, if possible, be managed without psychotropic drugs. The oral antipsychotics chlorpromazine and haloperidol, or a depot injection, are probably the safest if antimanic medication or prophylactic medication is needed when pregnancy is planned; there is a risk of transient EPS in the neonate if these are continued. Depression during pregnancy may be treated with a TCA or fluoxetine (see p. 264).

Fortunately, pregnancy is a time of much reduced risk for recurrence of bipolar disorder, but the 2 weeks after childbirth are a time of greatly increased risk in a mother with a history or family history of bipolar disorder. A quarter of bipolar patients develop postnatal psychosis with manic features at this time.

Lithium and mood-stabilising drugs should be stopped in pregnancy but restarted as soon as possible after childbirth. A woman who becomes pregnant while taking lithium or anticonvulsants should be counselled about the risks and offered high-resolution ultrasound screening and echocardiography at about 16–18 weeks for possible cardiac and other defects, with a view to termination.

If a woman has been taking lithium during pregnancy, the dose will need to be reduced after childbirth, when the glomerular filtration rate falls from a higher level back to normal. A foetus exposed to lithium in late pregnancy may be born with hypotonia (floppy baby) and hypothyroidism; but these should soon clear. A new-born infant getting breast milk from the mother taking lithium will be receiving a lithium dose that the infantile kidney has difficulty in excreting. Hypothyroidism and goitre are the main risks to the baby.

USEFUL CONTACTS

The Manic Depression Fellowship, 21 St George's Road, London SE1 6ES (tel: 0207 793 2600; website: www.mdf.org.uk).
Newcastle National Information Service on Drugs in Pregnancy, tel: 0191 232 1525.
The Perinatal and Reproductive Psychiatry Programme, Massachusetts General Hospital (http//:www.womensmentalhealth.org).

FURTHER READING

Manic–depressive illness

Goodwin, F. K. & Jamison, K. R. (1990) *Manic–Depressive Illness*. Oxford: Oxford University Press.

Goodnick, P. J. (ed.) (1998) *Mania: Clinical and Research Perspectives*. Washington, DC, & London: American Psychiatric Press.

Kessing, L. V., Anderson, P. K, Mortensen, P. B., *et al* (1998) Recurrence in affective disorder. I. Case register study. *British Journal of Psychiatry*, **172**, 23–28.

Kramlinger, K. G. & Post, R. M. (1996) Ultra-rapid and ultradian cycling in bipolar affective illness. *British Journal of Psychiatry*, **168**, 314–323.

DRUG TREATMENT

McTavish, S. F. B., McPherson, M. H., Harmer, C. J., *et al* (2001) Antidopaminergic effects of dietary tyrosine depletion in healthy subjects and patients with manic illness. *British Journal of Psychiatry*, **179**, 356–360.

Marneros, A. & Angst, J. (2000) *Bipolar Disorders: 100 Years after Manic–Depressive Insanity*. Dordrecht: Kluwer Academic Publishers.

Muller-Oerlinghausen, B. & Berghofer, A. (1999) Antidepressants and suicide risk. *Journal of Clinical Psychiatry*, **60**(Suppl. 2), 94–99.

Post, R. M., Rubinow, D. R., Uhde, T. W., *et al* (1989) Dysphoric mania: clinical and biological correlates. *Archives of General Psychiatry*, **46**, 353–358.

Secunda, S. K., Swann, A., Katz, M. M., *et al* (1987) Diagnosis and treatment of mixed mania. *American Journal of Psychiatry*, **144**, 96–98.

Stone, K. (1989) Mania in the elderly. *British Journal of Psychiatry*, **155**, 220–224.

Wehr, R. A., Sack, D. A., Rosenthal, N. E., *et al* (1988) Rapid cycling affective disorder: contributing factors and treatment responses in 51 patients. *American Journal of Psychiatry*, **145**, 179–184.

Personal accounts

Jamison, K. R. (1994) *Touched with Fire: Manic–Depressive Illness and the Artistic Temperament*. New York: Simon & Shuster.

—— (1995) *An Unquiet Mind: A Memoir of Moods and Madness*. London: Picador.

Treatment 'guidelines'

American Psychiatric Association (1994) Practice guideline for the treatment of patients with bipolar disorder. *American Journal of Psychiatry*, **151**(Suppl. 12), 1–36.

Francis, A. J., Kahn, D. A., Carpenter, D., *et al* (1998) The expert consensus guidelines for treating depression in bipolar disorder. *Journal of Clinical Psychiatry*, **59** (Suppl. 4), 73–79.

Antipsychotics in bipolar disorder

Cookson, J. (2001) Use of antipsychotic drugs and lithium in mania. *British Journal of Psychiatry*, **178**(Suppl. 41), S148–S156.

Rifkin, A., Doddi, S., Karajgi, B., *et al* (1994) Dosage of haloperidol for mania. *British Journal of Psychiatry*, **165**, 113–116.

Tohen, M., Sanger, T. M., McElroy, S. L., *et al* (1999) Olanzapine versus placebo in the treatment of acute mania. *American Journal of Psychiatry*, **156**, 702–709.

The place of luthium

Cookson, J. & Sachs, G. S. (1999) Lithium: clinical use in mania and prophylaxis of affective disorders. In *Schizophrenia and Mood Disorders: The New Drug Therapies in Clinical Practice* (eds P. F. Buckley & J. L. Waddington) Oxford: Butterworth Heinemann.

Mood stabiliser combination treatment

Freeman, M. P. & Stoll, A. L. (1998) Mood stabilizer combinations: a review of safety and efficacy. *American Journal of Psychiatry*, **155**, 12–21.

Pregnancy in bipolar disorder

Cohen, L. S., Sichel, D. A., Robertson, L. M., *et al* (1995) Postpartum prophylaxis for women with bipolar disorder. *American Journal of Psychiatry*, **152**, 1641–1645.

—— & Rosenbaum, J. F. (1998) Psychotropic drug use during pregnancy: weighing the risks. *Journal of Clinical Psychiatry*, **59**(Suppl. 2), 18–28.

Llewellyn, A., Stowe, Z. N. & Strader, J. R. (1998) The use of lithium and management of women with bipolar disorder during pregnancy and lactation. *Journal of Clinical Psychiatry*, **59**(Suppl. 6), 57–64.

Studies quoted

Muller-Oerlinghausen, B., Retzow, A., Henn, F. A. *et al* (2000) Valproate as an adjunct to neuroleptic medication for the treatment of acute episodes of mania: a prospective, randomised, double-blind placebo-controlled, multicentre study. European Valproate Mania Study Group. *Journal of Clinical Psychopharmacology*, **20**, 195–203.

Tohen, M., Jacobs, T. G., Meyers, T. M. *et al* (2000) Efficacy of olanzapine combined with mood stabilisers in the treatment of bipolar disorder. *The International Journal of Psychopharmacology*, **3**(Suppl. 1), S335.

Yatham, L. N. (2000). Safety and efficacy of risperidone as combination therapy for the manic phase of bipolar disorder: preliminary findings of a randomised, double blind study (RIS-INT-46). *The International Journal of Psychopharmacology*, **3**(Suppl. 1), S142.

13. THE MANAGEMENT OF SCHIZOPHRENIA

Although the clinical presentation of schizophrenia has changed little over the past century, our conceptualisation of the condition has evolved from Kraepelin, through Bleuler and Schneider, to the recent emphasis on groupings of positive and negative symptoms, and the importance of cognitive symptoms and depression.

Costs

Schizophrenia is one of the 30 leading causes of burden of disease worldwide, along with depression, bipolar disorder and alcohol. Because of its chronic and debilitating nature it constitutes a major public health problem. Direct costs of schizophrenia account for 1–3% of the total health budget, and the use of 25% of NHS beds. Only 5% of direct costs is spent on medication; the greatest proportion of cost is on residential care either in hospital or in supported hostels.

Patients with schizophrenia may show a great variety of behavioural and subjective symptoms and signs.

Positive, negative, cognitive and other symptoms

In understanding the effects of treatment, it is helpful to separate the symptoms of schizophrenia into positive symptoms (which cause abnormality by their presence) and negative symptoms (which represent the absence of normal function). A third group of symptoms of cognitive dysfunction is also increasingly recognised as important. In addition there are symptoms of general psychopathology such as depression, which commonly occur in schizophrenia.

The positive symptoms are mainly delusions, hallucinations, illogical thinking (formal thought disorder, conceptual disorganisation) and affective incongruity. For diagnostic purposes, particular significance is attached to the first-rank symptoms described by Kurt Schneider. But for treatment the negative and cognitive symptoms remain an important challenge.

The core or primary negative symptoms are poverty of speech, flatness of affect and a general lack of drive or motivation. These lead to lack of self-care and social withdrawal.

Cognitive symptoms

Schizophrenia is associated with cognitive deficits that develop from many years before the onset of psychosis, and may worsen as the psychosis proceeds. These include impairments of general IQ, attention and working memory. Poor attention results in difficulty remaining vigilant and in not getting distracted. Working memory is a system for temporary holding and manipulation of information, during tasks such as comprehension, learning and reasoning. The onset of acute psychosis is associated with a further deterioration in cognition, especially in attention.

The cognitive deficits overlap with negative symptoms, and together these are the most important determinants of the eventual long-term outcome with regard to social functioning, after the patient has had treatment. The cognitive impairments also contribute to lack of insight, and interfere with psychotherapies that rely upon verbal learning.

SYMPTOMS OF GENERAL PSYCHOPATHOLOGY

Other symptoms that are much less specific to schizophrenia may occur, for example depression and anxiety. Symptoms of catatonia are also among these, mainly affecting movement and volition but also speech; they include mannerisms, grimacing and posturing, waxy flexibility, negativism, echolalia and echopraxia.

SECONDARY NEGATIVE SYMPTOMS

Negative symptoms such as lack of self-care, active social withdrawal and muteness can develop in response to positive symptoms, and are then called secondary. Negative symptoms can develop further as a result of understimulation, for instance in households or wards where there is a lack of personal interaction or activities, or a barren environment. Overstimulation in an emotionally charged environment can also worsen both positive and secondary negative symptoms; hence the concept of high expressed emotion in homes and hostels.

Secondary negative features can also appear when the patient is depressed and can then be difficult to separate from the core negative symptoms. The EPS of Parkinsonism can present as akinetic depression in which lack of spontaneous movement and poverty of speech are parts, as is mental slowing or bradyphrenia. Other side-effects of medication that may contribute to negative symptoms are the sedation, dysphoria and mental dulling that patients report (see Box 13.1).

Box 13.1 Causes of negative symptoms

Core or primary negative symptoms
Secondary to positive symptoms
Understimulation, barren environment
Overstimulation
Secondary to depression
Secondary to extrapyramidal side-effects of antipsychotics
Secondary to sedative effects

DRUG TREATMENT

CLINICAL ASSESSMENT

A single clinical interview may not reveal the extent of either positive symptoms or, even more, the negative state. Therefore, independent accounts from those who see the patient every day, indicating how he or she has been behaving in different situations, may be essential to a good assessment. Some assessment of the home atmosphere is important, as high levels of expressed emotion in relatives or hostel workers are associated with an increased risk of relapse in chronic schizophrenia.

CLINICAL RATING SCALES

A rating scale that has been used in many recent clinical trials is the Positive and Negative Syndrome Scale (PANSS) devised by Stanley Kay (Kay *et al*, 1987). Box 13.2 shows the symptoms included in the PANSS, which is divided into the categories of positive, negative and general psychopathology. In this scale cognitive symptoms are included as symptoms of general psychopathology. Each item would be rated from 0 to 6 using defined anchor points, and total scores added for the three categories of symptoms.

EFFECTS OF ANTIPSYCHOTIC DRUGS

Antipsychotic drugs are very useful at alleviating positive symptoms, and to a lesser extent negative symptoms, but they are not curative,

---

Box 13.2 Positive and Negative Syndrome Scale (PANSS) items

Positive scale	Negative scale	General symptoms
Delusions	Blunted affect	Somatic concern/ delusions
Conceptual disorganisation	Emotional withdrawal	Anxiety
Hallucinations	Poor rapport	Guilt feelings
Excitement	Passive (apathetic) social withdrawal	Tension
Grandiosity	Difficulty in abstract thinking	Mannerisms/posturing
Suspiciousness/ persecution	Lack of spontaneity/ flow of conversation	Depression
Hostility	Stereotyped thinking	Motor retardation
		Uncooperativeness
		Unusual thought content
		Disorientation
		Poor attention
		Lack of judgement/insight
		Disturbed volition
		Poor impulse control
		Preoccupation
		Active social avoidance

and form only part of the management of the illness. They are important in four circumstances:

    (1) emergency control of acute disturbance (acute tranquillisation, see chapter 14)

    (2) relief of symptoms during the onset of the first episode of illness, or in relapses

    (3) continuing reduction of symptoms in the chronically ill

    (4) prevention of relapse of illness in those who have largely recovered.

The negative symptoms are improved much less by drugs than positive ones, so that emotional flatness and indifference, inertia and anergy, and poverty of interest and responsiveness persist in the form of a deficit or defect state after recovery from an acute illness. They may then form the major disability in a chronically ill patient, and can be responsible for an otherwise normal-seeming person proving unable to work or to maintain social relationships.

Atypical antipsychotics

This term is used for antipsychotics that produce less severe and fewer EPS than the conventional typical or classical drugs (see chapter 2). They have an obvious advantage for patients who have developed troublesome EPS that could not be resolved with an anticholinergic drug. This may involve as many as 30% of patients. They are discussed in detail in chapter 30.

Effects of antipsychotic drugs on cognition

Classical antipsychotics can initially worsen cognition. This is a transient effect on attention owing to sedation. In longer-term treatment attention usually improves quite markedly. But an additional cognitive impairment may arise accompanying Parkinsonian bradykinesia.

Atypical antipsychotics produce less Parkinsonism and less cognitive impairment than conventional drugs. Clozapine, risperidone and olanzapine produce less impairment of working memory than haloperidol, but long-standing deficits remain.

Anticholinergic drugs improve Parkinsonism but can themselves in high doses impair cognition, particularly in older patients, through effects on working memory and learning. Although some atypicals have anticholinergic effects, this does not appear to detract from their beneficial effects on attention and working memory.

Depression in acute schizophrenia

Depressive symptoms occur commonly in acute schizophrenia but are less obvious than the psychotic ones. Often the depression is only noticed or revealed when antipsychotic drugs have improved the psychosis. Severe depression may also appear for the first time after the psychosis has recovered (post-psychotic depression), and this is also the time that the patient recognises how ill he/she has been and confronts his/her problems more realistically.

Suicide in schizophrenia

Schizophrenia is associated with a high rate of completed suicide; rates of up to 13% have been found, but these have declined, probably as a result of better treatment. Risk factors include severe illness, a previous suicide attempt, current depression, recent discharge from hospital and drug or alcohol misuse.

Prognosis

This is assessed in terms of response of symptoms to medication, and the level of independence and return to normal social and occupational functioning. The large international study of schizophrenia (ISoS; Mason *et al*, 1997) found 12% of patients remained in hospital or a supported hostel after 15 years, but 16% had recovered and been drug-free for 2 years. Thus, the majority (72%) had required continued medication but maintained their independence.

Factors predicting a better prognosis are female gender, being older at onset, being married and having a more acute as opposed to gradual insidious onset. Patients with a longer history of untreated psychosis at the start have a worse prognosis. This seems largely owing to their having marked negative symptoms and cognitive deficits, neither of which would have benefited from earlier intervention with drugs.

Effective treatment of the psychosis reduces the high suicide rate.

Neuropharmacological theories of schizophrenia

Neurodevelopmental theory

The neurodevelopmental view of schizophrenia regards the condition as evolving from an early embryonic stage, when abnormal brain cytoarchitecture is determined. In a minority of patients with schizophrenia there are dysmorphic facial features, which are also thought to be determined at this embryological stage. In children who later develop schizophrenia there is evidence of increased ventricular volume, especially in the left temporal horn, low premorbid IQ, social aloofness or awkwardness (schizoid traits), odd postures and speech problems. The condition is eventually manifested as psychosis in adolescence or later.

Schizophrenia is associated with reduced brain size, especially in the temporal lobes, where the hippocampus is small and shows abnormal cellular architecture. There is reduced cerebral asymmetry. The cerebral cortex is diminished in volume, especially on the left side and near the speech areas (Broca's area and the planum temporale). These abnormalities, seen on neuro-imaging, do not progress at least up to 8 years after the first episode, and they too probably precede the onset of psychosis.

The connectivity hypothesis stresses the deficiency of synaptic connections, as measured by the marker proteins, synaptophysins and complexins. These deficiencies are found in most areas of the hippocampus and particularly in relation to glutamate neurons (complexin II). The neurons in layer III of the prefrontal and cingulate cortex are reduced in size, and synaptic vesicle protein is reduced in the frontal areas. The deep layer III pyramidal neurons have reduced dendritic spine density, a marker of excitatory inputs.

Genetic factors are important, with a heritability of 65–85%, though less so in those with a later age of onset; maternal virus infections and other obstetric complications may also contribute to the vulnerability.

Neuropsychological theories

The abnormalities of cytoarchitecture in the prefrontal and cingulate cortex may underly some of the neuropsychological deficits seen in schizophrenia, which include impairments in working memory and in motor planning. Also, the clinical syndrome of negative symptoms is associated with reduced blood flow in these areas of the brain (hypofrontality).

Other neuropsychological theories emphasise deficient sensory gating and a reduction in prepulse inhibition found in schizophrenia. Prepulse inhibition refers to a reduction in response to a strong startling stimulus (pulse), if this is preceded shortly by a prestimulus (prepulse), too weak to elicit a startle response itself.

Dopamine hypotheses

According to the original dopamine hypothesis (see p. 12), schizophrenia results from a functional overactivity of dopamine in certain areas of the brain. This hypothesis was founded upon two observations. First, drugs that stimulate dopamine pathways, such as amphetamines or direct dopamine agonists such as bromocriptine or the D_3 selective agonist pramipexole, can produce psychosis resembling paranoid schizophrenia when taken in large doses. Second, all known antipsychotic drugs have in common the ability to block dopamine receptors. However, there is little direct evidence in support of the hypothesis. Post-mortem studies show subtle changes in levels of dopamine and its metabolites in the brain – notably an asymmetry in amygdala dopamine levels, with an increase on the left. Dopamine receptor numbers are increased at post-mortem, but this may be entirely the result of previous exposure to antipsychotic drugs (up-regulation). Dopamine receptor numbers in the brains of unmedicated people with schizophrenia measured by PET scanning show no consistent increase, though there may be abnormal asymmetry with greater receptor numbers on the left side.

However, abnormally large increases in dopamine release in response to amphetamine have been detected in patients during acute exacerbations of psychosis but not during remissions.

A more integrated dopamine hypothesis suggests that there is a primary weakness in mesocortical dopamine function, associated with deficient activation of the prefrontal cortex, and compensatory activation of other dopamine pathways. This predicts that drugs blocking dopamine receptors would worsen the manifestations of hypofrontality, which may include cognitive deficits and some negative symptoms.

Glutamate hypotheses, dopamine and fronto-limbic circuitry

The findings of abnormal prefrontal and temporal cortex have focused attention upon the interconnections between these areas and the subcortical dopaminergic pathways. Glutamate is a transmitter that mediates excitatory effects from these cortical areas to the dopamine cell bodies, and to the dopaminergic nerve endings in the caudate-putamen and the nucleus accumbens.

The psychotomimetic effects of phencyclidine (PCP) result from blockade of NMDA-type glutamate receptors, and include both positive and negative symptoms resembling schizophrenia. A similar drug, the anaesthetic ketamine, can also produce a psychotic state, associated with activation of the prefrontal cortex.

Thus, it has been postulated that a deficiency in prefrontal cortical glutamate neurons contributes to the pathogenesis of schizophrenia. Indeed, there is evidence of fewer glutamate nerve endings in the regions of dopamine terminals in schizophrenia.

This deficiency of glutamate transmission is postulated to lead to diminished mesocortical dopamine release and hence to the core negative symptoms and cognitive deficits of schizophrenia.

The positive symptoms are associated with the activation of other brain areas, including the mesotemporal cortex and speech areas. It is postulated that as a result of mesocortical deficits there is dysregulation of dopamine release, which becomes more under control of the amygdala. This leads to excessive release in response to stress and to an impairment of sensory gating.

Alternative interpretations suggest that psychosis results from excessive glutamate release, and that PCP or ketamine, by blocking presynaptic NMDA-type glutamate receptors, increases glutamate release to act on non-NMDA-type glutamate receptors. It is also possible that excessive glutamate activity during acute relapses may have a neurotoxic effect upon the dopaminergic cells, resulting in the progression of negative symptoms.

TREATMENT

The disturbed patient: acute tranquillisation

Aggressive or disturbed behaviour is now the commonest reason for admitting patients with schizophrenia to hospital. With drugs, it is often possible to suppress hostility, dangerous behaviour and restlessness without complete sedation. Some patients, however, do require to be made to sleep, in order to be safely nursed. These uses are discussed in chapter 14. The antipsychotic drugs used in early treatment are usually given in combination with a benzodiazepine to reduce arousal and avoid the release of stress hormones that act on the heart. The combination allows lower doses of antipsychotics to be used. The oral route is preferable and syrup may be more acceptable; but intra-muscular, and occasionally even intravenous, injection may be needed. By the third or fourth day, as the patient improves, regular oral medication should suffice. However, the changeover requires care. A common error is to start off well and then lose control again through inadequate dosage. It is best to start the oral drug while continuing but gradually lessening the injected doses. Careful monitoring of change is required for the ensuing 2–3 weeks. After absorbing large quantities of drug during an acute phase, patients may suddenly develop marked side-effects, such as drowsiness or acute dystonic reactions. The latter can be mistaken for symptoms of the illness. Anti-Parkinsonian drugs may be needed, at times by injection, and antipsychotic drugs reduced.

Catatonic excitement

Catatonic symptoms during an excitement state or stupor may result from underlying schizophrenia or mania. They have a potentially ominous significance in that historically such conditions led to exhaustion and collapse, called malignant or lethal catatonia. Unfortunately modern antipsychotics do not always control such states and in some instances they worsen them by producing neuroleptic malignant syndrome (see p. 88). Benzodiazepines, such as lorazepam, are useful particularly for catatonic stupor.

Treatment of early phases: first episodes or relapses

Early intervention

There is growing recognition of the importance of early intervention in detecting and treating schizophrenia before severe damage has occurred to the person's health or social framework. There is also a view, established with less certainty, that by treating the illness early and avoiding relapses it is possible to prevent the more severe deterioration, with profound and irreversible negative symptoms, that used to be seen among large numbers of chronic patients in long-stay wards. The majority of the deterioration in functioning in schizophrenia occurs prior to and within the first 5 years of the onset of psychosis.

Prodromal signs

If there has been no previous psychotic episode, a family history may alert the clinician to the ominous significance of changes in temperament or personality, new oddities in talk or behaviour, or poor concentration and academic difficulties. The differential diagnosis from adolescent rebelliousness is often difficult. In the absence of obvious predisposing factors, it will usually be necessary for the person to display some of the positive symptoms listed above, or indeed one of the first-rank symptoms of schizophrenia, before antipsychotic medication can be recommended with confidence.

In a patient with a history of a previous acute schizophrenia-like episode, sufficient prodromal signs of relapse may be mild affective changes, undue anxiety, depression or insomnia before any delusions or hallucinations are apparent. These alone warrant starting or increasing antipsychotic medication.

Treatment of acute episodes

This may be in hospital or at home. For those who refuse treatment, a compulsory admission may be appropriate if his/her condition meets the criteria for a Section of the MHA (see chapter 10). Patients often improve, sometimes considerably, once away from the stresses of home and ordinary life, particularly if the hospital offers a simple, calm, routine. However, sustained improvement is unusual unless medication is taken.

DRUG TREATMENT

The milieu

Through their illness patients may suffer doubts and confusion about themselves, the world, and their relation to others; emotional relations with mothers and fathers may be particularly upsetting. A clear structure for a basic daily pattern of activities, including getting up, washing, shaving, make-up and other self-care, meals and manageable tasks, and either domestic or occupational therapy, helps them to return to reality and feel more effective. Permissiveness, on the contrary, may engender further confusion.

The initial contact with the patient and family may determine their attitudes to the psychiatric service for the future.

The ward should aim to be calm but sociable, and free of illicit drugs. This may be surprisingly difficult to achieve (see chapter 21). One or two nurses must make a special effort to befriend the patient; the establishment of a relationship even though, at times, seemingly tenuous, superficial or difficult, is therapeutic provided it does not become too close. This means that the ward staff must have constancy from day to day and week to week, and not be frequently replaced by agency staff, and they should be readily identifiable by patients.

The building of confidence allows the patient to enter positively into the life of the ward and to cooperate with treatment, largely free of attacks of distress or violence.

These objectives apply also to those treated in a day hospital or as out-patients, but efforts may be needed to persuade them to attend regularly. Supervision, by regular contacts with a CPN or other keyworker, is an invaluable part of out-patient treatment and home visits reveal more of their lives and enable family and friends to report progress or setbacks.

Assessment

Initial assessment of the patient means:

- making sure that the diagnosis is correct and that the illness is not an acute brain syndrome or an atypical manic–depressive disorder, for which the treatment and prognosis are different
- identifying symptoms – delusions, hallucinations, passivity feelings, poor concentration, thought disorder, paranoid thinking – that can be targets for medication. The decline of these symptoms will then serve as a guide to further treatment and dosage
- judging the contributory factors – recent stresses, the taking of illicit drugs (amphetamines, cannabis, cocaine, khat, etc.) and the presence of affective and other symptoms
- identifying family or social factors that may assist or retard recovery
- assessing whether antipsychotic medication has been successful in the past and whether cessation of treatment has contributed to the present episode
- establishing his/her level of understanding and consent to treatment and whether the powers of the Mental Health Act are needed.

Urine screening should be carried out in patients in whom there is doubt about their use of drugs. Hair analysis, where available, can detect illicit drugs used over previous months.

Commencing medication

If the patient is not distressed or agitated, give a non-sedative antipsychotic such as trifluoperazine or haloperidol, or an atypical antipsychotic such as sulpiride, risperidone or the slightly more sedative olanzapine. Within 1 or 2 weeks it should be clear whether the symptoms are lessening. If not, raise the dose gradually and review weekly.

In the distressed or agitated patient, drugs that are more sedative are used. Start with chlorpromazine, thioridazine or zuclopenthixol, twice daily, increasing to four times daily if necessary, to maintain sedation. Among the atypical antipsychotics, quetiapine is more sedative but less so than chlorpromazine. Again continue for 1 or 2 weeks and then review. With experience one learns to gauge from the severity of illness the dosage that will probably be required, and to increase it by steps.

Treating EPS

This is discussed in chapter 17 and chapter 29. With some drugs, such as trifluoperazine and haloperidol, EPS are so common that it is advisable to commence anticholinergic medication when starting the antipsychotic, in order to avoid distress for the patient. With others, such as chlorpromazine and thioridazine, the EPS are less common and can be treated if they arise. Patients should always be given an explanation about the possible occurrence of EPS. Alternatively, an atypical antipsychotic may be used.

The concomitant use of anticholinergics can delay the development of antipsychotic effects and the dose of anticholinergic drug should be adjusted to the lowest that is needed.

Doses: first episodes and drug-naive patients

The patient in a first episode requires lower doses of antipsychotic medication than in later relapses. There are three reasons for this. First, drug-naive patients, including those who relapse after a long period without medication, will have less hepatic enzyme induction and therefore less capacity to metabolise the drug. Secondly, there will not yet have been compensatory changes such as up-regulation of receptors that tend to overcome the effects of the initial doses of antipsychotics. Thirdly, the first episode represents an early stage in the evolution of psychosis and may require lower blood levels and lower degrees of dopaminergic receptor blockade to produce improvement. At the same time, these patients are more susceptible to side-effects that are normally associated with higher doses.

Thus, doses of haloperidol of 2–5 mg/day or doses of risperidone of 2–4 mg/day are often sufficient in a first episode and may be optimal.

Table 13.1 shows the lowest doses that may be effective in first-episode or drug-naive patients.

DRUG TREATMENT

Table 13.1 Lowest doses that may be effective at start of first episode schizophrenia and later (mg/day)

	Start of first episode	Later and in relapses
Classical antipsychotic drug		
Chlorpromazine	100–300	300–600
Trifluoperazine	5–15	10–30
Haloperidol	2–5	5–20
Atypical antipsychotic drug		
Risperidone	2–4	4–6
Olanzapine	5	10–20
Amisulpride	400	800–1200
Quetiapine	150	300–750
Ziprasidone		80–160

However, D_2 receptor up-regulation begins within a few days of starting treatment, and receptor numbers increase by, for instance, 40%. Thus, after a few weeks the doses may need to be higher. Also with continued treatment, hepatic enzyme induction occurs in patients on chlorpromazine, orphenadrine or carbamazepine. This will increase the metabolism of other drugs, including antipsychotics, and require higher doses.

The doses have been assessed more extensively in later relapses, particularly for haloperidol, trifluoperazine, fluphenazine, risperidone and olanzapine. The doses that are then required are generally higher: haloperidol 5–20 mg/day, trifluoperazine 10–30 mg/day, olanzapine 10–20 mg/day and risperidone 4–6 mg/day; for chlorpromazine the difference is greater, up to 600 mg/day, as a result of enzyme induction. Some patients require doses higher than these, but for others the use of higher doses simply increases side-effects and can worsen the overall clinical state. For example, haloperidol at 20 mg/day can produce a worse outcome than 10 mg/day.

Adjusting the dose

These drugs set in train a process of recovery that may not be obvious until 2 weeks have passed and it takes 4–8 weeks to approach the full effect on positive symptoms. Further improvement may develop over the next year, especially if the patient has been ill for a long time prior to treatment. During all this time nothing is usually gained, apart from additional sedation and other side-effects, by increasing the dose of medication above a certain level (for instance above 20 mg a day for trifluoperazine and 15 mg a day for haloperidol; or above 6 mg for risperidone, 750 mg for quetiapine and 1200 mg for amisulpride).

Start with lower doses and build up gradually because side-effects, for instance dystonia, hypotension and sedation, are more severe if time for adaptation is not allowed. As the patient improves, sedation becomes less (if at all) necessary and less sedative drugs may be preferable and more acceptable to the patient.

Once improvement is marked, the daily drug dose should be cautiously reduced by steps every 1–2 weeks, watching for the return of symptoms as a sign to return to a higher dose and then reduce the dose no further.

Reluctance to take medication

Some patients unwilling to take tablets are prepared to drink syrup, which is more quickly and regularly absorbed and cannot secretly be got rid of by a patient with persecutory delusions. To start with, all the day's dose can be given at night as it will aid sleep and some patients will accept this but refuse daytime drugs. More rarely, those who refuse tablets or syrup will be prepared to have intramuscular injections.

With tablets by mouth one can never be sure that the patient is taking them and this may be a reason when antipsychotics seem to fail in treatment. Even if the patient has not expressed concern, it is important to enquire after side-effects, but without alarming the patient. The rapidly dissolving 'Velotab' formulation of olanzapine can aid compliance because it is extremely difficult to spit out once in the mouth.

Blood level measurement and prolactin

Measurement of blood levels is sometimes available for haloperidol, clozapine and olanzapine, and can provide a rough guide to therapeutic level. With haloperidol there is a therapeutic window and higher levels lead to a worsening, with more EPS. Chlorpromazine has many metabolites and blood level measurement is not clinicallly helpful.

An indirect measure of dopamine receptor blockade can be obtained from plasma prolactin, but this relates to blockade of receptors in the pituitary rather than the limbic system. In drug-naive people prolactin is maximally raised by small doses of antipsychotics, but after a few weeks of treatment the level is sensitive over a higher range of doses and can rise further.

Further improvement

Early success in treatment is shown by modification of symptoms. Later assessment is by observing the patient's abilities to mix with others, to concentrate and to make realistic decisions, and his/her capacity to undertake work and persist at it. Observations made by nurses, occupational therapists and relatives are essential here. Do not increase the doses of medication further when these improvements appear.

Failure to improve

Failure of schizophrenia to improve successfully with an antipsychotic commonly arises because:

- the patient is not getting the drug
- the doctor has been overcautious and not prescribed big enough doses
- the doctor has not waited long enough, at least 2 weeks, for improvement to start
- the clinician is making a global assessment only of behavioural improvement, instead of watching for the decline of target symptoms (hallucinations becoming infrequent and less forceful, concentration improving, logicality returning, restlessness declining). Even if there is

no global improvement, the drug may have produced a change in the symptom pattern, which shows that it is doing something and can perhaps be used to better effect in a larger dose, on a different schedule or by a different route

- the illness is treatment-resistant.

Some patients who do poorly on phenothiazines, which are extensively metabolised, will do better with another class of drugs. In general, however, there is little evidence that one antipsychotic drug, in adequate doses, produces greater long-term improvement than another (except clozapine). If the patient seems not to improve, it may be because there is an admixture of affective symptoms, depressive, manic or mixed, or because he/she has treatment-resistant schizophrenia.

Treating affective symptoms in acute schizophrenia

For severe depression appearing in the post-psychotic phase, the addition of an antidepressant can improve both the depression and the overall clinical state. Imipramine has been proved to be effective in this role. Likewise lithium will help to reduce elation and other symptoms of mania. Carbamazepine has a similar role and both drugs may also reduce impulsive or aggressive behaviour in schizophrenia.

The atypical drugs, including olanzapine and risperidone, are associated with less depression than haloperidol, during follow up.

Treatment-resistant schizophrenia

The National Institute of Mental Health (NIMH) study found 75% of patients were much improved after 6 weeks on antipsychotic compared to 25% on placebo (Cole *et al*, 1964). About 50% of patients showed a good response and a further 25% showed moderate improvement. The term 'treatment-resistant' is applied to those in whom courses of adequate doses of three antipsychotics from different chemical classes, continued for a sufficient time, fail to produce moderate improvement. A course of 6 weeks' treatment is required to determine whether a patient is responding, whereas at least 6 months is needed to realise the full benefit. Thus a patient may remain ill for over a year before he/she is confirmed to be treatment-resistant. This consitutes 15–30% of people with chronic schizophrenia. Box 13.3 shows steps to be taken in treatment resistance.

If high doses have been reached and the patient still appears very disturbed, a reduction in dose may help, or even a temporary cessation under observation; this is particularly relevant if EPS are evident. High blood levels of antipsychotics can exacerbate psychosis. EPS and especially akathisia can worsen the mental state, as can high doses of anticholinergic drugs. When switching drugs or stopping treatment there may be a period of rebound from anticholinergic effects, with agitation and insomnia. Therefore, it is advisable to withdraw anticholinergics or low-potency antipsychotics slowly over up to a month.

Benzodiazepines are useful for short-term use (see acute tranquillisation, p. 156), but of limited benefit as longer-term adjuncts, because of the problems of tolerance, dependence and disinhibition.

Box 13.3 Management of treatment-resistant schizophrenia

Exclude substance misuse (dual diagnosis)
Check compliance
Treat extrapyramidal side-effects (EPS)
Ensure adequate dose, or use depot injection
If dose is high, try reduction
Review diagnosis, affective symptoms and cognitive impairment
Adjunctive antidepressant, lithium or carbamazepine
Change to atypical antipsychotic
Clozapine
Check electroencephalogram
Clozapine plus classical antipsychotic, e.g. sulpiride
Clozapine plus anticonvulsant: valproate or lamotrigine

For treatment-resistant schizophrenia, the first drug with proven advantage over others is clozapine (see p. 312). Because of the risk of agranulocytosis, weekly blood tests in a formal monitoring system are required. Both positive and some negative symptoms benefit, but the core negative and deficit symptoms including cognitive impairment change less. There is definite benefit in social functioning in 30–60% of patients, and the suicide rate is also reduced.

Although risperidone, olanzapine and other atypicals have advantages over haloperidol (see chapter 30), none as yet is as effective as clozapine in treatment-resistant schizophrenia.

The use of clozapine is discussed in chapter 30. For patients who show a partial response to it, another antipsychotic may be added, and sulpiride is useful as an adjunct. Patients with intractable psychosis often have other disorders that are comorbid (chapter14). Some have schizoaffective disorder, and some have cognitive impairment, which it is important to recognise as it interferes with the usual psychosocial therapies. Drug or alcohol misuse may also be a major contributory factor (chapter 21).

ECT with antipsychotics in schizophrenia

Rarely ECT is of value – in those patients who, despite adequate antipsychotic treatment, have persistent disturbing symptoms associated with destructive behaviour. Do not go beyond the maximum of five treatments unless improvement is clearly occurring. ECT by itself usually has only a temporary (48 hour) suppressant effect on symptoms. Combined with phenothiazines the effects last longer, but tend to disappear by 3 months. For these reasons ECT is not often used unless the psychosis is very severe or the patient is suicidal. However, it is effective for cases of acute catatonia, or when there is also severe depression. Deficit-state disabilities are not helped by ECT.

Duration of treatment after a first episode

After a first florid episode, drugs should be continued for at least 1 year. If the patient has remained well, he/she should then be gradually withdrawn and observed carefully for 3–12 months for the return of symptoms, and he/she remains at risk after that. Table 13.2 shows the results of two placebo-controlled studies of continued drug treatment after first episodes.

The rationale for continuing treatment is the much lower relapse rate in treated patients. The reason for limiting treatment to one year in patients who appear to do well is that as many as 59% of patients did not relapse on placebo within this time. However, the proportion who will relapse within 5 years is 85%, indicating the importance of cautious follow-up.

PLANNING DISCHARGE

Prior to discharge from hospital a plan of aftercare should be made following an assessment of needs in which the views of the patient, his/her CPN, social worker, relatives, GP and other professionals may contribute. This is formalised in the care programme for informal patients and in Section 117 of the MHA (1983) for patients who have been detained on a treatment order (see chapter 10).

The patient should be reviewed regularly, for example on a weekly basis at first, monthly later. Someone who lives with the patient should be asked regularly about him/her.

LONGER-TERM TREATMENT MANAGEMENT

After a first episode of schizophrenia a minority of patients become completely well. Others continue to require drugs to reduce their positive symptoms. In others the psychotic experiences remit but residual deficit symptoms persist. The majority are at risk of relapses.

Assessing residual symptoms

In assessing residual symptoms the negative symptoms of the illness itself must be distinguished from similar symptoms that can be caused by drugs (see Box 13.1). EPS are important to consider, because a switch to an atypical antipsychotic may be beneficial. The patient with schizophrenia with clinical depression may express feelings in an affectively flat way, and the usual disturbances of sleep and appetite may be masked by antipsychotic medication. Nevertheless, they can

Table 13.2 Continuation antipsychotic treatment in first-episode schizophrenia

Authors	Number	Duration (years)	Relapse (%) Drug	Relapse (%) Placebo	ARR (%)	Comments
Crow et al (1986)	120	1	38	63	25	Compliance varied
Kane et al (1982)	28	1	0	41	41	Depot treatment

ARR, absolute risk reduction.

benefit from antidepressants. Depression, anxiety or insomnia are often part of the prodrome of relapse and require an increase in antipsychotic medication. With modern treatments there is no evidence that long periods of hospitalisation are in themselves associated with higher levels of social withdrawal.

Treatment of relapses

If the acute episode is a recurrence, then treatment should follow the same principles until the symptoms are controlled. Then long-term treatment should be considered and depot medication offered, and in many cases encouraged.

RELAPSE PREVENTION AND LONG-TERM MEDICATION

Long-term use of antipsychotics requires careful consideration. They can produce harmful or unpleasant effects, tardive dyskinesia for instance, weight gain (see chapter 23) and mental dulling. In some patients their therapeutic value may seem limited. On the other hand, a schizophrenic illness can be so devastating that it is justifiable to go to great lengths to prevent or minimise it.

It has been firmly established that 60–70% of patients with chronic schizophrenia will relapse within 1 year of stopping medication, and 85% within 2 years. The most common time to relapse is the second 3 months after stopping. These figures are greatly reduced by drug treatment but 10% will still relapse each year even among those who adhere fully to treatment.

Adherence

The tendency to poor adherence and its management in patients with schizophrenia with compliance therapy is discussed in chapter 3. Taking tablets several times a day without fail can be difficult. Tablets that need to be taken only once a day are easier, but better still from this point of view are the long-acting depot injections of antipsychotics.

It is important to keep dose and side-effects to the minimum that is required to control the illness. This may be aided by using an atypical drug. However, these drugs are still relatively untested in long-term use; although patients often prefer an atypical rather than a classical antipsychotic, this preference does not necessarily translate into sustained adherence and prevention of relapse.

Education of the patient and his/her family about the illness and its treatment will help to improve adherence and facilitate a therapeutic alliance. For many patients the regular contact with a CPN provides the best hope, by encouraging adherence in a continuing relationship with a professional who can advise on local services, counsel about new problems and detect and respond to the early stages of relapse.

Depot medication

The development of depot formulations was one of the major advances in the treatment of schizophrenia. To be given as depot injections the drug must be highly potent and able to be esterified with a long-chain fatty acid (to increase its fat solubility), so a month's dose can be dissolved in a volume of vegetable oil small enough to be given by deep intramuscular injection. The available drugs are fluphenazine, flupenthixol, zuclopenthixol, haloperidol and pipothiazine. An injection every 1–6 weeks may suffice as maintenance treatment. Atypical antipsychotics will soon be available in long-acting microsphere or depot formulations. The advantages and disadvantages of depot medication are listed in Box 13.4.

Efficacy of depot prophylaxis

The justification for persuading patients to continue taking medication, despite side-effects, for many years is illustrated in Table 13.3, which summarises the placebo-controlled trials.

With an ARR of up to 58%, the advantage of continued treatment corresponds to an NNT of only two. Patients discharged more recently are at higher risk of relapse. Effectiveness in routine practice is also established (see chapter 3, p. 27).

Doses for maintenance treatment

The doses of antipsychotic medication that are effective in maintenance treatment have been studied in trials comparing low, standard and

---

Box 13.4 Advantages and disadvantages of depot injections of antipsychotics

Advantages

Medical – it is possible to recognise non-adherence immediately, and to encourage resumption. Decisions about changes in dose can be made with more confidence, in the light of information about adherence.

Nursing – regular contact with a community psychiatric nurse (CPN), who administers the injection, facilitates the role of the nurse as keyworker, supervision of progress and recognition of relapse.

Stigma and expressed emotion – patient and relatives are relieved of worry about daily tablet taking.

Pharmacokinetic – more steady blood levels, with less frequent peaks, are associated with fewer acute side-effects, drowsiness and dizziness.

Convenience – many patients come to regard injections as convenient and value particularly the contact with the CPN.

Cost – in urban settings a depot injection clinic is highly cost-effective.

Disadvantages

Injection may be viewed as painful, inconvenient and humiliating.

Patients lacking insight may refuse injections while claiming to be willing to take tablets.

Extrapyramidal side-effects (EPS) still require oral medication.

Peaks of blood level can occur for a day immediately after the injection, and may cause side-effects then.

Cost of nurse's time, especially in rural settings where distances to travel are long.

Table 13.3 Relapse prevention in schizophrenia with depot injections

Authors	Number	Duration (months)	Relapse rate (%)		ARR (%)	Comment
			Drug	Placebo		
Hirsh et al (1973)	74	12	8	66	58	Previously well-maintained
Rifkin et al (1977)	73	9	10	68	58	Previously well-maintained
Wistedt et al (1981)	41	6	27	62	35	Recently discharged

ARR, absolute risk reduction.

high doses. Above a certain dose no additional improvement or protection from relapse is obtained.

The most common dose of fluphenazine decanoate in a group of outpatients is 25 mg a fortnight. Younger male patients require more, whereas patients over 60 years or those who have been free of relapse for 3 years manage with less. In the elderly a dose as low as 5 mg a fortnight may be beneficial. People with a first onset of delusional disorder in old age manage with even lower doses than those who graduate into old age having already been ill when younger. The reduction with age in the dose required is less pronounced with flupenthixol decanoate. For haloperidol decanoate the most common effective dose is 150 mg every 4 weeks, although doses as low as 50 mg every 4 weeks are sufficient in some patients; these correspond to oral daily doses of 7.5 mg and 2.5 mg, respectively.

Pharmacokinetics of depot medication

Depot medication causes blood levels of drug that decline slowly, as if they had a half-life of 1–3 weeks. All prescribers should note the effects of the time taken to reach steady-state plasma levels. After 2 to 3 months of regular dosing, plasma levels may be four times higher than after the first dose. Thus dose increases during this time are usually unnecessary. Indeed, it may be preferable to give an early larger loading dose to achieve the desired steady-state plasma level sooner. Otherwise it takes about 12–16 weeks for a steady-state blood level to be reached after a change of regular dose.

Reviewing medication

The care of schizophrenia is a long-term job and the CPN or social worker who is usually the keyworker will need the support of a regular clinical review, with medical input, not by a succession of junior doctors but by a consultant accompanied by doctors in their training. These team reviews should be conducted at least once a year for even the most stable patients and at shorter intervals for less stable patients.

When reviewing long-term treatment, look back over the history, the early symptoms before treatment started, the early signs of relapse, the circumstances of the last admission and evidence about previous relapses (the relapse fingerprint) when the dose has been reduced below a certain level. After controlling a relapse it is possible to reduce medication gradually over the next 3 years.

Obviously the patient whose hallucinations and paranoid outbursts are suppressed but not removed by drugs should continue to take them. A problem arises in the person with a chronic disability, with predominant negative symptoms but no current positive symptoms. Should they be on long-term treatment? The answer lies in deciding whether there has been previous experience of the patient relapsing when medication was reduced further. In such patients long-term treatment is helpful in maintaining improvement and preventing relapses.

The best strategy for long-term drug treatment is gradually to reduce the dose of medication to the lowest that keeps the patient free of relapse. Remember that after reducing the dose of the depot the blood level will not reach the new steady state until about 3–4 months later, and relapses related to earlier dose reductions can occur up to 18 months afterwards.

Attempts to discontinue medication and then to identify the earliest symptoms of relapse are generally less successful and place the patient at greater risk.

Choose the time for managing without drugs with great care so that if, by ill chance, a relapse does occur it will not fall at a critically upsetting time for the patient. For example, a student who has a schizophrenic breakdown should be carried through his/her exams and well into his first job before considering drug withdrawal. Remember that a schizophrenic illness can have a disastrous effect on the course of a person's life, for instance the prospects of a career and marriage.

Polypharmacy

Too many patients are continued on a multiplicity of drugs, sometimes for years, for example an oral as well as a depot antipsychotic, benzodiazepine and anti-Parkinsonian drugs, and perhaps an antidepressant as well. Medication should be cut down on a rational basis. Very few patients require both oral and depot antipsychotics in long-term treatment and the tablets should be converted to depot equivalents and phased out. Anti-Parkinsonian drugs may no longer be necessary, having been started in other circumstances. Benzodiazepines, useful at an earlier stage, should not be required later and have no long-term benefit. To demonstrate what the regime is actually doing, alterations may be needed, while looking for changes – either good or bad – in the patient.

CBTs

Specific behavioural techniques may be useful in patients with particular behavioural difficulties, for instance attention-focusing for poverty of speech, relaxation training for screaming or aggressive behaviour, over-correction for urinary incontinence or enuresis. Intensive psychosocial interventions can exacerbate schizophrenia, especially in patients on low-dose medication. But training on medication management, symptom management, social problem-solving and skills of daily living can improve social adjustment provided the patient is on medication. Other approaches have been tried to improve the outcome, but claims for specific efficacy must take account of the possibility that any benefits are the result of improved adherence to medication, rather than other psychological changes in the patient or family.

Care in the Community

Current practice leads to many patients with substantial impairments living outside hospital. They are vulnerable to exploitation and social pressures, and may have difficulty making friends; they are often poor at looking after their own domestic and business interests, failing to shop and cook for themselves or to claim money to which they are entitled. A balance has to be struck between interference in the life of the disabled and encouragement to further independence. However, there have been too many examples of people with schizophrenia losing contact with the psychiatric services, missing their medication and coming back into treatment only after being arrested.

Collaboration with voluntary bodies such as the National Schizophrenia Fellowship can provide a network of support and advice to patients and their relatives (tel: 020 8547 3937; advice line: 020 8974 6814). SANE (Schizophrenia A National Emergency) offers telephone advice (SANE line: 020 7724 8000). Patients discharged from hospital often take time to recover their full capacity for self-government. After-care hostels should be available, providing appropriate levels of support, and the hostel staff should work with the patient's keyworker to encourage medication and plan the next stage of rehabilitation. Day centres and drop-in centres are useful in providing daytime activity at a level appropriate for the patient's needs.

FURTHER READING

Overview

Johnstone, E. C., Humphreys, M. S., Lang, F. H., *et al* (1999) *Schizophrenia: Concepts and Clinical Management*. Cambridge: Cambridge University Press.

Reveley, M. A. & Deakin, J. F. W. (eds) (1999) *The Psychopharmacology of Schizophrenia*. British Association of Psychopharmacology Monograph Series. London: Arnold.

Dopamine and glutamine

Anand, A., Charney, D. S., Oren, D. A., *et al* (2000) Attenuation of the neuropsychiatric effects of ketamine with lamotrigine: support for hyperglutamatergic effects of N-methyl-D-aspartate receptor antagonists. *Archives of General Psychiatry*, **57**, 270–276.

Moore, H., West, A. R. & Grace, A. A. (1999) The regulation of forebrain dopamine transmission: relevance to the pathophysiology and psychopathology of schizophrenia. *Biological Psychiatry*, **46**, 40–55.

Cognition

Goldberg, T. E., Greenberg, R. D., Griffin, S. J., *et al* (1993) The effect of clozapine on cognition and psychiatric symptoms in patients with schizophrenia. *British Journal of Psychiatry*, **162**, 43–48.

Green, M. F., Marshall, B. D., Wirshing, M. D., *et al* (1997) Does risperidone improve verbal working memory in treatment-resistant schizophrenia? *American Journal of Psychiatry*, **154**, 799–804.

DRUG TREATMENT

Harvey, P. D. & Keefe, R. S. E. (2001) Studies of cognitive changes in patients with schizophrenia following novel antipsychotic treatment. *American Journal of Psychiatry*, **158**, 176–184.

Sharma, T. (1999) Cognitive effects of conventional and atypical antipsychotics in schizophrenia. *British Journal of Psychiatry*, **174**(Suppl. 38), 44–51.

First episode

Meeham, K. M., Aitchison,. K. J. & Murray, R. (1997) *First Episode Psychosis*. London: Martin Dunitz.

Kopala, L., Kimberly, P. G. & Honer, W. G. (1997) Extrapyramidal signs and clinical symptoms in first-episode schizophrenia: response to low-dose risperidone. *Journal of Clinical Psychopharmacology*, **17**, 308–313.

Maintenance treatment

Davis, J. M. (1975) Overview: maintenance therapy in psychiatry, I: schizophrenia. *American Journal of Psychiatry*,**132**, 1237–1245.

Placebo-controlled depot studies

Crow, T. J., MacMillan, J. F., Johnson, A. L., *et al* (1986) A randomised controlled trial of prophylactic neuroleptic treatment. *British Journal of Psychiatry*, **148**, 120–127.

Hirsch, S. R., Gaind, R., Rohde, P., *et al* (1973) Outpatient maintenance of chronic schizophrenic patients with long-acting fluphenazine: double-blind placebo trial. *BMJ*, **1**, 633–637.

Kane, J. M., Rifkin, A., Quitkin, F., *et al* (1982) Fluphenazine vs placebo in patients with remited, acute first-episode schizophrenia. *Archives of General Psychiatry*, **39**, 70–73.

Rifkin, A., Quitkin, F., Rabiner, C. J., *et al* (1977) Fluphenazine decanoate, fluphenazine hydrochloride given orally, and placebo in remitted schizophrenics. *Archives of General Pychiatry*, **34**, 43–47.

Wistedt, B. (1981) A depot neuroleptic withdrawal study. *Acta Psychiatrica Scandinavica*, **64**, 65–84.

Treatment-resistant schizophrenia

Barnes, T. R., McEvedy, C. J. & Nelson, H. E. (1996) Management of treatment resistant schizophrenia unresponsive to clozapine. *British Journal of Psychiatry*, **169**(Suppl. 31), 31–40.

Shiloh, R., Zemishlany, Z., Aizenberg, D., *et al* (1997) Sulpiride augmentation in people with schizophrenia partially responsive to clozapine. A double-blind placebo-controlled study. *British Journal of Psychiatry*, **171**, 569–573.

Malignant catatonia

Mann, S. C., Caroff, S. N., Bleier, H. R., *et al* (1986) Lethal catatonia. *American Journal of Psychiatry*, **143**, 1374–1381.

Benzodiazepines in catatonia

Bush, G., Fink, M., Petrides, G., *et al* (1996) Catatonia. II. Treatment with lorazepam and electroconvulsive therapy. *Acta Psychiatrica Scandinavica*, **93**, 137–143.

Studies quoted

Cole, J. O., Goldberg, S. C. & Klerman, G. L. (1964) Phenothiazine treatment in acute schizophrenia. *Archives of General Psychiatry*, **10**, 246–261.

Mason, P., Harrison, G., Croudace, T., *et al* (1997) The predictive validity of a diagnosis of schizophrenia. A report from the International Study of Schizophrenia (ISoS) coordinated by the World Health Organization and the Department of Psychiatry, University of Nottingham. *British Journal of Psychiatry*, **170**, 321–332.

Wahbeck, K. (1999) Evidence of clozapine's effectiveness in schizophrenia: a systematic review and meta-analysis of randomised trials. *American Journal of Psychiatry*, **156**, 990–999.

Walburn, J., Gray, R., Gournay, K., *et al* (2001) Systematic review of patient and nurse attitudes to depot antipsychotic medication. *British Journal of Psychiatry*, **179**, 300–307.

Goff, D. C. & Coyle, J. T. (2001) The emerging role of glutamate in the pathophysiology and treatment of schizophrenia. *American Journal of Psychiatry*, **158**, 1367–1377.

Scale quoted

Kay, S. R., Fiszbein, A. & Opler, L. A. (1987) Positive and Negative Syndrome Scale (PANSS) for Schizophrenia. *Schizophrenia Bulletin*, **13**, 261–276.

DRUG TREATMENT

14. VIOLENCE: ASSESSING RISK AND ACUTE TRANQUILLISATION

Violence is the exercise of physical force so as to cause injury or damage to oneself, others or property. Aggression is the threat of violence.

ASSOCIATION WITH MENTAL DISORDER

Until recently many researchers were sceptical about any relationship between mental illness and violence and some professionals ignored the association, because perceived dangerousness and unpredictability can contribute to the stigma of mental illness. However, recent studies demonstrate an increased risk of violence in certain groups. Only a minority of patients with mental disorders are violent, but personality disorder, schizophrenia and alcoholism show increased rates compared to the general population. The risk is particularly high when there is a combination of previous violent behaviour, alcoholism and antisocial personality, or of untreated schizophrenia with alcoholism or substance misuse.

Compared to the general population the odds ratios for violent behaviour in men ranges from four in schizophrenia without alcoholism to 11 in alcoholism and 17 in schizophrenia with alcoholism. The highest odds ratios were in released forensic psychiatric patients in their first year outside hospital (see Table 14.1).

MANAGEMENT

A traditional way of coping with the violence of those with mental illness was by physical restraint: chains, the strait waistcoat or seclusion in the padded cell. Then, in the early 19th century, came the

Table 14.1 Risk of violence compared with general male population

Diagnosis	Odds ratio	95% C.I.
Released homicide offender	254	145–442
Antisocial personality disorder	12	10–14
Alcoholism	11	9–12
Schizophrenia[1]	4	0.9–12
	8	6–10
Schizophrenia with	17	12–24
alcoholism	25	6–97
Discharged forensic patients (first year)	293	119–724

1. Data from two seperate studies.
Reproduced with permisssion from Eronen et al, 1997.

demonstration in England that calm, friendly concern for the individual and simple psychological management made much of restraint unnecessary. Drugs, bromides, chloral, hyoscine, paraldehyde, morphine, and later barbiturates, became the compellers of peace, in effect by heavy sedation, or partial anaesthetisation or, in some cases, by inducing a toxic-confusional state (see chapter 1).

Modern psychotropics with more subtle effects calm without necessarily making the person unconscious or even unduly drowsy, and psychological handling has again become an important component of management. The violent patient presents the most extreme challenge to the psychiatrist of how to combine psychology and pharmacology and compassion and safety in effective proportion. In the general hospital ward the psychiatrist may be asked to help not only with the violent, but in some cases with lesser degrees of disturbance involving complex problems of diagnosis or management, and not necessarily to arrange removal of the patient.

What the psychiatrist offers is:

- a skill in gaining the patient's confidence, and sensitivity to pointers in the history or behaviour suggesting an organic as well as a psychological origin of symptoms
- a systematic assessment of mental state, covering all main mental functions
- pursuit of a detailed reliable history, with awareness of the relevance of social and interpersonal factors on the one hand and of the impact of physical illness and toxic effects of prescribed medicines or illicit drugs on the other
- the ability at times to wait and observe further before drawing conclusions
- continuity of care, with only one doctor in charge, keeping medication to the minimum and maintaining, with nurses and other staff, a clear and consistent approach to problems
- skills in the involvement of relatives or friends to gain the patient's confidence
- keeping a record of medication and behavioural change.

It is important to be wary of clever labels and glib interpretations and to be prepared to seek advice from colleagues with more experience. Spend time with nurses, who bear the brunt of difficult behaviour and often have considerable skills in its management.

THE ACCIDENT AND EMERGENCY DEPARTMENT

Violent and dangerous behaviour is common. People intoxicated with alcohol and those with severe personality disorders are often quickly recognised and deflected towards the police. But beware of too ready use of such nuisance labels and of overlooking mania, schizophrenia, drug-induced psychosis, head injury or post-epileptic state, any of which may occur in a person previously known to drink heavily or to have a difficult personality. Some degree of altered consciousness may be detectable and of importance in diagnosis, even if no history is available.

DRUG TREATMENT

Assessing the patient

It is important to have an adequate and defined space for the interview, so that the patient can move about and not feel restricted. Do not ignore the potentially violent person. It is essential that the doctor should appear as calm and neutral in manner as possible and adopts a relaxed, friendly stance. Speak calmly and in a low tone. Non-verbal communication matters. Ask for any weapons to be put down (and later handed over); also any hot drinks and cigarettes. Try to establish a relationship of trust; allow him/her to verbalise his/her concerns. Do not promise anything that cannot be carried out (except in a situation of immediate danger), and if it cannot, tell the patient why. Body language is important. Keep one's hands down; maintain eye contact without staring. Stay at arm's length, sit between the patient and the door. Be aware of how to call for help.

It is impossible to feel confident unless there is adequate back-up. Do not interview alone but have one or two nurses present and try to do without police. Two nurses are not threatening to an excited person, especially if they are seen as carers rather than authority figures. Large numbers of helpers can be threatening.

Resist pressure to make decisions based on inadequate information. Be prepared to listen for 30 minutes or more to a patient's stream of complaints. Appear interested in them and do not give meaningless reassurances; interpretations and arguments do not help at this stage. It is always possible to move from contentious areas of conversation to less emotionally charged matters. Ask for the facts of problems, and encourage reasoning.

Drug treatment

Drugs are used both to treat the underlying mental disorder (mania, schizophrenia, etc.) and to reduce aggression and arousal.

Rapid or acute tranquillisation

Whatever the cause, if violent or disturbed behaviour continues or is threatened it may need to be controlled rapidly.

Antipsychotics and benzodiazepines

Consistency is important and many hospitals have a local protocol or guidelines for the use of drugs for acute disturbance, prepared in collaboration with the pharmacist to assist ward doctors. These may list a variety of options with their advantages and risks, or may suggest a flow chart. The aim of acute tranquillisation is to calm or sedate the patient sufficiently to minimise the risk posed to the patient and to others. Often it is used for sedation, but sometimes it addresses also the underlying illness, particularly mania. Schizophrenic symptoms tend to respond more slowly.

In some cases medication that is rapidly eliminated is preferred, for instance the benzodiazepine lorazepam. Until 2001, the short-acting sedative butyrophenone droperidol was used in some centres (see p.

298). However, the patient may remain severely disturbed when the medication wears off, in which case longer-acting drugs are preferable, for instance the benzodiazepine diazepam, and the antipsychotics haloperidol, zuclopenthixol or chlorpromazine. The intravenous route offers the most rapid method of sedation. A high peak concentration of the drug is achieved; but this may have cardiovascular side-effects, and the early sedation wears off quickly as the drug is redistributed. Intramuscular injection gives a more gradual rise in blood concentration, but in individuals with low muscle blood flow there is a risk of successive doses accumulating in muscle and then being released to the circulation in unexpectedly high concentrations. Intramuscular use of diazepam should be avoided. It is very painful; also this drug is absorbed more quickly orally and the intravenous route is more reliable and safer than the intramuscular route.

For patients who continue to refuse oral medication, the use of a longer-acting intramuscular injection of clopenthixol as acetate ('Acuphase') helps to reduce the need for frequent injections (see below).

The greatest concern about acute tranquillisation is that sudden deaths have been reported, particularly in young males, and sometimes with modest doses of medication. Both cardiac arrhythmias and respiratory depression may be involved. When the patient requires higher doses than usual, it is advisable to check the electrocardiogram (ECG), and to use benzodiazepines rather than antipsychotics, especially if there is evidence of QT prolongation. When sedated the patient should be kept under constant nursing observation, with attention to the respiration, pulse and blood pressure. Staff should be familiar with cardiopulmonary resuscitation techniques and equipment. The drug flumazenil should be readily available to counteract respiratory depression caused by benzodiazepines: its effects in blocking benzodiazepines are short-lived and staff should be aware of this. An apparently alert patient may quickly lapse again into respiratory depression as the effect of flumazenil wears off.

If there is uncertainty about the diagnosis, it may be desirable to avoid the use of antipsychotic drugs and to use benzodiazepines in the first instance. Lorazepam (2–4 mg orally, 1–2 mg intramuscularly or slowly intravenously) is usually very effective and safe; 1 mg of lorazepam is roughly equivalent to 10 mg of diazepam. Diazepam may be given intravenously (10–30 mg slowly, about 2.5 mg per 30 seconds), orally (20–40 mg) or rectally. These drugs may need to be repeated 2 hourly up to 80 mg or more of diazepam in 24 hours or 8 mg or more of lorazepam (the *BNF* maximum is 4 mg).

When an antipsychotic is used, haloperidol is often the drug of first choice. Five to 10 mg may be given intramuscularly for the first injection and repeated every half hour to 1 hour until the patient is sedated, up to a maximum of 100 mg in 24 hours. Intravenous haloperidol may be given, 5–10mg, repeated after 15 minutes if necessary. These should then be changed to an oral dose of 2–10 mg three times a day (the *BNF* maximum for haloperidol has been reduced to 18 mg per day intramuscularly and 30 mg orally).

Chlorpromazine is also a sedative antipsychotic and may be given orally as tablet or syrup 100–200 mg, 2 hourly up to a maximum of 1 gm in 24 hours. It may also be given by intramuscular injection in doses of 50–100 mg every 4 to 6 hours; however, this method can cause local pain, acute hypotension and occasionally a sterile painful abscess. This route of administration avoids first-pass metabolism, which can be substantial in patients previously exposed to treatment over long periods; high blood levels can be reached unless the dose is lowered for drug-naive patients. It may also have a higher risk of inducing seizures. For these reasons it should not be the first-line treatment, and some authorities avoid its use.

The elderly, particularly those with cognitive impairment or acute psychosis, should be given much lower doses, e.g. chlorpromazine 10–25 mg orally or haloperidol 0.5–1 mg orally or intramuscularly with careful monitoring of blood pressure and physical state. Lewy body dementia is renowned for sufferers' exceptional sensitivity to the EPS of antipsychotics.

The atypical antipsychotic ziprasidone is effective similarly to haloperidol in acute psychotic disturbances, but is better tolerated, not causing EPS. Olanzapine may be given intramuscularly, 10 mg being as effective as 7.5 mg of haloperidol over the course of 2 hours.

Other sedatives

The barbiturate sodium amylobarbitone ('Amytal') (250 mg) given intramuscularly as an adjunct to sedative antipsychotics and benzodiazepines can be very effective for sedation. Careful nursing observation is important because of the risk of respiratory depression, hypotension and chest infections. 'Amytal' may also be given orally 200 mg when required. It should be born in mind that there is no pharmacological antagonist for barbiturates, as there is for benzodiazepines (see p. 366).

Depot medication

If excitement or aggression persist and repeated injections are required (because the patient refuses oral medication), zuclopenthixol acetate ('Clopixol Acuphase') has an effect lasting for about 3 days; 50–150 mg is given by deep intramuscular injection. The onset of action takes 2–8 hours, during which time another drug may be required. The injection should not be repeated for 24 hours, and the maximum amount for a course of zuclopenthixol acetate is 400 mg in total. Subsequently the longer-acting zuclopenthixol decanoate may be used, with a duration of 1–2 weeks. The maximum dose of zuclopenthixol decanoate is 600 mg weekly. (see p. 299)

Administering medication

Establish the patient's legal status and follow MHA procedures. Under common law (established by cases and not statute), restraint and sedative medication can be used even without consent if it is needed in order to prevent imminent harm to the patient or others. Such use of common law must be documented and justified in the medical notes.

It should be explained to the patient why and how medication is to be given. Two or three nurses (of either sex, but with special training in restraint) working as a team can control and inject a patient without causing injuries. The less acutely disturbed patient may be confronted and offered a choice of either oral medication or injection. Some patients will accept oral medication in the knowledge that an injection will otherwise be given. The whole procedure, if carefully done, will usually not be resented by the patient later on. Blood can be taken for analysis at the same time, including for glucose (in case of hypoglycaemia), electrolytes and alcohol level. Rapid effective control by medication reduces behaviour that is distressing to the patients themselves, and it results in the possibility of discussion and co-operation in further management. Patients generally prefer this to seclusion or prolonged periods of restraint.

Drugs used in this way demand close supervision and reassessment every few hours. The search for a firm diagnosis, and the causes, must be pursued as this will determine where to place the patient for further treatment (for mania, delirium tremens and drug-induced psychosis, see under these headings elsewhere).

Always check that laboratory investigations have been adequate and complete. If the patient is pyrexial, a full blood count and CPK level may be very helpful in identifying infection or incipient NMS (see p. 88). Urine analysis for drugs is useful where illicit drugs are suspected, to identify cannabis, amphetamines, cocaine, opiates, Ecstasy, phencyclidine and khat. Blood analysis is important when toxicity is suspected, for instance with phenytoin, tricyclics, barbiturates or aspirin through deliberate or accidental overdose. Generally, patients suffering from toxic effects of drugs should be treated on medical wards by physicians with expert knowledge, assisted by psychiatric advice for control of disturbed behaviour. Additional information is available, day and night, from regional poisons information services (see *BNF* for telephone numbers).

PSYCHIATRIC INTENSIVE CARE UNITS

Acute behavioural disturbance, associated with onset or relapse of a psychotic illness or a drug-induced state, usually settles after a few days with the regime outlined above. During this time the patient may be best managed in a secure psychiatric intensive care unit (PICU), with high nursing levels. Continuing with regular antipsychotics at a reduced level may then maintain stability. The structural features of a PICU should include safety, space, privacy, cleanliness, ease of observation and facilities for exercise and personal interactions, including phone calls and visits. There should be a policy for the management of substance misuse, including the role of the local police.

The National Association of Psychiatric Intensive Care Units (NAPICU) holds conferences (Pathways, Goodmayes Hospital, Barley Lane, Goodmayes, Ilford, Essex IG3 8YB; tel: 020 8970 5808; website: http://www.napicu.org.uk) and its chairman is Dr S. Pereira.

RISK ASSESSMENT AND DE-ESCALATION OF VIOLENCE

The staff should be trained in recognising warning signs of violence and in break-away techniques (to release oneself from holds). For staff

DRUG TREATMENT

Box 14.1 Risk factors for violence

Risk factors for future violence	Risk factors for imminent violence
Personal history	
History of violence	Increased arousal, restlessness
Young, male	Loud speech, erratic movement
Threats of violence	Angry appearance
Violent subculture	Social withdrawal
Clinical	
Alcohol, drug misuse	Unclear thought processes
Active schizophrenia or mania	Violent content to delusions, hallucinations
Agitation, suspiciousness	Aggressive gestures, threats
Delusions, command	Signs noted in previous episode
hallucinations	Reports violent feelings
Preoccupation with violence or a	
potential victim	
Situational	
Low social support	Carers sense danger
Availability of weapon	
Relationship to potential victim	

Adapted from Royal College of Psychiatrists (1998) *Management of Imminent Violence. Clinical Practice Guidelines to Support Mental Health Services.* Occassional Paper OP41.

working in specialised areas such as PICUs, there are courses in control and restraint. Risk factors for imminent violence include restlessness, tension, unpredictability, loudness, discontent, withdrawal, muddled thinking, angry feelings and a violent content to delusions or hallucinations. Signs from earlier episodes of violence may be recognised, for instance reports of particular delusional thoughts. Despite these lists, violence is notoriously difficult to predict, and the carer's intuitive sense of danger remains important (see Box 14.1).

The reasons and procedure for restraint should be explained to the patient; any confrontation should take place with staff appropriate to the patient's age, gender and size. Physical restraint should be used in a coordinated manner, using secure grip, minimising pain, protecting the patients head and neck and air supply, and avoiding unnecessary pressure on the back or chest. It should also attempt to maintain dignity.

Most acute wards cope with violent behaviour without a specially designed seclusion room. Seclusion (isolation) can be justified only as a last resort, when all other methods have failed, and then for the shortest possible time. Hospitals are expected to have a clear protocol for the use of seclusion.

LONGER-TERM MANAGEMENT

A small group of patients do not improve with high doses of the common antipsychotics and show persistent or intermittent dangerous behaviour for months or years. Unlocked acute or long-stay wards are ill-suited to provide care for these patients: PICUs usually take patients with acute mental illness for a period of days or weeks, and medium secure units serve patients with a forensic history or those judged most immediately dangerous. Thus, such patients have been labelled difficult to place. Some districts set up small special care units and others use private specialised units. Ideally these units are secure, provide spacious areas for a range of activities and allow good observation. Staff are highly trained, with a high ratio per patient and include a range of disciplines. The multi-disciplinary approach reflects the limits of drug therapy, the often multiple handicaps of these patients and the need for patients to develop skills and to change unwanted behaviour before preparing for more independence.

A small number of these patients have devastating schizophrenic illnesses with active symptoms and serious secondary deficits, which have not responded to medication. Here the aim is to prevent deterioration in behaviour and residual abilities, while exploring new, possibly more effective, antipsychotics such as clozapine (see Treatment-Resistant Schizophrenia: p. 144). On the other hand, the majority of the patients present a complex problem with an interplay of fluctuating psychotic states, mood disturbance, unstable personality, mental impairment or brain damage and drug misuse. Close observation may reveal a repetitive pattern and identify likely triggers, and thus with foresight florid episodes may be avoided.

Their multiple handicaps often lead to polypharmacy, the use of several medications in combination. Weight gain from long-term high doses of medication will add to patients' problems, worsening diabetes, cardiovascular and respiratory difficulties and lowering self-esteem. Good practices in prescribing are necessary. For example, minimise the use of several drugs of the same class (e.g. phenothiazines), ensure that adequate amounts of a particular antipsychotic are given (and that the patient is receiving it) before discarding its use, make only one change in treatment at a time and give a period of some weeks before coming to a conclusion. Before using a new drug identify the target symptoms, obtain a baseline and then monitor regularly. In addition to antipsychotics, lithium or carbamazepine may lessen mood changes and impulsive or aggressive behaviour. The patients may have depressive or obsessional symptoms, requiring antidepressants including SSRIs. The risks of pharmacokinetic interaction should be considered. Excessive doses of antipsychotics may cause akathisia and also worsen the mental state. Anticholinergics can worsen psychosis or cause confusion in high doses, and are prone to abuse. Tardive dyskinesia may develop and impair speech and swallowing. Benzodiazepines are often started either for insomnia or in an attempt to calm behaviour; there is a greater risk of dependence with personality disorders, and any benefit from benzodiazepines may be shortlived. The overall aim is to suppress distressing symptoms or destructive behaviour with the least amount of drug to achieve this end, which also allows the patient to be alert and mobile. This allows inputs from psychologists, occupational therapists, teachers and social workers to be effective.

DRUG TREATMENT

AFTER A VIOLENT INCIDENT

The incident should be documented and discussed as soon as possible at a meeting of those staff involved, with a view to learning from it rather than to apportion blame. Could the incident have been predicted or averted? Were there warning signs in the patient, such as unusual quietness, sullenness, abusiveness or impulsivity? Had he/she been more restless? Were medicines, drugs or alcohol involved? Had there been some provocation? Do any members of staff feel hostile to the patient, and if so are they prepared to discuss this, and does it affect their behaviour? Does the layout of the ward help or worsen the situation? Tattiness and faulty technology can provoke destructive behaviour.

Plans should be made as to how to avoid a further incident, including changes in the level of nursing observation and in medication. The hospital should have a written policy for the prevention and management of violence.

FURTHER READING

Beer, D., Pereira, S. M. & Paton, C. (2001) *Psychiatric Intensive Care*. London: Greenwich Medical Media.

Cookson, J. (1996) Management of an acutely disturbed new admission. *Advances in Psychiatric Treatment*, **2**, 55–60.

Eronen, M., Tiihonen, J. & Hakola, P. (1997) Psychiatric disorders and violent behaviour. *International Journal of Psychiatry in Clinical Practice*, **1**, 179–188.

Kerr, I. B. & Taylor, D. (1997) Disturbed or violent behaviour: principles of treatment. *Journal of Psychopharmacolgy*, **11**, 271–277.

Macpherson, R., Anstee, B. & Dix, R. (1996) Guidelines for the management of patients with acutely disturbed patients. *Advances in Psychiatric Treatment*, **2**, 194–201.

Rabinowitz, J. & Mark, M. (1999) Risk factors for violence among longstay psychiatric patients. *Acta Psychiatrica Scandinavica*, **99**, 341–347.

Royal College of Psychiatrists (1996) *Assessment and Clinical Management of Risk of Harm to Other People*. London: The Royal College of Psychiatrists.

—— (1998) *Management of Imminent Violence. Clinical Practice Guidelines to Support Mental Health Services*. Occasional Paper OP41. London: The Royal College of Psychiatrists.

Steadman, H. J., Mulvey, E. P., Monahan, J., *et al* (1998) Violence by people discharged from acute psychiatric facilities and by others in the same neighbourhoods. *Archives of General Psychiatry*, **55**, 393–401.

Taylor, P. & Buckley, P. (2000) Treating violence in the context of psychosis. In *Schizophrenia and Mood Disorders – The New Drug Therapies in Clinical Practice* (eds P. F. Buckley & J. L. Waddington), pp. 297–316. Oxford: Butterworth Heinemann.

15. ANXIETY STATES: PANIC DISORDER, SOCIAL PHOBIA, OCD, PTSD AND BDD

Fears, anxieties, panics, brief bouts of depressive feelings, obsessionality, suspiciousness, irritability, tension headaches and nausea are experienced on occasion by nearly everyone, usually in a stressful situation or after an event that justifies such feelings as normal. But in some people symptoms occur where the situation does not seem to call for it, or often with greater severity or greater frequency than in the majority. These feelings, which may be termed neurotic, may be associated with sweating, rise in pulse rate, palpitations, indigestion, disturbed breathing, urinary frequency or diarrhoea – well-recognised physical correlates of emotional arousal.

These physical symptoms result from arousal in the autonomic nervous system with sympathetic dominance, combined with skeletal muscular tension – the 'fight or flight reaction' described by Walter Cannon (1929). Apart from the unpleasantness, which may lead to the patient seeking relief, the symptoms are usually associated with disturbing thoughts and with some disability in free behaviour. The patient is blocked in some way and cannot undertake certain acts in family, social or sexual relationships or in daily work in spite of a wish to do so – one person cannot go outside the front door and becomes very anxious if trying to do so; one becomes anxious, possibly impotent, in sexual situations; another starts to get episodes of sudden panic after a workmate has died; and another with promotion at work beyond his/her abilities gets incapacitating headaches.

In meeting someone with symptoms of this sort, the first question is diagnosis. Is this patient abnormal, over-sensitive in the situation and, if so, in what way? Are these symptoms the tip of the iceberg and others will be admitted on questioning? How do they change over time? Is this the reaction of an abnormal personality to stress or an episode of depressive illness in which depressive mood has not yet appeared, but other signs of biological depression are there: early-waking insomnia, loss of appetite, impaired concentration or lack of energy. Is alcohol or another substance involved? Is this the beginning of a schizophrenic illness? Anyone over 40 in whom 'neurotic' symptoms are appearing for the first time is probably suffering either from an attack of depressive illness or from some hidden organic disease, possibly a presenile dementia, temporal lobe epilepsy or a carcinoma. However, does the person have an abnormal personality and, through a sort of emotional colour-blindness, keeps running into social and emotional difficulties and reacting in an upset, angry or depressed way? Occasionally, this seems to be a pattern from an early age. In some cases, unusual earlier experiences and mistaken learning seem to exert a powerful influence in the present. The patient cannot run away from some current experience or face it and act, but remains in inner conflict over what to do. These people may be classified as neurotic or suffering from a personality disorder.

If one identifies what situation provokes the anxiety or other symptoms, one can help the patient to avoid it without shame or, better, it may be possible to change it for him/her so that it no longer challenges and upsets. But one can also lessen the patient's degree of self-concern, which will have built up on top of the original difficulties. Giving him/her sufficient interview time conveys that the therapist values him/her and encourages him/her to feel better about him-/herself. He/she learns that he/she is not alone, that others have troubles like his/hers, that one can talk openly about them and not be criticised or condemned. No guilt or shame attaches to them. He/she also begins to learn to understand his/her troubles, not to interpret symptoms as always indicators of physical illness but sometimes of internal emotion or unhelpful reactions to stresses that have become established over the years. Freud's term 'signal anxiety' is indicative of an underlying conflict. He/she sees factors at work that he/she previously ignored or of which he/she was unaware. The human mind hungers for explanation and he/she may need to be given this to explain his/her own hypersensitivity in terms of a present illness, past mis-education or family dynamics. Patients may also appreciate an account of the disturbed physiology that leads to such distressing somatic symptoms, and reassurance that they are not going mad.

Feeling that the therapist understands his/her case raises hope for the future. Hope may lessen symptoms and milder or less frequent symptoms may allow spontaneous improvement to follow, as illness is not reinforced by more attacks. In some cases, a single hour with the therapist can be enough to start recovery. Suppression of symptoms with a drug may also be helpful. It brings the patient relief, it displays the therapist's power to help, and it stops reinforcement of the illness. Except in someone who is using illness to protect him-/herself from something he/she wants to avoid, removal of symptoms does not result in new complaints but in general benefit.

Psychotherapy of a more advanced kind, whether analytical, cognitive or behavioural, individual or group or family, is an attempt to re-educate the patient, and sometimes his/her close family, too, so that earlier and partly buried misconceptions cease to inhibit or to create conflict. Cognitive therapy can prove very effective in some patients selected on the basis of their personality, cooperation and intelligence.

These methods may be time consuming and not suitable for everyone; fortunately a good deal can be done in other ways. Counselling and support of a more general kind can help. Drugs may relieve distressing and incapacitating symptoms and allow the patient to be more accessible to a psychological approach. They should not be withheld on some theoretical or moral ground stemming from the belief that psychological problems can only be treated by psychology or that only the patient's own efforts are valid. The aim must be to spare suffering and increase the person's freedom to act as he/she wishes within the law.

Obviously, where neurotic symptoms are part of depressive illness, schizophrenia or organic disease, medication of the main illness will be important. But where they are localised in a small maladaptive segment of the patient's total behaviour, with very limited symptomatology, medication plays a smaller and usually short-term role. Planning a treatment, and expectations from it, must be appropriate to the pattern of illness and distinction made between acute, acute becoming chronic and the very chronic picture.

SITUATIONAL ANXIETY

Someone becoming anxious and panicky before an important job interview, a student with worry and insomnia before an exam and a patient awaiting the dentist are examples of acute trouble, where a hypnotic or a daytime sedative, in either case in single dose, may be helpful. The hypnotic must be effective, without hangover, and may need to be repeated for 2 or 3 nights at most. The sedative is taken half to 1 hour before the feared experience and it is very advisable to try it out beforehand to get the dose and timing right, so that it is neither too strong nor too weak at the time its support is wanted. The person who becomes upset at having to eat in a public restaurant, or at being a passenger in an aeroplane, can be helped in the same way, though other treatments may be more curative in the long-run for them. Short-acting hypnotics such as zopiclone, zolpidem or chlorpromazine 25–50 mg, by mouth, or a sedative antidepressant are three hypnotics that may be considered. Bear in mind, though, that stopping a hypnotic often means a poor night or more following, until normality is reasserted.

For daytime use, diazepam 2 or 5 or even 10 mg once only an hour beforehand may be helpful, and can be repeated only before later stressful events of the same character. Oxazepam 10 mg or 15 mg is another alternative, though its onset of action is slower, or chlorpromazine 25 mg.

Beta-blockers can reduce the somatic symptoms of anxiety but not the psychic symptoms. For example, propranolol taken before an exam can reduce tremor, tachycardia and palpitations, which might otherwise interfere with writing the exam. This action on somatic symptoms might also be helpful in reducing the vicious circle whereby worry about physical symptoms heightens the psychic anxiety and causes further arousal.

Abnormal reactions to situations can be the result of some frightening incident in the past, which may have been forgotten. Abreaction is sometimes helpful in bringing it out. Relaxed by intravenous drug (see chapter 40) the patient (in a more suggestible condition) can be induced to talk frankly about relevant emotional experiences and to recall exceptionally potent events. Talking about them into full consciousness may remove their force. Dissociative amnesia and paralysis may be relieved in this way.

ANXIETY DISORDERS

The classification of anxiety disorders is less clear than that of the psychoses, and a mixture of different syndromes is common, as well as comorbidity with other problems such as depression, personality disorder and substance misuse.

Pathophysiology

Current neuropharmacological models of anxiety disorders emphasise the role of intact 5-HT pathways from the raphe nuclei in modulating the response to aversive stimuli, and the role of noradrenalin pathways from the locus coeruleus in mediating arousal.

Panic attacks are viewed as a spontaneous activation of mechanisms close to the respiratory chemoceptor area that normally mediate the response to suffocation. Panic attacks can be triggered, but only in susceptible individuals, by a range of agents including infusion of lactate or bicarbonate, breathing carbon dioxide, caffeine and cholecystokinin analogues.

Theories about post-traumatic stress disorder (PTSD) emphasise the effects of hormones and neuromodulators upon conditioned learning. It is suggested that learning in highly stressful situations becomes over-consolidated and that peptides including ACTH and vasopressin, which are known to consolidate memory, are opposed by opioid peptides and oxytocin, which favour the extinction of conditioned responses. Oxytocin is also postulated to support bonding.

The DST (see p. 105) shows hypersensitivity in the hypothalamic-pituitary-adrenal axis in PTSD, in contrast to depression.

In social phobia, there is a definite but modest genetic contribution, and limited evidence of abnormal dopamine function with reduced levels of D_2 receptors and dopamine transporter.

In OCD neuroendocrine challenges of 5-HT function are less consistently abnormal than in depression, and suggest that 5-HT function may be increased in OCD as a partial adaptive reaction.

Tryptophan depletion (see chapters 24 and 25) has been tested in these conditions. It does not result in relapse of OCD after improvement on SSRI. However, injection of the 5-HT agonist mCPP worsens OCD. mCPP is an agonist at 5HT-1, -2A and -2C receptors and can cause anxiety, probably by stimulating 5HT-2C receptors.

Simple phobia

The irrational fear and avoidance of specific stimuli such as spiders, cats or dogs or closed spaces occasionally requires treatment. Desensitisation by gradual exposure is the most effective. A benzodiazepine will allow the person to endure closer contact with the feared object, whereas a beta-blocker such as propranolol will reduce his/her tremor and tachycardia but not allow him/her to make closer contact. Neither of these drugs is useful for this condition in the long term.

Generalised anxiety disorder

Some patients develop free-floating anxiety, not obviously related to any situations, though it often waxes and wanes over periods of weeks. They are tense, irritable and worried, sleep badly, overreact and are jumpy. There may be circadian variations in symptoms, and usually a degree of depression. It may be present on and off at least from adolescence, or it may start in adult life at a time of stress and then continue for a long period. It can be made worse by an environment that cannot be evaded: noise, crowded children in a cramped home, or an unpleasant office where work must go on. Relaxation can be taught, attempts made to clarify the historical origins of the disturbance and durability, and the principles of CBT or IPT applied. But it may be humane, or essential, to suppress the symptoms if the patient is to continue at work; psychological methods may fail and other treatment may be demanded.

Benzodiazepines are only of use in the short term, for 2–4 weeks. Thereafter the benefit diminishes and dependence develops, with a rebound exacerbation of anxiety when the drug wears off and a crop of unpleasant withdrawal symptoms if the patient tries to discontinue it. If used, benzodiazepines should be given in the lowest effective dose and on a time schedule that recognises that some of these drugs are metabolised to longer-acting forms. Thus, diazepam has an acute effect over 4 hours, but a chronic effect owing to its metabolites thereafter and this effect may build up slowly, day by day, so that less drug is needed; for example, give diazepam 5 mg three times daily and then perhaps 2 mg three times daily, though it is best not to choose a rigid schedule of this sort but to tailor one to the patient's life. Oxazepam is not metabolised in this way and may be preferable because of its shorter duration of action.

For longer-term treatment an antidepressant, either an MARI (chapter 24) or an MAOI (chapter 27), should be tried in doses similar to those used for depressive illness. SSRIs are of some help (chapter 25).

Buspirone is a different class of drug. It has weak anxiolytic properties that develop over 2–3 weeks. It does not relieve benzodiazepine withdrawal symptoms.

Antipsychotic drugs have little role in the treatment of anxiety but small doses may be used in severe cases resistant to other treatments.

Panic disorder

The term 'panic attack' is often used by patients, but is best reserved for sudden episodes of intense anxiety with a feeling of impending disaster accompanied by somatic manifestations of anxiety. These usually last for minutes, occasionally hours. Some patients present to casualty departments or to their GP, fearing that they may be having a heart attack or other serious illness. Skill is required to convince the patient of the nature of the illness, explaining it in terms of physiological dysfunction. It may be noticed that the person is hyperventilating and needs advice about this. Hyperventilation can lead to additional symptoms, including paraesthesiae and headache and may also contribute to the depersonalisation that is liable to occur.

Patients who have panic attacks become afraid of having an attack outdoors or in public, where they would feel helpless or self-conscious. This leads to the development of agoraphobia or social phobia. It is then common to experience anticipatory anxiety, similar to panic, when they are called upon to go outdoors or meet people (avoidance conditioning). Behavioural treatments are not always successful. Relaxation techniques and cognitive psychotherapy may be of some help, but panic disorder may become chronic.

Beta-blockers are usually ineffective in panic disorder. Although benzodiazepines give some initial relief, this does not endure. With a shorter-acting drug such as lorazepam, the patient develops panic as each tablet wears off and this intensifies his/her dependence.

Imipramine was the first antidepressant shown to reduce the intensity and frequency of episodes; it is no longer the first choice. But if used, it should be started in low doses (25 mg daily) and increased slowly over 4 weeks to 150–200 mg daily. Other sedative MARIs, for instance amitriptyline or dothiepin, are also useful.

The remarkable discovery that the SSRI fluvoxamine improves this condition, whereas the NRI maprotiline does not, was followed by a series of well-designed mainly positive placebo-controlled studies of SSRIs in panic disorder. MAOIs, for instance phenelzine, are also beneficial.

The outcome in panic disorder should be measured not simply in terms of the number of panic attacks, but the overall (global) condition of the patient, which results from anxiety, depression and phobic avoidance, as well as from panic attacks.

There is good evidence that fluvoxamine, paroxetine, citalopram and sertraline are effective (and they are licensed for this use). They reduce the frequency and severity of panic attacks, and lead to global improvement (see Table 15.1), though they have less obvious effects on anticipatory anxiety. The effect is additive in patients already receiving CBT. By comparison, the broader-spectrum TCA clomipramine is less well tolerated and no more effective than the SSRIs in panic disorder.

However, the use of fluoxetine in panic disorder leads to many early dropouts because of jitteriness (perhaps in part akathisia), increased anxiety and shakiness. At a dose of 20 mg/day fluoxetine has not been found to reduce the frequency of panic attacks, but brings about only slight overall improvement, with reductions in anxiety and depression.

When using an SSRI in panic disorder, the drug should be started in lower doses and increased slowly because patients may at first feel more anxious, and may require encouragement to continue the treatment long enough. For instance, 10 mg paroxetine is started in the first week and increased in 10 mg steps, week by week.

Dose-finding studies have shown an increased rate of response with doses of paroxetine up to 50 mg daily. With sertraline there is no added benefit from doses greater than 50 mg daily in panic disorder.

The duration of treatment may need to be up to 1 year in the first instance; discontinuation sooner than that carries a high risk of relapse.

Night terrors

Children and some adults experience episodes of intense fear, occurring from slow-wave sleep in the first third of the night, and for which they have little recollection the following day. During an attack they may lash out and hurt themselves or others. Paroxetine 20–40 mg a day shows benefits within a few days of starting treatment.

Social phobia

When first described in the 1960s it was thought to be a rare condition, but social phobia is now thought to affect as many as 3% of people at any one time, most often single people of reduced financial means. For some the fears relate to specific situations such as speaking or eating in

Table 15.1 Efficacy of SSRIs in panic disorder: number needed to treat (NNT)

Treatment	Duration	Criterion of improvement	ARR drug–placebo (%)	NNT	Reference
Fluvoxamine 300 mg/day (including depressed)	8 weeks	No panic attack (1 week)	23	4.3	Black et al, 1993
		Much improved or very much improved (CGI)	51	2	
CBT plus paroxetine 20–60 mg/day	12 weeks	1 or 0 panic attacks (3 weeks)	20	5	Oerberg et al, 1995
		Much improved or very much improved (CGI)	31	3.2	
Paroxetine 40 mg/day	10 weeks	Panic-free (2 weeks)	36	2.8	Ballenger et al, 1998
		Improved or very much improved (CGI)	30	3.3	
Sertraline 50–200 mg/day	10 weeks	Panic-free (1 week)	16	6.3	Londborg et al, 1998
Citalopram 20–30 or 40–60 mg/day	8 weeks	Panic-free (2 weeks)	17–25	4–6	Wade et al, 1997
		Global improvement (PHYGIS)	13–20	5–8	
Fluoxetine 20mg/day	10 weeks	Panic-free	NSD		Michelson et al, 1998
		Much improved or very much improved (CGI)	8.6	12	

ARR, absolute risk reduction; CBT, cognitive–behavioural therapy; CGI, clinical global impression; PHYGIS, physicians general impression scale; NSD, not statistically significant.

169

> **Box 15.1 Comorbidity with generalised social phobia**
>
> Panic disorder
> Agoraphobia
> Major depression
> Alcohol misuse
> Benzodiazepine dependence
> Substance dependence
> Obsessive–compulsive disorder
> Eating disorders

public (non-generalised); for others the fear is generalised to almost all social situations. The majority of sufferers with the generalised form show comorbidity with other conditions (see Box 15.1).

Social phobia affects men and women about equally. The generalised form tends to be manifest from adolescence or earlier and to run a chronic course. This early onset can cause serious developmental and educational problems, and the condition affects their prospects of work. There is also an increased risk of suicide.

Fear and avoidance of the scrutiny of others, especially in small groups, are the core features and may be present from childhood. The person may, for instance, have been unable to read in class or stand in view in front of others at school, because of embarrassment. Many have had anxiety-based school refusal. Situations that they avoid include meeting people, performing in public, using the telephone, eating in restaurants and using public transport or public toilets. There may be a particular fear of blushing (erythrophobia) or of vomiting in public.

The comorbid conditions add greatly to the distress and disability and the suicide risk. They tend to develop after the onset of social phobia, and alcohol and substance misuse seem often secondary and perpetuating. Patients are more likely to seek help for the comorbid conditions than for the social phobia.

Treatment of social phobia

The early onset and interference with the development of normal coping strategies indicates the importance of early and effective treatment. Many sufferers receive inappropriate therapy, for instance counselling and benzodiazepines, and few are given treatments of proven efficacy – SSRIs, MAOIs and CBT (see Table 15.2).

Treatment should be considered when the condition is causing significant impairment of personal and social functioning. Scales are available to assess the severity and monitor progress. Besides psychoeducation with instructions on self-exposure and cognitive–behavioural group therapy (CBGT), drug treatment is of proven value.

Beta-blockers

Non-generalised social phobia is associated with high levels of sympathetic arousal that does not adapt, is distracting and causes

Table 15.2 Placebo-controlled studies in social phobia: efficacy and number needed to treat (NNT)

Treatment dose	Duration	Criterion	Drop-out (%)	Improvement (%)	ARR Drug–placebo (%)	NNT (95% CI)	Reference
Phenelzine (n=31) Max 90 mg/day	12 weeks	Marked or moderate improvement	16	65	32	4 (2–12)	Heimberg et al, 1998
Group CBT (n=36)			22	58	25	4 (3–45)	
Education support (n=33)			21	27		NSD	
Placebo (n=33)			18	33			
Phenelzine (n=25) Av. 76 mg/day	8 weeks	CGI much or very much improved	13	55	34	3 (2–12)	Liebowitz et al, 1992
Placebo (n=26)			13	21			
Atenolol (n=23) Av. 98 mg/day			13	25	4	NSD	
Paroxetine (n=139) Av. 35 mg/day	12 weeks	CGI much or very much improved	25	66	34	3 (3–5)	Baldwin et al, 1999
Placebo (n=151)			28	32		3 (3–5)	
Gabapentin (n=34) Av. 2,100 mg/day	14 weeks	CGI much or very much improved	38	38	21	6 (3–22)	Pande et al, 1999
Placebo (n=35)			49	17			

ARR, absolute risk reduction; Av., average; CBT, cognitive–behavioural therapy; CGI, clinical global impression.

worry that it will be noticed. Propranolol 20 mg taken 30 minutes before a feared performance or situation can reduce the autonomic symptoms and prevent the development of panic.

Generalised social phobia is associated with subjective anxiety often without autonomic arousal, and beta-blockers are of little help. The addition of pindolol does not augment the effect of paroxetine in social phobia.

MAOIs

Phenelzine is more effective in the generalised form and will lessen symptoms in about 60–70% of patients, compared with 20–30% on placebo. Start with 10 mg daily, increasing if necessary to 90 mg daily over 4 weeks. The response to CBGT is slower and smaller but tends to be more sustained after stopping. The combination of drug and CBGT may offer the best hope, and the drug may need to be continued.

RIMAs

Moclobemide (up to 600 mg daily) is better tolerated than phenelzine but less effective. The full effect of treatment develops over 16 weeks. Another RIMA, brofaromine, seems more effective but is not licensed in the UK.

SSRIs

Studies with paroxetine, fluvoxamine, sertraline and fluoxetine have shown efficacy, but the most data is available for paroxetine, which is licensed for use in social phobia. With doses of up to 50 mg daily, the size of the effect in generalised social phobia is comparable to that with phenelzine, and improvement develops from 1 to 12 weeks.

Gabapentin

This anticonvulsant improves social phobia, though the size of effect is smaller than with SSRIs.

Conclusion

For the generalised form, drug treatment should be with an SSRI or MAOI. Patients with comorbid OCD may respond better to MAOIs than to SSRIs. For the non-generalised form, a beta-blocker may be tried first; intermittent use of a benzodiazepine may be tried but carries a risk of dependence. Clonazepam has been found to be helpful. An antidepressant may also be tried. If there has been improvement with an antidepressant, an attempt should be made to taper off after 9 months, and periodically thereafter. In contrast to benzodiazepines, a rebound exacerbation of the condition will not then occur.

OCD

Obsessional rituals can sometimes be treated with a few hours of CBT using exposure to the trigger, and response prevention. Some patients are too anxious or distressed to cooperate. In other patients obsessional thoughts dominate the picture. For these groups drug treatment is often helpful, and CBT may be tried again later.

The SSRIs that are licensed for use in OCD are fluvoxamine, fluoxetine, sertraline and paroxetine. They are more effective than the noradrenergic drug desipramine (desmethyl imipramine). However, clomipramine, which affects both 5-HT and noradrenalin, may be more effective than the SSRIs, albeit with more side-effects.

Compared with placebo, SSRIs reduce the amount of time engaged in obsessional thinking and compulsive behaviour, but the size of the improvement is relatively small (see Table 15.3). Higher doses of fluoxetine (up to 60 mg per day) are associated with an increased rate of response and of side-effects. With paroxetine, 40 and 60 mg doses are more effective than 20 mg, but with sertraline (as in panic disorder) there is no advantage in increasing the dose above 50 mg daily. In the case of fluvoxamine the dose is usually increased towards 300 mg per day. The time course of improvement is usually slower than in depression, up to 2 months.

For compulsive rituals, SSRIs add little to the effect of CBT, unless the patient is depressed. For obsessional thinking, CBT is of limited value, and the addition of an SSRI confers significant added benefit.

If there is improvement, treatment should continue for 6 months and then an attempt to taper it should be commenced. For most people, medication must be continued indefinitely, because relapse rates of 80–90% within 3 months follow discontinuation of successful treatment. The improvement is maintained if treatment is continued, at least for 2 years.

Adjunctive antipsychotic

Antipsychotic treatment alone has not been shown to be effective. Unfortunately many patients achieve only a partial improvement on an SSRI. After 2 months, adjunctive treatment with an antipsychotic drug may be given, for example sulpiride 200–800 mg daily. This is more likely to help if the patient has tics, or schizotypal personality, in addition to OCD. Alternatively a combination of SSRI with lithium may be tried, although the supportive evidence is weak.

In the case of new atypical drugs, clozapine, risperidone and olanzapine have all been found occasionally but not always to worsen obsessional symptoms or to induce them in patients with schizophrenia. On the other hand, the addition of risperidone or quetiapine to OCD patients with only partial response to an SSRI has been found to lead to further improvement in almost half. Sexual side-effects tend to worsen.

For those who do not respond to the above, an MAOI may be tried. Otherwise refer to a specialist behavioural unit.

Tourette's syndrome

Tourette's syndrome was first described by Jean Itard in 1825 but named after Georges Gilles de la Tourette, a French neuropsychiatrist who described a case in 1885, emphasising the triad of multiple tics, echolalia and coprolalia. Current research suggests that Tourette's

Table 15.3 Selective serotonin reuptake inhibitors in obsessive–compulsive disorder (OCD): efficacy and number needed to treat (NNT)

Diagnosis	Treatment (n)	Duration	Criterion	Improvement (%)	ARR (%)	NNT (95% CI)	Reference
OCD	Fluoxetine 20–60 mg/day (266)	13 weeks	35% reduction in Y–BOCS	29	21	5 (4–8)	Tollefson et al, 1994
	Placebo (89)			8			
OCD (including depression)	Fluvoxamine plus CBT (24)	9 weeks	35% reduction in Y–BOCS	88	28	4 (2–34)	Hohagen, 1998
	Placebo plus CBT (25)			60			

ARR, absolute risk reduction; CBT, cognitive–behavioural therapy; Y–BOCS:Yale-Brown OCD Scale.

syndrome is not really rare; the cited prevalence of 1/2000 is an underestimate. Males are more often affected (3–4:1). The family history is frequently positive. Tourette's syndrome usually begins with facial tics such as excessive blinking; the median age at onset is 7 years. Associated features include attention-deficit hyperactivity disorder (ADHD) and obsessive–compulsive behaviours. Treatment is with antipsychotics (for tics and OCD); some cases benefit from fluoxetine. Clonidine is used for associated ADHD (also see p. 195).

Somatoform disorders

Patients presenting with abnormal thoughts and anxiety about their appearance present difficulties in diagnosis. In some, the thoughts have an obsessional quality, in others they are overvalued or even delusional.

Body dysmorphic disorder (BDD) is separated as involving a non-delusional preoccupation with some imagined or slight defect in appearance. It occurs in about 10% of people seeking cosmetic surgery. Its classification as between the OCD spectrum and somatoform disorders is controversial. SSRIs seem helpful in some cases, and in combination with CBT. Clomipramine is more effective than the noradrenergic desipramine, and even in some who are delusional. Improvement occurs slowly over 8 weeks and longer. However, others benefit from antipsychotic treatment.

Pimozide is used for monosymptomatic delusional hypochondriasis, a paranoid disorder; trifluoperazine is also helpful in cases with delusions of smelling.

PTSD

This condition is recognised as a disabling reaction to a very severe stress, often of a life-threatening kind, which would cause distress in anyone. The symptoms overlap with those of anxiety, depression, simple phobia and OCD. It may be helpful to encourage the patient to talk about and relive the experience (debriefing) soon afterwards. Antidepressants, including amitriptyline, imipramine or phenelzine, can all be of benefit when continued for 8 weeks. The symptoms of anxiety, depression and intrusive thoughts all improve. However, more severe cases seem less responsive.

The SSRIs are also of value, especially for the avoidance symptoms and intrusive thoughts. Short-term efficacy has been demonstrated for paroxetine, sertraline and fluoxetine, and paroxetine is licensed for PTSD. However, the benefits appear less than from older TCAs. Improvement develops over 2–8 weeks, but symptoms specific to PTSD improve less than the overall condition.

Borderline personality

A small group of patients, often female, pose a severe problem in diagnosis and management. The condition is usually phasic, with periods of relative stability followed by complex patterns of depression, paranoia, behavioural disturbance with injury to self and to others, and abnormal eating continuing for weeks or months. Psychotic-like symptoms may appear temporarily. A variety of diagnostic labels are applied but often as problems persist personality disorder is added. Lithium carbonate or carbamazepine may lessen instability of mood, which in some cases amounts to brief recurrent depression or rapid-cycling bipolar disorder. Low-dose antipsychotics, especially as a depot to ensure adherence, can alter the picture of out-of-control feelings and behaviour to a more stable state. Flupentixol decanoate can reduce self-injurious behaviour. But such medication must be linked with a consistent and firm overall plan of psychological management. Particular care is needed to stop drugs that have proved ineffective and avoid prescribing multiple additional medications that may exacerbate the condition. SSRIs have not proved helpful in brief recurrent depression, and antidepressants may worsen rapid cycling. The role of SSRIs in treating borderline personality requires further study, particularly as such people can be made more tense and irritable by fluoxetine.

CONTACT

National Phobics Society, tel: 0870 770 0456.

FURTHER READING

References

Cannon, W. B. (1929) *Bodily Changes in Pain, Hunger, Fear and Death*. New York: Appleton.

Marks, I. M. (1987) *Fears, Phobias and Rituals*. New York: Oxford University Press.

Bagdy, G., Graf, M., Anheuer, Z. E., *et al* (2001) Anxiety-like effects induced by acute fluoxetine and sertraline or m-CPP are reversed by pretreatment with the 5HT-2C receptor antagonist SB-242084 but not by the 5HT-1A receptor antagonist WAY-100635. *International Journal of Neuropsychopharmacology*, **4**, 399–408.

Panic disorder and agrophobia

Bell, C. J. & Nutt, D. J. (1998) Serotonin and panic. *British Journal of Psychiatry*, **172**, 465–471.

Johnson, M. R., Lydiard, R. B. & Ballenger, J. C. (1995) Panic disorder: pathophysiology and drug treatment. *Drugs*, **49**, 328–344.

Marks, I. M. , Swinson, R. P., Basoglu, M., *et al* (1993) Alprazolam and exposure alone and combined in panic disorder with agoraphobia. A controlled study in London and Toronto. *British Journal of Psychiatry*, **162**, 776–787.

Social phobia

Stein, M. B., Liebowitz, M. R., Lydiard, R. B., *et al* (1998) Paroxetine in the treatment of generalised social phobia (social anxiety disorder). *JAMA*, **280**, 703–713.

Versiani, M. (2000) A review of 19 double-blind placebo-controlled studies in social anxiety disorder (social phobia). *World Journal of Biological Psychiatry*, 1, 27–33.

OCD

Hoehn-Saric, R., Ninan, P., Black, D. W., *et al* (2000) Multicentre double-blind comparison of sertraline and desipramine for concurrent obsessive–compulsive and major depressive disorders. *Archives of General Psychiatry*, **57**, 76–82.

Lawrence, T. P., Jefferson, J. W. & Greist, J. H. (1997) Obsessive–compulsive disorder: treatment options. *CNS Drugs*, **7**, 187–202.

McDougle, C. J., Goodamn, W. K., Leckman, J. F., *et al* (1994) Haloperidol addition in fluvoxamine-refractory obsessive-compulsive disorder: a double-blind, placebo-controlled study in patients with and without tics. *Archives of General Psychiatry*, **51**, 302–308.

——, Epperson, C. N., Pelton, G. H., *et al* (2000) A double-blind placebo-controlled study of risperidone addition in serotonin uptake inhibitor-refractory obsessive-compulsive disorder. *Archives of General Psychiatry*, **57**, 794–801.

Stein, D. J., *et al* (1997). Risperidone augmentation of serotonin reuptake inhibitors in obsessive–compulsive and related disorders. *Journal of Clinical Psychiatry*, **58**, 119–122.

Adult night terrors

Wilson, S. J., Lillywhite, A. R., Potokar, J. P., *et al* (1997) Adult night terrors and paroxetine. *Lancet*, **350**, 185.

PTSD

Connor, K. M., Sutherland, S. M., Tupler, L. A., *et al* (1999) Fluoxetine in post-traumatic stress disorder. Randomised double-blind study. *British Journal of Psychiatry*, **175**, 17–22.

Davidson, J. R. T., Malik, M. L. & Sutherland, S. N. (1997) Response characteristics to antidepressants and placebo in post-traumatic stress disorder. *International Clinical Psychopharmacology*, **12**, 291–296.

Davidson, J., Pearlstein, T., Brady, K. T., *et al* (2001) Efficacy of sertraline in preventing relapse of posttraumatic stress disorder: results of a 28-week double-blind, placebo-controlled study. *American Journal of Psychiatry*, **158**, 1974–1981.

Body dysmorphic disorder

Hollander, E., Allen, A., Kwon, J., *et al* (1999) Clomipramine vs desipramine crossover trial in body dysmorphic disorder: selective efficacy of a serotonin reuptake inhibitor in imagined ugliness. *Archives of General Psychiatry*, **56**, 1033–1039.

Personality disorder

Dolan, M., Anderson, I. M. & Deakin, J. F. W. (2001) Relationship between 5-HT function and impulsivity and aggression in male offenders with personality disorders. *British Journal of Psychiatry*, **178**, 352–359.

Stein, G. (1992) Drug treatment of personality disorders. *British Journal of Psychiatry*, **161**, 167–184.

Studies quoted

Baldwin, D., Bobes, J., Stein, D. J., *et al* (1999) Paroxetine in social phobia/social anxiety disorder. Randomised, double-blind, placebo-controlled study. Paroxetine Study Group. *British Journal of Psychiatry*, **175**, 120–126.

Ballenger, J. C., Wheadon, D. E., Steiner, M., *et al* (1998) Double-blind, fixed-dose, placebo-controlled study of paroxetine in the treatment of panic disorder. *American Journal of Psychiatry*, **155**, 36–42.

Black, D. W., Wesner, R., Bowers, W., *et al* (1993) A comparison of fluvoxamine, cognitive therapy, and placebo in the treatment of panic disorder. *Archives of General Psychiatry*, **50**, 44–50.

Heimberg, R. G., Liebowitz, M. R., Hope, D. A., *et al* (1998) Cognitive behavioural group therapy vs phenelzine therapy for social phobia: a 12-week outcome. *Archives of General Psychiatry*, **55**, 1133–1141.

Hohagen, F., Winkelmann, G., Rasche-Ruchle, H., *et al* (1998) Combination of behaviour therapy with fluvoxamine in comparison with behaviour therapy and placebo. Results of a multicentre study. *British Journal of Psychiatry*, **173**(Suppl. 35), 71–78.

Liebowitz, M. R., Schneier, F., Campeas, R., *et al* (1992) Phenelzine vs atenolol in social phobia. A placebo-controlled comparison. *Archives of General Psychiatry*, **49**, 290–300.

DRUG TREATMENT

Londborg, P. D., Wolkow, R., Smith, W. T., *et al* (1998) Sertraline in the treatment of panic disorder. A multi-site, double-blind, placebo-controlled, fixed-dose investigation. *British Journal of Psychiatry*, **173**, 54–60.

Michelson, D., Lydiard, R. B., Pollack, M. H., *et al* (1998) Outcome assessment and clinical improvement in panic disorder: evidence from a randomized controlled trial of fluoxetine and placebo. The Fluoxetine Panic Disorder Study Group. *American Journal of Psychiatry*, **155**, 1570–7157.

Oehrberg, S., Christiansen, P. E., Behnke, K., *et al* (1995) Paroxetine in the treatment of panic disorder. A randomised, double-blind, placebo-controlled study. *British Journal of Psychiatry*, **167**, 374–379.

Pande, A. C., Davidson, J. R., Jefferson, J. W., *et al* (1999) Treatment of social phobia with gabapentin: a placebo-controlled study. *Journal of Clinical Psychopharmacology*, **19**, 341–348.

Tollefson, G. D., Rampey, A. H., Potvin, J. H., *et al* (1994) A multicentre investigation of fixed-dose fluoxetine in the treatment of obsessive-compulsive disorder. *Archives of General Psychiatry*, **51**, 559–567.

Wade, A. G., Lepola, U., Koponen, H. J., (1997) The effect of citalopram in panic disorder. *British Journal of Psychiatry*, **170**, 549–553.

16. ACUTE AND CHRONIC BRAIN SYNDROMES: DELIRIUM AND DEMENTIA

Acute brain syndrome is also called toxic confusional state, acute confusional state, or delirium. It occurs most commonly at both extremes of life and is usually potentially reversible. Drugs and drug withdrawal can be important contributory factors. Most readers will have distant memories of mild acute confusional states in the context of febrile childhood illnesses. Chronic brain syndromes, which are normally progressive and irreversible, are also referred to as dementias. People with dementia are particularly vulnerable to super-added acute confusional states.

Impairment of memory and other intellectual functions, partial or complete disorientation in time and place or even person, perceptual disorders, especially visual, and poor self-care are key signs of brain dysfunction from organic disease. These features may be mild, moderate or severe, and (particularly in acute brain syndromes) may fluctuate from day to day or even hour to hour. Sometimes an acute attack is superimposed on a chronic illness as yet so mild as to be hardly noticeable.

Acute brain syndromes arise from many physical causes, and several potentially reversible conditions may masquerade as dementias. Every patient presenting to medical services with an apparent brain syndrome requires a careful physical examination and appropriate laboratory tests to try to identify potentially treatable causes or contributory factors. Subsequent management has three main aims: treatment of the underlying causal condition, if identified; control of symptoms if these are troublesome; and the long-term management of residual symptoms and handicaps. Identifying the role of family or other informal carers, and the stresses and burdens placed upon them, is an essential part of the assessment.

ACUTE BRAIN SYNDROMES

Patients with confusional symptoms of recent acute onset often present during treatment for some other condition – medical, surgical or psychiatric – in the home, in casualty or in hospital. Patients in intensive care or after eye operations are particularly liable to become confused.

Causes of acute brain syndromes are many and various. As stated above, acute febrile illnesses are the most common causes of acute confusion in young children. In teenagers and younger adults, experimentation with drugs of misuse (euphoriants, illicit drugs or hallucinogenic plants such as cannabis, khat and magic mushrooms) are the most common causes. Such misuse can often be identified through urine screening. HIV infection (both directly and via the cerebral effects of intercurrent infections) is a further important cause of both acute and chronic brain syndromes in younger people.

Dependence on barbiturates, opiates or alcohol may cause delirium at any age if the customary drug intake is not kept up, for example following admission to hospital. Patients may be unaware of the degree of their own dependency, and even if they are, they may not reveal what they feel to be a shameful habit.

Prescribed drugs are also an important cause of acute confusion at any age. Psychotropic drugs are particular culprits. Tricyclic antidepressants such as amitriptyline or imipramine and antipsychotics including chlorpromazine and thioridazine (because of their antimuscarinic potency) are examples of psychotropic drugs that can provoke an acute brain syndrome. Others include the antimuscarinic drugs such as procyclidine and benzhexol, lithium and the benzodiazepines. Confusion may be precipitated not only by excessive doses but (particularly in the elderly) even by doses within the therapeutic range. It must be borne in mind that individuals vary greatly in blood levels generated by a given drug dose. Impaired renal or hepatic function (common in older subjects) may, in particular, increase drug accumulation. Acute brain syndromes may, in susceptible individuals, occur in the context of therapeutic blood drug levels.

Drugs used for common medical conditions may also precipitate acute confusion, again particularly in older patients and in those with pre-existing cognitive impairment. In this context, common culprits include diuretics, digoxin and opiate analgesics. When searching for a cause, prescribed drugs should be suspected and stopped if medically possible.

Thiamine (B1) deficiency, arising through alcoholism, malnutrition or excessive vomiting, may present as an acute confusional state. Associated specific neurological signs (nystagmus, double vision, external ocular palsy, ataxia, cerebellar signs and peripheral neuropathy) indicate the diagnosis of Wernicke's encephalopathy. This is an emergency requiring thiamine injection to prevent or attenuate the subsequent development of Korsakoff's syndrome, characterised by severe impairment of short-term memory.

Serious infection, congestive heart failure, anaemia, renal failure, hepatic failure, hyper- or hypoglycaemia, profound electrolyte disturbance and space-occupying cranial lesions may all present with an acute brain syndrome. In older subjects, urinary tract and respiratory infections and subdural haematomas (which may be otherwise clinically silent) are particularly common causes. ECT can lead to a spontaneously resolving post-ictal confusional state (as indeed can idiopathic epileptic fits). Post-ECT confusion most commonly occurs in elderly patients.

To discover the causal disease may require a search for subdural haematoma, a cerebrovascular accident, an endocrine disturbance or recognition of an unadmitted drug overdose. Residual cognitive deficit usually indicates a pre-existing dementia that may not only have increased vulnerability to the acute episode but is also likely to need further evaluation and management (see below).

The first principles of management of acute confusional state are calm and reassurance (patients are often extremely anxious and distressed) and the early identification and management of the underlying cause. Physical restraint should be avoided if possible, and it must be remembered that cot sides do little apart from increasing the height from which patients can fall.

If patients are restless, noisy, frightened, aggressive or unable to cooperate in their care, immediate physical treatment may be essential before the definitive cause has been identified. Antipsychotics are usually drugs of first choice; those relatively free of alpha-adrenergic blockade and resultant postural hypertension (such as haloperidol 2.5–5 mg intramuscularly or intravenously, repeated if necessary every 2–4 hours) should be used. Augmentation with lorazepam 0.5–2 mg intramuscularly can be effective. Diazepam 2–20 mg intravenously (preferably as 'Diazemuls' emulsion, which is substantially less irritant) 4 hourly may be sufficient. For elderly or frail patients, smaller doses should be used in the first instance, and the intravenous route should be used only with caution. In situations of less pressing urgency, oral medication is preferable. Syrup preparations are often more acceptable than tablets. Nursing care of confused patients is important. Confused patients may have great difficulty in identifying members of staff. Good lighting is helpful; the minimum practicable number of staff members should be involved, and nurses and doctors alike should identify themselves positively and make themselves known, by touch as well as voice, each time they do something for the patient.

Delirium caused by alcohol withdrawal is considered on p. 205. Delirium caused by antimuscarinic drugs may be relieved by injection of the cholinesterase inhibitor physostigmine (2 mg). The duration of action is about 1 hour.

Most acute brain syndromes are short-lasting and resolve spontaneously in 3–10 days even without drug treatment, but regular daily assessments are needed. Patients whose acute syndrome takes a quieter path – an episode of partial disorientation and muddle, a sudden unexpected bed-wetting, some strange behaviour or a sudden occurrence of hallucinosis – should, if possible, be nursed appropriately and observed closely without recourse to drug treatment until any underlying cause is identified and appropriate specific management initiated.

CHRONIC BRAIN SYNDROMES

Chronic brain syndromes or dementias are characterised by progressive loss of higher mental functions. Changes in behaviour, loss of complex daily living skills and altered personality usually accompany and may be more prominent than cognitive decline. Psychotic phenomena (delusions, often persecutory in nature, and auditory or visual hallucinations) are also quite common. Abnormalities of mood are frequently found; these include apathy, anxiety, irritability and lability. More consistent features of depression are also common.

The most common types of dementia are Alzheimer's disease, vascular dementia, dementia with Lewy bodies and alcoholic dementia. Alzheimer's disease is usually gradually progressive, the initial picture usually being one of prominent impairment of short-term memory. In

DRUG TREATMENT

vascular dementia progression is often step-wise, cognitive impairment is patchy and other features of vascular disease such as focal neurological signs, hypertension and ischaemic heart disease are apparent. In dementia with Lewy bodies the characteristic features are of fluctuating cognitive function, falls, features of Parkinson's disease and prominent visual hallucinations. Less common causes of dementia include chronic inflammatory conditions or systemic lupus erythematosus, the effects of trauma, transmissible degenerative disorders like Creutzfeld-Jakob disease and genetic conditions, such as Huntington's chorea. Subdural haematomas, benign cerebral tumours such as meningiomas and normal pressure hydrocephalus (characterised by apathy, gait disturbance and inappropriate micturition) are potentially reversible dementia-like syndromes.

Acute confusional states (see above) and severe depression, in which apparent deterioration in functioning (pseudodementia) may be more obvious than the characteristic features of the depression itself, are important differential diagnoses. The possibility of depressive pseudo-dementia should always be considered, since it is often responsive to antidepressant drugs or ECT.

Principles of management

As in acute confusional states, potentially treatable underlying causes should be identified and treated. The range of problems affecting both patient and carers should be delineated and appropriate further multi-disciplinary assessment and management initiated. Behavioural problems such as wandering and insomnia often respond well to environmental change (such as provision of safe, e.g. courtyard, space to wander in) or to behavioural programmes. The latter may include sleep hygiene programmes, increased organised daytime activities and support of staff in avoiding situations associated with undesirable behaviours.

Appropriate management of coexistent physical problems may have an impressive effect on mental state and behaviour. Urinary infection, gastrointestinal upset and respiratory infection are common causes of super-added acute confusion and should always be suspected if a patient with known dementia presents with sudden worsening of cognition or behaviour. Poorly controlled pain (even when secondary to as simple a problem as constipation) may be associated with marked behavioural disturbance. More serious medical conditions such as diabetes or cardiac failure may be uncovered by an appropriate medical assessment.

The only specific treatments for dementia currently available are the cholinesterase inhibitors (tacrine, donepezil, galantamine and rivastigmine; see chapter 33). These are licensed specifically for use in Alzheimer's disease and have some (usually modest) effects on cognition and probably also on psychotic phenomena, daily living skills and abnormal behaviours. Antioxidants, such as vitamins E and C, may have some role in protecting against the development of Alzheimer's disease and in modifying its course. Non-steroidal anti-inflammatory drugs and oestrogens may also prove useful in this context. Modification of stroke risk factors (control of hypertension, statins, low-dose aspirin, etc.) are probably useful both in preventing vascular dementia and in slowing its progression.

Pharmacological treatments may be useful for specific symptoms, but the increased vulnerability of older patients (particularly those with dementia) to drug side-effects (particularly neurotoxicity) should always be borne in mind. Antipsychotics may be helpful in controlling agitation, wandering, aggressive or sexually disinhibited behaviours and psychotic phenomena. Dementia and increasing age are, however, important vulnerability factors for antipsychotic-induced tardive dyskinesia, which is often irreversible. Patients with dementia with Lewy bodies are particularly vulnerable to anitpsychotic side-effects that may even be fatal. Antipsychotics should be avoided if at all possible in patients with dementia with Lewy bodies. The utility of cholinesterase inhibitors in dementia with Lewy bodies is currently being evaluated.

The newer atypical antipsychotics may be less hazardous, particularly in people with dementia with Lewy bodies. Benzodiazepines may be a useful alternative to antipsychotics, although they may accumulate in older people and cause ataxia as well as increased confusion. Depressive symptoms and signs in people with dementia often remit spontaneously. Persistent depression may warrant the use of antidepressants. SSRIs and moclobemide appear effective and may be preferred to tricyclics, whose anticholinergic effects are likely to worsen cognitive function.

DRUG TREATMENT

FURTHER READING

Ballard, C., Holmes, C., McKeith, I., *et al* (1999) Psychiatric morbidity in dementia with Lewy bodies: a prospective clinical and neuropathological comparative study with Alzheimer's disease. *American Journal of Psychiatry*, **156**, 1039–1045.

Lindesay, J., Macdonald, A. & Starke, T. (1990) *Delirium in the Elderly*. Oxford: Oxford University Press.

Extrapyramidal reactions are important side-effects of psychotropic drugs, especially antipsychotics and, more rarely, high doses of certain antidepressants, especially SSRIs or lithium. Other dopamine-blocking drugs such as the anti-emetic metoclopramide can also cause them. These neurological side-effects should be readily recognised by psychiatrists, but this may not be the case with clinicians in other specialties. Signs vary from the barely noticeable to the very obvious. Four types of reaction are described: acute dystonia, Parkinsonism, akathisia (which usually, but not always, occurs early in the course of treatment and is termed acute) and tardive dyskinesia, which develops later on.

Dystonia is a distortion of posture caused by a spasmodic involuntary contraction of one or more muscle groups. Acute dystonia comes on suddenly. It occurs early in the course of drug treatment, sometimes after the first dose, and is more common in young males. Spasm of the muscles of the jaw, neck, spine or eyeball can occur and cause trismus, torticollis, opisthotonos or an oculogyric crisis, depending on the muscle groups affected. The patient may writhe, twist, protrude or bite the tongue, or have difficulty swallowing, breathing or speaking. It is sometimes painful and often frightening. So bizarre are these symptoms that hysteria can mistakenly be diagnosed. The patient may present as an emergency in casualty, or it may be an alarming new symptom in the course of a psychiatric illness.

Akathisia is the name given to a compulsive motor restlessness, especially of the legs, usually accompanied by an unpleasant sense of mental agitation. The word means an inability to sit down, reflected in the term 'the jitters'. The patient with akathisia will stand, alternately lifting one leg and then the other, or, when sitting down, swing or cross and uncross the legs with a greater than usual frequency. Pacing and fidgeting may also be signs of akathisia. The continual activity and apprehension can mislead the doctor, so that more drug, not less, is prescribed for control. Akathisia is a common reason for patients to discontinue medication themselves. It may also be linked to aggression, suicidal urges and behavioural disturbance.

Parkinsonism shares some features with postencephalitic Parkinson's disease (e.g. excessive salivation and seborrhoea). Because the cause is a drug, the term pseudo-Parkinsonism is sometimes used. Tremor, unusual early on, becomes more common later. Severity varies from the barely perceptible absence of facial expression and stiffness of posture or gait to complete immobility. Cog-wheel rigidity, especially in the wrists, is a sensitive sign. Drug-induced Parkinsonism is the most frequently encountered of the EPS. Weeks may elapse between the start of drug treatment and symptom onset. It is more common in older patients and females. The diagnosis is readily overlooked, the clinical picture being mistaken for apathy or even depression or schizophrenia. This akinetic depression responds to anti-Parkinsonian drugs. Some degree of Parkinsonism may have to be tolerated because of the antipsychotic drug dosage required to maintain control of a psychosis, although this view has diminished since the introduction of atypical drugs.

Atypical antipsychotics are less likely to cause acute EPS. Of the group, risperidone and amisulpride are definitely associated with EPS, particularly at higher doses (e.g. above 6 mg/day for risperidone). Placebo-level reactions are said to be seen with clozapine and quetiapine. Note that this does not mean that EPS do not occur, but that their frequency and severity are statistically no higher than with placebo in clinical trials. Acute reactions are often seen with placebo, especially after switching from an active drug and stopping the anti-cholinergic drug at the same time. Olanzapine produces these side-effects at higher doses (e.g. 30 mg/day) and clozapine may do so occasionally.

Tardive (delayed) dyskinesia occurs with increasing exposure to years of antipsychotic treatment. Involuntary movements of choreiform or athetoid type affect the orofacial and laryngeal muscles. Smacking of the lips, grimacing, tongue protrusion, grunting and blepharospasm are often striking. Less commonly the trunk and limbs are affected, resulting in abnormal posture and gait, sometimes grotesque in severity. Symptoms vary considerably, even from day to day. Old age, brain damage and female gender appear to predispose to tardive dyskinesia that develops in a persistent form to the extent of about 2.5–5% of patients per year during long-term (up to 8 years) treatment. In the elderly 10% or more develop this condition within 1 year of treatment, and it is found in as many as 40% of chronically ill patients with schizophrenia who are aged over 65. Patients who develop Parkinsonism or akathisia early in treatment are more at risk of later tardive dyskinesia. Similar abnormal movements may also occur spontaneously in older people.

Tardive dyskinesia affecting the larynx interferes with speech, which becomes slurred and shows spasmodic dysphonia; it can also affect the oesophagus, causing difficulty in swallowing – a problem that can lead to choking on food, particularly in older patients.

Cases of tardive dyskinesia have been reported in people with schizophrenia who have not received antipsychotics, presumably resulting from brain pathology. It appears from recent studies in populations who have never received antipsychotics that many people with schizophrenia develop symptoms of tardive dyskinesia. This is particularly evident in older people. The range of disordered movements suggests that tardive dyskinesia is not a single entity. The term 'tardive dystonia' describes more severe cases with blepharospasm, postural abnormalities and repetitive twisting limb movements; it can develop in young males and then has a faster onset. It is more distressing and disabling than tardive dyskinesia. Tardive akathisia has also been described, but its cause and pathology are obscure.

DIFFERENTIAL DIAGNOSIS

Anxiety, agitation and depression can be excluded with greater certainty if the doctor is aware that the patient either has taken recently, or continues to receive, a drug that can produce EPS. Hysteria, encephalitis, Parkinson's disease and Huntington's chorea may be diagnosed in error. Trismus or lock-jaw may suggest tetany, especially if the patient is hyperventilating. Dystonia and tardive dyskinesia might also suggest tetanus, but the relaxation between spasms, the relative absence of pain and the normal movement of other muscles distinguish these drug-induced conditions from tetanus.

If the conditions are mistaken for partly controlled mental illness, there is a danger of antipsychotic drugs being prescribed with a worsening of side-effects. If in doubt about whether the signs are those of mental illness or side-effects, the effect of an intravenous injection of procyclidine (5–10 mg) should be observed. Alternatively the antipsychotic drug should be reduced or stopped and the patient observed. Patients should be warned of the possibility of these side-effects before commencing treatment in order to reduce anxiety and avoid a delay in their seeking help.

Particularly problematic is the association between akathisia and aggressive behaviour or suicidal impulses. This cause of disturbed behaviour is difficult to detect. Of diagnostic value, however, is the observation that increasing doses of antipsychotics worsen behavioural problems.

PATHOPHYSIOLOGY

Extrapyramidal side-effects result from the blocking action of antipsychotics at dopamine receptors in particular areas of the brain, especially the basal ganglia, including the corpus striatum. Within the caudate-putamen, dopamine acts as an inhibitory transmitter on a variety of post-synaptic neurons, especially cholinergic ones. Thus, antipsychotics produce a release of acetylcholine, and anticholinergic drugs are needed to relieve acute dystonia and Parkinsonism and to a lesser extent they relieve akathisia. On the other hand, tardive dyskinesia seems to develop in a way resembling denervation hypersensitivity (see p. 66) during long-term blockade of dopamine receptors. It can be revealed on reducing antipsychotic medication, and temporarily suppressed by increasing the dose. Anticholinergic drugs may worsen it, as do dopamine agonists such as L-dopa and bromocriptine, and perhaps SSRIs.

Interestingly the occurrence of acute dystonia corresponds to the time of increased release of dopamine from nigrostriatal neurons, because of blockade of feedback inhibition (see p. 66). During long-term treatment those dopaminergic neurons eventually become quiescent, so that there is less dopamine released while dopamine receptors remain blocked. This phenomenon – which does not occur with clozapine – may correspond to the delayed development of Parkinsonism.

More recently, sophisticated imaging techniques have brought some clarity to our understanding of acute EPS. PET and single photon emission computerised tomography (SPECT) are modern *in vivo* experimental methods that use radio-labelled ligands with an affinity for specific receptors. Dopamine-D_2 receptor ligands include raclopride and epidepride. Using these compounds, it can be shown that typical antipsychotics occupy 70% or more of the D_2 receptors in the striatum at normal clinical doses.

This level of occupancy seems to be the threshold for the emergence of acute EPS. Atypical drugs such as clozapine, olanzapine and quetiapine appear to show lower striatal occupancies and this may account for their low incidence of acute reactions. Atypical drugs are also potent inhibitors of 5-HT-2A receptors. Again, this can be shown using PET and SPECT. The propensity to block central 5-HT-2A receptors is thought to reduce the incidence and severity of EPS. Some atypical drugs (e.g. sulpiride, amisulpride) are thought to affect selectively a subtype of D_2 receptors (perhaps D_3 that predominates in limbic areas), while sparing striatal D_2 receptors. Evidence for this limbic selectivity is not yet conclusive, largely because different techniques and ligands give different estimates of receptor binding activity (see also chapter 30, p. 323–324). Akathisia may result from cortical release of dopamine. An alternative view is that serotonin is involved. A small dose of the antidepressant mianserin (15 mg) can improve akathisia, perhaps by blocking 5HT-2 receptors.

TREATMENT

Acute dystonia can be reversed in 15 minutes or so by procyclidine 5–10 mg given intravenously or intramuscularly or by 1–2 mg of benzotropine, followed by oral procyclidine, orphenadrine, benzotropine or benzhexol, until control is established. The effect of an acute dystonic reaction on patient confidence should not be underestimated. Some clinicians prefer to prescribe atypical drugs first-line, so as to avoid or lessen the risk of acute dystonia. Others use prophylactic anticholinergics with certain older drugs such as haloperidol or trifluoperazine, in order to avoid acute dystonia, which undermines the patients' confidence in their treatment.

Akathisia can be controlled or lessened with oral anticholinergic drugs, but there is limited evidence to indicate that they are only useful if akathisia forms part of an acute EPS (Parkinsonism). Alternatively, a beta-blocker such as propranolol 30–80 mg daily may be helpful. Should they fail, then a reduction in dose should be considered. For short-term treatment, a benzodiazepine such as diazepam may be tried, but it is not usually helpful. Again, atypical drugs are a worthwhile option in those suffering from akathisia, and both quetiapine and olanzapine are relatively free of this side-effect.

An attempt to control or lessen Parkinsonism by altering dose frequency or reducing the dose of antipsychotic should be considered before prescribing anti-Parkinsonian drugs. For example, 25 mg fluphenazine decanoate every 2 weeks could be given weekly as 12.5 mg, which reduces the peak levels occurring in the blood soon after the drug is given; or the period between doses may be extended to 3-4 weeks. Reducing the dose of antipsychotic carries a risk of relapse of mental illness in order to relieve EPS, and so many clinicians prefer to switch to an atypical drug rather than risk relapse.

DRUG TREATMENT

If Parkinsonian symptoms are distressing or if they persist after adjustment of the dose, then anticholinergic drugs should be prescribed. Patients should be advised that they can keep the dose to a minimum by adjusting it themselves, but they should not stop anticholinergic drugs abruptly as this leads to transient unpleasant feelings (see p. 304). Anticholinergic drugs are often not required after switching to an atypical antipsychotic, and should be tapered while the previous drug leaves the body (which may take 10 days). L-dopa and bromocriptine, which are valuable in Parkinson's disease, are not useful in drug-induced Parkinsonism and may worsen psychosis.

Tardive dyskinesia can be worsened by anticholinergic drugs but is not caused by them. If early signs appear, then anticholinergic medication should, if possible, be reduced, and a reduction of the antipsychotic should also be considered. However, the latter increases the risk of relapse, which must be balanced against the disability of the dyskinesia. Frequent review of the need for long-term or high-dose antipsychotic medication is an important part of good practice. For instance, all patients on long-term maintenance treatment should be reviewed at least once a year, and the less stable ones more often. Treatment with clozapine reduces the severity of pre-existing tardive dyskinesia. Olanzapine and quetiapine may share this property.

Tardive dystonia is also difficult to treat. A high dose of benzhexol may help, perhaps through the dopaminergic effect of this drug, which blocks dopamine reuptake at high doses. Switching the patient to clozapine can also lead to improvement. There is no specific treatment for the condition. Tetrabenazine 75–200 mg a day may help but, as with an increase in the dose of antipsychotic, the suppression of dyskinesia is usually transient, and as the drug may cause depression it is now rarely used.

When using depot injections, anticholinergic drugs may be needed for only a few days immediately after each injection, when serum levels are increased. The patient may be the best judge of need, dose and frequency of anticholinergic. Intramuscular anticholinergics given with the depot injection as an alternative to oral drug give cover for 24–48 hours, but in some cases this may be too short a time to cover peak antipsychotic plasma levels.

Routine prescribing of anticholinergic drugs at the commencement of treatment with antipsychotics is considered undesirable by some because not all patients develop EPS. However haloperidol and trifluoperazine are particularly liable to cause dystonia and Parkinsonism and these should usually be combined with an anticholinergic drug. Higher doses of haloperidol used in mania seem less liable to cause dystonia than lower doses. Chlorpromazine (and thioridazine) has intrinsic anticholinergic properties that are are less liable to produce early EPS. The newer atypical antipsychotics also are less liable to produce early EPS.

Tolerance to Parkinsonian side-effects of antipsychotics does develop and then anticholinergic drugs may no longer be required. Their gradual withdrawal, by several dose reductions, should be tried from time to time; sudden withdrawal may provoke more severe Parkinsonism as the nervous system may have developed some physical dependence.

Some patients experience a buzz, especially with benzhexol or procyclidine, and develop dependence with a desire for higher doses. Their requests for extra anticholinergic medication should be carefully recorded to avoid double prescribing; these drugs should not be continued unless there is definite evidence that the patient is indeed experiencing EPS.

Prescribers should also be aware that nursing staff might be unclear about the purpose of anticholinergic medication. Many believe that such drugs treat all adverse effects (they are known as side-effect medications) and it is not unusual for procyclidine, say, to be given to a patient complaining of dry mouth.

REFERENCES

Barnes, T. R. E. & McPhillips, M. A. (1996) Antipsychotic-induced extrapyramidal symptoms: role of anticholinergic drugs in treatment. *CNS Drugs*, **6**, 315–330.

Braude, W. M., Barnes, T. R. & Gore, S. M. (1983) Clinical characteristics of akathisia. A systematic investigation of acute psychiatric inpatient admissions. *British Journal of Psychiatry*, **143**, 139–150.

Chaplin, R. & Kent, A. (1998) Informing patients about tardive dyskinesia. Controlled trial of patient education. *British Journal of Psychiatry*, **172**, 78–81.

Owens, D. G. (1990) Dystonia – a potential pitfall. *British Journal of Psychiatry*, **156**, 620–634.

Horiguchi, J., Shingu, T., Hayagashi, T., *et al* (1999) Antipsychotic-induced life-threatening 'esophageal dyskinesia'. *International Clinical Psychopharmacology*, **14**, 123–127.

Lieberman, J. A., Saltz, B. L., Johns, C. A., *et al* (1991) The effects of clozapine on tardive dyskinesia. *British Journal of Psychiatry*, **158**, 503–510.

McCreadie, R. G., Thara, R., Kamath, S. *et al* (1996) Abnormal movements in never-medicated Indian patients with schizophrenia. *British Journal of Psychiatry*, **168**, 221–226.

Marsden, C. & Jenner, P. (1980) The pathophysiology of extrapyramidal side-effects of neuroleptic drugs. *Psychological Medicine*, **10**, 55–72.

Poyurovsky, M., Shardorodsky, M., Fuchs, C., *et al* (1999) Treatment of neuroleptic-induced akathisia with the 5-HT2 antagonist mianserin. Double-blind, placebo-controlled study. *British Journal of Psychiatry*, **174**, 238–242.

DRUG TREATMENT

18. DISORDERS OF CHILDHOOD

Many psychological disturbances are a normal part of development. Transient fears of strangers, animals and imaginary monsters are all appropriate at certain ages; a degree of defiance and recklessness is an expected part of the acquisition of independence. Parents or teachers rather than the child present the complaint; referrals to a clinic may therefore stem from the difficulties of a depressed, obsessional, inexperienced or rejecting adult in coping with an essentially normal child. Assessment must therefore be directed to the child's home and school as well as to the individual child, in determining whether psychopathology is present and the use of psychopharmacological treatment is justified.

A child's need for treatment is based on an evaluation of the following features:

- the duration of symptoms – a short-lived tendency to isolation during a time of stress might wisely be regarded as benign and self-limiting; persistent and prolonged social withdrawal probably means something is wrong
- the developmental stage of the child – wetting the bed in a 4-year old is probably not an indication for treatment, but if frequent in a 10-year old it very likely is
- the number and severity of symptoms – minor rituals and compulsions are unremarkable, but pervasive and severe obsessions causing suffering need treatment
- the impairments that the symptoms impose on normal psychological development – hyperkinetic behaviour in a child from a normal home may disrupt learning as well as developing relationships with peers and adults. This warrants treatment with stimulant drugs. In contrast, for a child in a deprived environment, over-activity may be the only way to get adult attention – representing an adaptive behaviour in an adverse environment.

THE PLACE OF DRUGS

A decision to use drugs as a part of the treatment plan depends on balancing several factors: the effectiveness of a drug; its side-effects; and the likelihood of successful symptom control by psychological treatments alone, without a drug. Drug treatment, as in adults, is usually symptomatic, and will not alter pathological processes at the aetiological level.

In general, be slower to prescribe for children than for adults. Nevertheless, serious psychiatric symptoms are such a barrier to normal development that, when psychological or social treatments have failed, useful medication must not be withheld, least of all for ideological reasons.

Drugs should only be given for definite indications and form one part of a management programme. They should be supported by careful explanation and by discouraging the child or the parents from placing the responsibility for the child's conduct solely on medication. Many parents, teachers and social workers are apprehensive of doctors using medication in children. A sensitive and understanding discussion of its value can encourage cooperation and ensure compliance.

The pharmacokinetics of psychotropics is often not as thoroughly studied in children as in adults. Children metabolise most drugs more rapidly than adults do, and hence the dose–response relationship differs. The intended action of a drug for a child may differ from that of an adult. For these reasons, it is not safe to calculate the child's dose from the adult dose corrected for body weight. Wide variations between individuals and therapeutic windows of dose are often observed in practice. Careful dose titration for each individual child is often required. Start the drug in a low dose and then assess the effects of increasing the dose gradually. The most common indications for psychotropic drugs are nocturnal enuresis, disorders of sleep, hyperactivity, Tourette's syndrome, depression, mania, psychosis, anxiety and conduct problems. Medicating children with learning disabilities warrants a separate discussion.

NOCTURNAL ENURESIS

Bedwetting does not usually get medical intervention before the age of 6 years, at which age 80% of children are dry. Some children are ashamed of wetting and distressed by their apparent weakness, for others bedwetting is a focus for rejection by exasperated parents. Nocturnal enuresis is usually simple to treat symptomatically.

Initial assessment should include identifying other problems, and appraising the child's psychological strengths and weaknesses and those of the family. Urine should be cultured, especially in girls, and any infection investigated and treated. Childhood sexual abuse can sometimes present as secondary enuresis or recurrent urinary tract infection. When there are symptoms of PTSD or other psychosocial risk factors, specialist opinion should be sought. For boys, urinary tract infection is rare, and usually indicates underlying congenital malformations that may lead to renal failure when left untreated. Urinary tract infection in boys should therefore always be followed up by specialist paediatric urological investigations.

Treatment should start with a behavioural programme. A diary record of dry and wet nights – as a star chart – should be kept by child and parent. Sometimes this alone is sufficient treatment. The safest and most effective treatment is the enuresis alarm (bell and pad apparatus): the bell conditions the child to associate waking with the sensation of a full bladder. The child soon learns to wake and pass urine when the bladder is full. If the alarm fails or is impractical owing to family circumstances, such as overcrowding, then tricyclic antidepressants, such as imipramine, in low doses of 0.5 to 1.5 mg/kg can be tried. The action of TCAs is rapid; they usually reduce wetting within a week. Relapse, however, is common when treatment is stopped. If 50 mg given 2 hours before bed is not effective, there is no point in trying higher doses. If the handicap from persistent enuresis justifies other treatment, then intranasal desmopressin (20–40 μg) at bedtime is an alternative short-term remedy. If these fail, more complex behavioural approaches for teaching continence are available.

Other TCAs should be avoided because of case reports of sudden death in children and adolescents, presumably due to cardiac dysrhythmia. Tricyclics can be toxic drugs and should not be given lightly or to exceptionally young children. If drug treatment is to be prolonged, then cardiovascular status should be monitored. A special hazard is accidental overdose of the palatable elixir by very young children. Thus precautions must be taken when there are other young children living in the same household. The three-year old is particularly inquisitive and vulnerable.

The anticholinergic oxybutynin is useful only in those enuretic children refractory to imipramine treatment, and who have neurogenic bladder (unstable detrusor) or are found in urodynamic studies to have 'inadequate bladder storage function' (IBSF). It is not recommended for routine use.

SLEEP DISORDERS

Simple sleeplessness is often transient, requiring little intervention. The disturbance to parents may be much greater than any to the child. It is usually a better goal to train the wakeful child to play quietly in his or her own room than to extend sleeping hours by hypnotics. However, when an established sleep rhythm has been disrupted, for example by a period of distress, a short course of a hypnotic drug may help to re-establish a normal cycle.

The use of benzodiazepines as hypnotics in children is controversial. Children absorb and metabolise them more quickly than adults. They are associated with multiple problems: tolerance, withdrawal rebound, relapse, dyscontrol of aggression, disinhibitions, dependency and withdrawal-related seizure, especially with high-potency and short-acting ones. The short-acting ones should definitely be avoided, for reasons of withdrawal-induced seizures, as well as dependency. The long-acting ones can cause irritability and drowsiness, thereby impairing learning in the daytime. The medium-acting ones, some authors suggest, can be used, but only for short term – that is, 12 weeks maximum, followed by gradual withdrawal. Most clinicians prefer to avoid benzodiazepines altogether. If a child relapses after withdrawal or develops tolerance, one may become pressurised by the parents to prescribe more, thereby exacerbating the original problem in the long run.

Sedative antihistamines, such as trimeprazine, are therefore preferred by some child psychiatrists for short-term use. Chloral in a dose of 40 mg/kg is sometimes effective. For hyperkinetic children, low-dose clonidine may also be helpful (such as 25–50 μg at night). Be cautious to ensure that micrograms, not milligrams, are dispensed, as both formulations are available. Though these may be regarded as somewhat old drugs, child psychiatrists prefer to stay with well-tried medications than to use new drugs that have only recently been marketed. The reason is safety: children's brains are still developing and the potential of adverse effects on the developing human brain of many new compounds is largely unknown.

Night terrors are to be distinguished from nightmares. In night terrors, the child screams in a panic from deep sleep and does not remember the episode. Night terrors have no sinister significance but may be associated with other rather benign problems of stage IV sleep such as sleepwalking. Reassurance for the parents is usually all that is required. When night terrors do cause suffering or handicap, diazepam in a dose of 0.1 to 0.3 mg/kg will reduce the frequency and diminish the proportion of time spent in stage IV sleep – one of the few indications to use a benzodiazepine in children. Paroxetine may also be useful (see p. 168).

ADHD

Many children are boisterous and energetic and may be described as overactive by harried carers; but these are not grounds for formal diagnosis or treatment. Such children should not be labelled as having hyperkinetic disorder or ADHD, despite pressure from parents to do so.

Hyperkinetic children, however, are pervasively and persistently inattentive, hyperactive, impulsive, chaotic and disorganised. The North American diagnostic system (DSM–IV) sub-classifies ADHD into (1) pure inattentive; (2) pure hyperactive and (3) combined subtypes. All three are responsive to drug treatments. The behaviours of these children are ill-regulated, interrupting normal development in learning, recreation and family lives, as well as relationships with peers, siblings and adults. It is a serious but treatable condition. Left untreated, it is associated with significant impairments and serious adverse long-term outcomes. These children must therefore be offered appropriate evidence-based treatments. Treatment is guided in part by the pattern of symptoms and their severity, and also by, if any, comorbid psychiatric conditions. Hence, a thorough and well-informed assessment is essential.

Medication is most helpful for the core ADHD symptoms of inattentiveness and disinhibited and disruptive behaviour. This is regardless of whether brain damage is the cause. The core ADHD disorder should be treated by stimulants. About 60% of children will respond to the standard regime, with a further 30% requiring fine-dose adjustment. The remaining 10% – usually complicated by comorbid psychiatric conditions – needs sub-specialist management that may entail monotherapy with second- or third-line drug treatments, or combination therapy. The MTA trial (MTA Cooperative Group, 1999) found individually tailored dose regimens more effective than using a standard dosage. This suggests a high individual variation in dose–response.

If comorbid defiant, aggressive and oppositional behaviours are present, additional behavioural modification techniques and/or parenting training would be indicated. For comorbid specific learning disorders, psychometry or specialist language testing would be required to delineate the profile of deficits, and thence the appropriate remedial teaching should be instituted. For a child with poor self-esteem, individual counselling may have a part to play in counteracting the sense of failure, which may have arisen. If other neuropsychiatric conditions (such as autism or Tourette's syndrome) are present, special consideration in selecting psychotropics (sometimes, second- or third-line anti-hyperactivity medication) may become relevant.

The first choice in drug treatment is a stimulant, preferably methylphenidate at a daily dose of 0.3–0.7 mg/kg body weight. Dexamphetamine is an alternative. Stimulants reduce hyperactivity and improve performance on laboratory tests of sustained attention, motor control and reaction time. These are not paradoxical effects, as similar effects could be seen in normal adults and children. The effect of methylphenidate is short-lived, with an average half-life of 2–4 hours only, thus requiring twice or thrice daily dose. There are wide inter-individual differences in dose–response for these drugs; hence careful dose titration for each individual child is essential to obtain the optimal response.

A starting dose of 5 mg twice daily can be doubled after 3 days to 10 mg twice daily; then to the 10 mg (a.m.), 10 mg (noon) and 5 mg (p.m.) regime; then increasing in 5 mg increments to the optimal dose for the individual. Daily dose should exceed 60 mg per day only in exceptional cases. Monitoring of weight, height, blood pressure and pulse should be routinely carried out. Peripheral vasodilatation induces reflex tachycardia, hence both hyper- and hypotension are recognised side-effects. Hypertension has been identified as a particular risk for children of African-Caribbean parentage in a recent meta-analysis, probably due to genetic factors.

The most common unwanted effects are appetite suppression, tearfulness and insomnia, usually transient and dose-related. Growth retardation can take place with long-term, high-dose medication, possibly due to endocrine changes unrelated to appetite suppression. Methylphenidate can lower the threshold for epileptic seizures; dexamphetamine is therefore preferable for epileptic subjects. Misery and irritability, especially in those with brain injuries, may be another stimulant side-effect. Stimulants are legally controlled substances, and some children may find that they can sell their medications. Addiction has not been reported as a consequence of taking prescribed drugs in therapeutic doses. Despite recent negative publicity, outcome studies all point to the same pattern. That is, later substance misuse is more correlated with pre-existing conduct disorder (or externalising problems) and the presence of psychosocial risk factors, such as low parent monitoring and high use of drugs in the peer-group.

Different psychological processes respond to different doses of stimulants: concentration often improves at a lower dose than overactive behaviour. The need for careful monitoring of response is thus all the greater. Indeed, a dose that is optimal for restless behaviour may actually lead to deterioration in the ability to attend. Both need to be assessed. The treatment target should be clearly defined at the outset. Otherwise, one may find oneself continuing to alter the dosage to meet the ever-changing goalpost of varying targets.

Benzodiazepines should be avoided in ADHD: they are useless and can be harmful, especially when they induce disinhibition that unleashes aggression.

For stimulant treatment-refractory cases, a tricyclic antidepressant, such as imipramine, as a second-line agent, in low dosage of 1.0 mg/kg may reduce hyperactivity, but without improving cognitive performance. They carry a higher incidence of side-effects, especially cardiovascular ones (see enuresis). ECG monitoring is recommended. Third-line agents include clonidine, buproprion, slow-release methylphenidate and antipsychotics. Clonidine at low dose of 2–5 µg/kg/day can be used, especially for controlling impulsivity. Rebound hypertension is a possible serious complication if clonidine is abruptly withdrawn. Novel MARIs are being investigated in ADHD.

Typical, or preferably atypical, antipsychotics can control wildly overactive behaviour when stimulants fail, but this is usually at the price of compromising the ability to learn. Low-dose risperidone can be started at 0.5 mg daily, then twice daily, then titrate, up to the maximum dose of 3 mg twice daily, for an adolescent according to response. Tardive dyskinesia, neuroleptic malignant syndrome and weight gain are side-effects of risperidone. Weight gain is a more marked side-effect of olanzapine. Substantial weight gain is associated with fatty liver changes and liver function should be monitored in these individuals. Alternatively, haloperidol in a dose of 0.02–0.08 mg/kg can be used. For example in a 25 kg child aged 7, 0.25 mg daily or twice daily, then 0.5 mg titrating up to 2 mg twice daily and higher doses in specialist centres. The potential benefit of antipsychotics must be weighed against possible risks. Prescribing second- and third-line treatments is therefore not recommended outside sub-specialist clinics.

TOURETTE'S SYNDROME

The common age of onset of Tourette's symptoms is around 7–9 years. It is a condition characterised by combined vocal and motor tics, and is associated with ADHD, OCD, autism spectrum disorders, conduct disorders and later substance misuse. Clonidine represents the first-line treatment, again titrating dose up to a maximum of 10 µg/kg. For non-responsive cases, SSRIs, risperidone, amisulpiride, sulpiride and haloperiol can be tried. For some children, haloperidol remains the most effective drug and its use has to be balanced between the risks and benefit. Tourette's syndrome is known to follow a fluctuating clinical course. It is essential to reduce the dosage of medications after an increment to control acute exacerbation. Otherwise escalation of dosage may accumulate over time.

AFFECTIVE STATES

Depressive conditions can occur in children before puberty, but presentation can differ from that in adults. In children aggressive and defiant conduct, decline in school performance and unexplained somatic pains may indicate depression.

The prevalence of both major depression and dysthymia increases dramatically in adolescence. These conditions incur serious morbidities including the recurrent and prolonged course of functional impairments, and in some cases result in a fatal outcome such as

DRUG TREATMENT

suicide. Depression must never be regarded as expected adolescent turmoil. As educational systems often impose tightly timed structures upon adolescents to meet attainment targets, an untreated young person with depression who underperforms may miss life opportunities, which may permanently alter his/her life trajectory. Depression, therefore, represents an important medical condition that requires prompt assessment and effective treatment.

The first goal of treatment is rapid resolution of the acute episode. The second goal is to prevent future recurrence, and if it recurs, to reduce the severity of its adverse impacts. Double-blind placebo-controlled trials have not demonstrated the efficacy of tricyclic antidepressants in adolescent major depression, although there is a high rate of placebo response in this group. Despite earlier studies showing improvement on 100–200 mg/day of imipramine (81% on imipramine v. 47% on placebo), more recent studies and meta-analysis have failed to replicate the benefit over placebo. Because of the significant adverse effects, reported cardiotoxicity and sudden death, there is no indication to prescribe this class of drugs for childhood and adolescent depression unless in exceptional cases. Likewise there is little evidence that typical reversible MAOIs are useful. Furthermore, dietary restrictions in children and adolescents can be impossible to maintain.

Currently, the strongest evidence for efficacy and tolerability exists for SSRIs, in the initial double-blind placebo-controlled trials of fluoxetine (see Table 18.1) and paroxetine. An SNRI such as venlafaxine is another potentially useful medication, but its efficacy has not yet been firmly established.

Bipolar disorders can occur in adolescence, and less frequently in childhood. The first episode is usually depression. Hence, follow-up should be provided for those who present with early onset major depression (between ages 6 and 12), and especially for those with a strong family history of mood disorders. The prevalence of bipolar disorder in children has been subjected to debate in the recent years: some authors are ready to attribute aggression and unruly conduct to underlying bipolar disorder, and promote the use of atypical antipsychotics and/or mood stabilisers, even when adult criteria are not fully met. Such practice is more common in North America, where there is a greater interest in integrating psychotropic treatment throughout the life cycle, but it remains controversial in other countries.

Full-blown bipolar disorder, with or without psychotic symptoms, is rare in children and its management should be mostly confined to sub-specialist centres. The principles of treatment are guided by experiences and practice in adults. Lithium, sodium valproate and carbamazepine have been used successfully.

ANXIETY, SCHOOL REFUSAL AND OCD

Children may refuse to attend school, especially during primary and secondary school transitions. School refusal is merely a clinical symptom; and, when prolonged, its underlying psychiatric diagnosis (such as phobia, abuse, depression or anxiety disorder) should be sought. In refractory cases, when depression or pathological separation

Table 18.1 Placebo-controlled studies in children

Diagnosis	Drug (n)	Duration	Drop-outs (%)	Criterion of improvement	Response (%)	ARR (%)	NNT (95% CI)	Reference
Depression in childhood	Fluoxetine (48)	8 weeks	29	CGI much or very much improved	56	23	5 (3–28)	Elmslie et al, 1997
	Placebo (48)		46		33			
	Fluoxetine (48)		29	Complete remission	31	8	13 (NSD)	
	Placebo (48)		46		23			
OCD	Sertraline, child (53)	12 weeks	20	CGI much or very much improved	42	16	7 (4–39)	Marsh et al, 1998
	Adult (39)				26			
	Placebo, child (54)		14					
	Adult (41)							

ARR, absolute risk reduction; NNT, number needed to treat; CGI, clinical global improvement; OCD, obsessive–compulsive disorder; NSD, not statistically significant.

anxiety are involved, medication can be used, but in combination with family counseling and graded reintroduction to classroom study.

Benzodiazepines are seldom effective in reducing anxiety, and carry the hazard of impairing concentration and learning. There is a trend for child psychiatrists to use an SSRI to reduce anxiety instead. Some clinicians use paroxetine or sertraline for anxiety. For some children, fluoxetine may be too activating and may cause agitation. Propanolol, reducing tremors and palpitations and being a fast-acting agent, can be used to reduce discrete anxiety episodes, such as performance anxiety, panic or hyperventilation attacks. Short-term, small open-label studies suggest that buspirone can be used for anxiety and irritability.

For the treatment of childhood and adolescent OCD clomipramine, sertraline (see Table 18.1) and fluvoxamine have been granted a product licence in the US. They, and fluoxetine too, are effective in reducing the severity of symptoms. Careful and slow-dose titration is required, especially for children. There may be a narrow therapeutic window in children. Some clinicians prefer fluoxetine or fluvoxamine for the practical reason that their dose can be finely titrated. Fluoxetine is available in syrup form, easy for titration in children. Few child psychiatrists use clomipramine.

Autism

The symptoms of infantile autism place a serious handicap upon a child, and are usually chronic. An appropriate educational placement has most to offer, yet most parents will need support in coping with the difficulties of daily care. Antipsychotic treatment has a small role in controlling short-term agitation or aggression, using relatively low doses, for instance chlorpomazine 50–150 mg daily, but only for short-term use. In open trials, SSRIs are effective in reducing three types of autism-related difficulties: (1) stereotypic repetitive behaviour; (2) anxiety symptoms and (3) anxiety-driven aggression, triggered for example by the disruption of rigid routines. The reported efficacy of secretin, which has attracted much media attention, has not been confirmed by recent double-blind placebo-controlled trials.

Psychosis

Schizophrenia can begin in adolescence and occasionally in childhood. Psychosis can be overdiagnosed, if one fails to appreciate that there is frequently blurring between fantasy and reality in normal childhood and that children with autism and learning difficulties commonly misreport their thoughts as voices.

The first presenting symptom may be a suicidal attempt, which appears to 'happen out of the blue' – that is without external precipitants, triggers or stressors – mostly likely as a response to delusions or hallucinations. Childhood psychosis may be preceded by a discrete episode of obsessive and compulsive behaviours. Characteristically, florid positive symptoms emerge only after a prolonged non-specific prodrome (lasting 1–2 years) of obsessive–

compulsive symptoms accompanied by withdrawal, personality deterioration and change of affects. Atypical, but not classical, autism is associated with early-onset schizophrenia.

When the diagnosis is confirmed, typical or preferably atypical antipsychotics should be prescribed, following similar principles to those governing adult treatment, particularly the need for low doses in first-episode or drug-naive patients. Specialist units, with access to in-patient facilities, should manage these young people at their presentation. Children are more prone than adults to acute dystonia but less likely to develop Parkinsonian symptoms. NMS and long-term dyskinesias have also been reported. Clozapine has been shown to be effective in some cases of treatment-refractory psychosis in children and adolescents.

CONDUCT DISORDERS IN THOSE WITH MENTAL IMPAIRMENT

Prescribing for those with learning disability is discussed in the following chapter.

Antipsychotics sometimes quieten aggression but carry high risks of causing movement disorders, especially in those with brain damage. Anti-cholinergic side-effects – such as the discomfort of a dry mouth or blurred vision – may induce fears, which manifest as aggressive behaviours in children with mental impairment, who are unable to comprehend the cause or verbally express their distress. Akathisia can also cause aggression. Large doses can reduce attention and learning, in already impaired children. Surveys show that, in spite of these hazards, long-term phenothiazines are prescribed for children with learning disabilities living in institutions. This practice is not sound. Behavioural programmes following a functional analysis often achieve good results without medication.

A common mistake is to prescribe benzodiazepines as sedation, especially in low dose. They are contraindicated for the risks of disinhibition and confusion that frequently exacerbate aggression.

However, some handicapped children express their psychoses and mood disorders with altered behaviour: aggression is the most troublesome. Here careful use of antipsychotics, antidepressants, carbamazepine or lithium can assist behavioural and social programmes of care.

Doses in childhood

Titration of dose against response is the soundest way of prescribing. The doses recommended here are guides to deciding a starting dose based on mg/kg body weight. Individual differences in children at each age are so great that weight is a better guide to dose than age. The approximate average weight of a 6-year-old child is 20 kg (3 st 3 lb), a 10-year old 30 kg (4 st 10 lb) and a 15-year old 50 kg (7 st 12 lb). As adulthood is reached and metabolism slows, the dose per kilogram of some drugs, if used long term, may need to be reduced.

The following dose–weight schedule is a guide. Imipramine, 0.5–1.5 mg/kg for enuresis. Methylphenidate, 0.3–0.7 mg/kg and dexamphetamine, 0.1–0.5 mg/kg. Chlorpromazine, 1.5–3.5 mg/kg for psychoses. Haloperidol, 0.02–0.08 mg/kg for hyperactivity; 0.1–0.5 mg/kg for control of psychotic symptoms. Sertraline start at 25 mg and then increase by 12.5 mg steps. Risperidone start at 0.5 mg daily, then twice daily, then increase by 0.5 mg steps. Clonidine 50–100 µg at night or twice daily for ADHD or related insomnia; for Tourette's syndrome titrate up to 10 µg/kg daily.

FURTHER READING

American Psychiatric Association (1994) *Diagnostic and Statistical Manual of Mental Disorders* (DSM–IV). Washington, DC: APA.

Disney, E. R., Elkins, I. J., McGue, M., *et al* (1999) Effects of ADHD, conduct disorder, and gender on substance use and abuse in adolescence. *American Journal of Psychiatry*, **156**, 1515–1521.

Emslie, G. J., Rush, A. J., Weinberg, W. A., *et al* (1997) A double-blind, randomized, placebo-controlled trial of fluoxetine in children and adolescents with depression. *Archives of General Psychiatry*, **54**, 1031–1037.

Geller, B., Cooper, T. B., Sun, K., *et al* (1998) Double-blind and placebo-controlled study of lithium for adolescent bipolar disorders with secondary substance dependency. *Journal of the American Academy of Child and Adolescent Psychiatry*, **37**, 171–178.

——, Craney, J. L., Bolhofner, K., *et al* (2001) One-year recovery and relapse rates of children with a prepubertal and early adolescent bipolar disorder phenotype (brief report). *American Journal of Psychiatry*, **158**, 303–305.

Gillberg, I. C., Hellgren, L. & Gillberg, C. (1993) Psychotic disorders diagnosed in adolescence: outcome at age 30 years. *Journal of Childhood Psychology and Psychiatry*, **34**, 1173–1185.

Hazell, P., O'Connell, D., Heathcote, D., *et al* (1995) Efficacy of tricyclic drugs in treating child and adolescent depression: a meta-analysis. *BMJ*, **310**, 897–901.

Marsh, J. S. , Biederman, J., Wolkow, R., *et al* (1998) Sertraline in children and adolescents with OCD: multicenter randomized controlled trial. *JAMA*, **280**, 1752–1756.

MTA Cooperative Group (1999) A 14-month randomized clinical trial of treatment strategies for attention-deficit/hyperactivity disorder. Multimodal Treatment Study of Children with ADHD. *Archives of General Psychiatry*, **56**, 1073–1086.

Reichart, C. G., Nolen, W. A., Wals, M., *et al* (2000) Bipolar disorder in children and adolescents: a clinical reality? *Acta Neuropsychiatrica*, **12**, 132–135.

Impairment of mental development from birth or early years used to be called mental deficiency, mental handicap or mental retardation. Learning disability, a term introduced by the Department of Health, is now commonly used in Britain for those needing special services, but mental impairment, the term used in the MHA 1983, though clinically ambiguous, is also used.

People with learning disability are far more likely than other people to suffer from mental illness. Pooled results of studies suggest that 2–6% have schizophrenia and 3–8% have affective disorders. Half of those in hospitals have neuroses or behaviour disorders such as hyperkinesis, autism, hysteria or anxiety states, and some 25–40% have epilepsy. But hospitalised patients reflect a highly selected group and do not indicate the prevalence in the overall population.

These coexisting disorders may benefit from drug treatment. Symptoms and signs of mental disorder in such patients are similar to those in other people, although greater significance has to be given to non-verbal clinical signs and behaviour. That is, mental illness can be expressed as altered or unusual behaviour such as deterioration in adaptive skills, altered sleep or eating patterns, and aggression or self-injury. In those with severe learning disability a diagnosis of schizophrenia may be impossible to make. In this situation a formulation of the clinical problem in terms of conduct, including the influence of the immediate social environment, is essential. Drugs can then be prescribed for a defined purpose and preferably for a stated period when their effectiveness can be reviewed. Avoid long-term prescribing for non-specific sedation or behavioural problems. Screening questionnaires have been developed to help staff assess psychopathology in adults with learning disability. Organic causes of disturbed behaviour must also be ruled our before treatment with antipsychotics commences.

An acutely disturbed person, for instance, may be sedated for a few days as a way of breaking up a fraught situation, with the aim of commencing a programme of social contacts, reassurance and occupation from a calmer baseline. Anxiety may be relieved by day-time sedation, a depressive illness or impulsive behaviour by an antidepressant and schizophrenia-like illnesses treated with antipsychotics. Naltrexone has been found helpful in the treatment of self-injury in individuals with severe learning disability. Instability of mood, repeated explosive outbursts or persistent behavioural disturbance may respond to either lithium carbonate or carbamazepine or valproate. Drug treatment should be used as part of a planned programme of behavioural management, psychotherapy perhaps and environmental manipulation. However, few randomised controlled trials have been conducted in this group and treatment has to be based on that for people of normal intelligence, but taking account of the possibility of drug interactions, particularly with anticonvulsants.

Responses to drugs are altered by an abnormality or damage to the brain's structure, and hence side-effects may readily appear. Be cautious with the size of dose until experience with the person has taught what is tolerated. Barbiturates, especially, may make the patient irritable, and therefore phenobarbitone and primidone are unsuitable as anticonvulsants. Because of limitations of memory and reasoning, the patient with a learning disability may not be able to manage his/her own medication or report side-effects, even after training programmes, especially those living outside hospital. To get the best out of treatment everyone – parents, relatives, social workers and nurses – must understand and agree with what is planned.

Drug therapy aimed at a specific psychiatric disorder is justified, and its efficacy should be assessed in relation to identified target symptoms. Too readily, however, long-term psychotropic drugs are given to suppress behavioural disorder by sedation. This impression is confirmed if there is no diagnosis of a psychiatric illness. This contributes largely to the high proportion of people with learning disabilities who receive such drugs, especially those residing in an institution. Such untargeted medication is poor practice. It should also be remembered that individuals with brain damage are prone to tardive dyskinesia with long-term typical antipsychotics. Only use medication for such behavioural control when there are clear and short-term aims. Once a crisis has passed, consider psychological ways of encouraging the patient to develop more adaptive behaviour. That approach requires skilled staff, applying a plan of treatment with patience and consistency. As with all long-term disabilities, drug therapy should be reviewed every 3–6 months, as to its aims and the grounds for continuing it.

ANTIPSYCHOTICS

Typical antipsychotics are rarely the first choice because of the greater risk in these patients of EPS, tardive dyskinesia and epilepsy. Atypical antipsychotics are increasingly used.

For those who do not have a psychosis, a systematic attempt to reduce the use of antipsychotic drugs should be conducted from time to time, at a rate of, for example, 20% every month.

ANTIDEPRESSANTS

Tricyclic antidepressants and fluoxetine can be useful to reduce self-injurious behaviour and irritability, as well as overt depression. Stereotyped behaviours can also be improved. However, there is also an occasional association between SSRIs and the emergence of aggression and sleep disturbance.

ANTICONVULSANTS

Anticonvulsants are widely prescribed for people with learning disabilities for the treatment of epilepsy and for the control of behavioural problems. The likelihood of having epilepsy is greatest in those with a severe or profound degree of learning disability and cerebral palsy. The special features of the epilepsy in this group include a greater likelihood of suffering multiple seizure types, absence seizures, myoclonic jerks and for the seizures to remain refractory to treatment. Concerns have frequently been expressed about polypharmacy and overmedication with anticonvulsants, with limited benefit on the quality of life of the patient. Benzodiazepines frequently cause disinhibition and irritability in people with organic brain impairments, and other anticonvulsants should be used if possible. Valproate can cause liver damage, especially in young people, and liver function should be monitored in the initial stages of its use.

Challenging behaviours are also a feature of people with learning disabilities. These include aggression, self-injury, destruction to property, verbal abuse, temper tantrums, repetitive and obsessional behaviours and a wide range of unacceptable habits. Whether these behaviours are caused by difficulties in learning acceptable behaviours or have a biological origin is unclear. Anti-epileptic drugs are frequently prescribed and sometimes found to be helpful for the control of such behaviours.

Treatment could appear to be successful for a number of reasons. For example, the behaviour could be caused by an undetected epileptic abnormality resulting from the brain damage suffered by the person. Alternatively, it could be associated with the overt epilepsy suffered by the person; or the person could be suffering from a mood disorder that, because of communication problems, presents as a maladaptive behaviour. In addition, the anticonvulsant could be interacting with other psychotropic drugs to enhance the effectiveness of the other drug, or the anticonvulsant could be exerting a sedative effect.

These uncertainties about both the cause of the behavioural abnormality and the mode of action of the drug treatment, and the reliance on the opinions of carers rather than the patient about the benefits and the side-effects, make rigorous assessment vital in order to avoid the accumulation of psychotropic drug prescriptions.

STIMULANTS

Drugs such as methylphenidate are more effective for symptoms of ADHD in those with mild rather than more severe learning disabilities. They may worsen epilepsy, anxiety and tics. There is a dearth of information on the use of these drugs in adults with hyperactivity and learning disability.

DRUGS TO REDUCE SEX DRIVE

Sexual offences are commonly committed by people with a learning disability. When psychiatric help is requested it should focus on sex education and a social skills programme to redirect inappropriate sexual behaviour, but antilibidinal drugs such as cyproterone, goserelin and depot provera (see chapter 39) can be of benefit.

DRUG TREATMENT

A SYSTEMATIC APPROACH TO TREATMENT

Important ethical issues are raised, particularly from the point of view of information and consent. A systematic approach may help by identifying the target symptoms, relating them to possible diagnoses, attending to legal issues over consent, integrating medication with other treatments, considering drug interactions and side-effects, and monitoring changes during treatment by simple ratings of severity carried out by staff familiar with the patient and by planning reductions of dose carefully. The references below offer some assistance.

FURTHER READING

Ahmed, Z., Fraser, W., Kerr, M. P., *et al* (2000) Reducing antipsychotic medication in people with a learning disability. *British Journal of Psychiatry*, **176**, 42–46.

Casner, J. A., Weinheimer, B. & Gualtieri, C. T. (1996) Naltrexone and self-injurious behaviour: a retrospective population study. *Journal of Clinical Psychopharmacology*, **16**, 389–394.

Clarke, D. J. (1989) Antilibidinal drugs and mental retardation: a review. *Medicine Science and Law*, **29**, 136–146.

—— (1998) Psychopharmacology of severe self-injury associated with learning disabilities. *British Journal of Psychiatry*, **172**, 389–394.

Cooper, A. J. (1995) Review of the role of two antilibidinal drugs in the treatment of offenders with mental retardation. *Mental Retardation*, **33**, 42–48.

Einfeld, S. L. (2001) Systematic management approach to pharmacotherapy for people with learning disabilities. *Advances in Psychiatric Treatment*, **7**, 43–49.

Fraser, B. (1999) Psychopharmacology and people with learning disability. *Advances in Psychiatric Treatment*, **5**, 471–477.

Tyrer, S. (1997) The use of psychotropic drugs. In *Seminars in the Psychiatry of Learning Disability* (ed. O. Russell), pp. 205–222. London: Gaskell.

20. ALCOHOL: THE AGENT AND ITS PROBLEMS

People can enjoy alcoholic drinks and may, on occasion, become drunk without being alcoholics. Alcoholism is a form of substance dependence. Physical dependence is recognised when abstinence for any reason results in the appearance of withdrawal symptoms – tremor or shaking, nausea, weakness, irritability and insomnia. Psychological dependence has no simple set of agreed signs, but displays itself as uncontrolled drinking. Different definitions describe alcoholism in terms of the distress expressed or observed, the damage to physical health, the difficulty in cutting down or giving up drinking altogether, or the damaging effects to working, social or family life.

The aetiology of problem drinking can be understood as an interaction between alcohol as the agent (or drug), the predisposition of the individual drinker and his/her environment (family, peer group and culture, including availability and cost).

THE AGENT

The quantity of ethyl alcohol being consumed is usually defined in terms of the number of units, one unit being 10 ml or 8 g, roughly equivalent to half a pint (284 ml) of ordinary strength beer or lager, 1 glass (125 ml) of average strength wine, 1 glass (25 ml) of fortified wine, e.g. sherry, or 1 measure (25 ml) of spirits. However, a can (440 ml) of strong lager contains 4 units, and a litre of strong cider contains 8.4 units.

Metabolism

Ethyl alcohol is rapidly absorbed to a peak blood level after about 1 hour, and is metabolised mainly in the liver, with a small amount being excreted in urine and breath. Alcohol dehydrogenase in cytoplasm is the main enzyme, but microsomal enzymes (CYP IIE1) and catalase in peroxisomes play a small part. These form acetaldehyde, which is further oxidised by mitochondrial acetaldehyde dehydrogenase (ALDH) to acetic acid, which enters the Krebs cycle. The metabolism of large amounts of ethanol has effects on intermediary metabolism and can cause acidosis, and alterations in glucose, lipid and steroid metabolism. At the same time, the absorption of vitamins may be reduced. Thiamine (vitamin B1) deficiency is especially important, and the prescription of thiamine to heavy drinkers is a priority.

ALDH has two main isoforms, one of which has a less active mutation occurring as an autosomal dominant in 40% of South-East Asians, but in far smaller proportions of other ethnic groups. People with this form experience unpleasant flushing, caused by acetaldehyde, after consuming small amounts of alcohol.

Women reach about 8% higher blood levels than men after ingesting alcohol because they have a smaller body water compartment. Ethanol is eliminated with zero-order kinetics (see p. 53), at a rate of 7–10 g (about 1 unit) per hour. Chronic alcohol misuse results in induction of microsomal enzymes and faster metabolism of ethanol.

The legal limit for driving in the UK is 80 mg/100 ml, and the blood level declines at about 20 mg/100 ml every hour.

Pharmacodynamics

Being lipid soluble and taken in large amounts, ethanol has properties in common with general anaesthetics and can result in unconsciousness. In lower concentrations it interferes with receptors in cell membranes. Thus, it activates GABA-A receptors, increasing chloride permeability, reducing anxiety and causing sedation. It may also block glutamate receptors, thus triggering psychosis in some people. It is thought to release and deplete catecholamines and serotonin, causing elation initially and leading subsequently to depression.

THE PROBLEMS

Concentrations as low as 20 mg/100 ml impair coordination and judgement, increase aggression in the predisposed and cause accidents and injuries. This corresponds to a single unit. This risk increases progressively with higher blood levels or consumption and is the greatest cause of morbidity and mortality. Other risks include violence, breakdown of relationships, liver disease, cardiovascular disease, stroke, cancer, neurological damage, foetal damage and numerous other physical complications.

Mortality and morbidity

A consensus opinion of Royal Colleges in the 1980s was that a weekly intake of less than 21 units in men and 14 units in women carried a "low overall risk" to the health. However, alcohol is popular and supports a huge industry with annual sales in the UK of some £17 billion. In 1995, the Government published a review stating that regular consumption of 3–4 units a day in men and 2–3 units a day in women would not accrue a significant health risk. It also recognised that alcohol consumption of 1–3 units a day in middle-aged men and 1–2 units a day in post-menopausal women conferred protection from coronary heart disease. There is also a particular protective effect of moderate consumption of wine upon the risk for cancer of the upper digestive tract. A J-shaped curve relates total mortality rates to alcohol consumption. The lowest risk is in those drinking an average of 1–2 units a day, but above this the protective effect on coronary disease becomes outweighed by other increased risks. The higher figures have not been accepted as guidelines by the professions. In 1994, 27% of men and 14% of women drank in excess of the recommended low-risk levels.

Social and psychological problems

The social consequences include domestic violence, child neglect and abuse, inefficiency and absenteeism at work, unemployment, criminal offences, marital breakdown, poverty, vagrancy and homelessness.

Psychiatric presentation

'Problem drinkers' come to psychiatric notice for three main reasons: withdrawal symptoms, referral for the treatment of alcoholism and longer-term effects such as psychosis or brain damage. Withdrawal symptoms and even delirium tremens may begin at home, or after admission for any reason to a medical, surgical or psychiatric ward, or after remand in custody – situations where the supply of drink is removed. Out-patient referral for treatment of alcoholism is usually on the urging of someone else because of the social effects on the person or on other people.

There is a high comorbidity between excessive alcohol consumption and psychiatric illness, particularly phobic anxiety (panic attacks or social phobia), depression and paranoid psychoses including morbid jealousy and schizophrenia. In some, alcohol misuse starts as a symptom of the mental illness; it should always be enquired about, together with the reasons leading the person to drink. During withdrawal, anxiety and depression are at first exacerbated, as may be alcoholic hallucinosis. This encourages the person to think that alcohol relieves his/her problems, rather than worsening them, which is more likely. Alcohol-induced paranoid states worsen rapidly when the person drinks. Depression is more likely to be a consequence of the drinking, especially in men, and there is a very strong link between depression, alcohol misuse and suicide. Reducing or stopping drinking is a priority in treating people with these illnesses.

TREATMENT

Studies of interventions to help problem drinkers show a high rate of response in the control group. This suggests that the recognition of an alcohol problem and its explanation to the patient can play an important part in management for many people.

Drugs play an important part in detoxification, and the treatment of delirium tremens, but they play only a small part in preserving abstinence from further drinking, where management is largely psychotherapeutic and social. Long-term damage causing Korsakoff's syndrome is not relieved by specific drugs, but Wernicke's encephalopathy requires urgent medical treatment with thiamine (see p. 384).

Pathological intoxication is associated with severe excitability, and aggression, and subsequent amnesia. It is controlled with benzodiazepines, but barbiturates may exacerbate it.

Attempts to decriminalise drunkenness resulted in detoxification centres being opened by voluntary organisations. Management is in the hands of staff specially experienced in treating detoxification, with medical care supplied by GPs, and in liaison with a hospital physician. Schemes for detoxification in the person's own home have more recently been recommended.

Drug treatment in detoxification

Withdrawal symptoms may be slight or lead to epileptic fits or full-blown delirium tremens. Management often requires hospital admission, especially for the severely affected, where there is a risk of death. The principal psychiatric symptoms are insomnia, tremor, weakness, nausea, irritability, confusion, tactility, visual and auditory hallucinations and terror. Withdrawal fits are common. Acute circulatory collapse, hypothermia and infection may occur and require urgent action. The patient may be dehydrated and hypoglycaemic.

Out-patient treatment is more risky because people may drink while taking medication that is potentiated by alcohol, and they may become dependent on the prescribed drug. Chlormethiazole is particularly dangerous in these regards. Daily supervision is usually necessary with this drug, but also with benzodiazepines.

The aim of treatment is the control of psychological symptoms, the prevention of fits and the care of the patient's physical health. Make sure the patient has no secret supply of alcohol or sedative drugs. Experienced physical nursing and close medical supervision are needed. Temperature, pulse and blood pressure must be noted four-hourly and fluid balance recorded. Serum electrolytes and blood glucose need to be checked.

Suppression of psychological symptoms (and prevention of withdrawal fits) can be accomplished with chlordiazepoxide, diazepam or chlormethiazole, the dose depending on age, weight and severity of symptoms. This use of chlormethiazole is described in chapter 35 and of diazepam and chlordiazepoxide in chapter 34. Chlorpromazine 200–300 mg daily or haloperidol can also be used where disturbance is severe. When symptoms start to wane these drugs should be steadily reduced, to zero over a total of 7–10 days. Because heavy drinkers have a poor diet, and are at risk of Wernicke's encephalopathy, a course of intramuscular vitamins ('Pabrinex') should be given (p. 384).

The sedative drugs used to control symptoms must be reduced and then stopped as soon as withdrawal symptoms are over, because diazepam, chlordiazepoxide and chlormethiazole are, like alcohol, drugs of dependency to the susceptible and should not be used for chronic treatment. Chlormethiazole should not be prescribed to patients who are still drinking; the combination can lead to fatal respiratory depression. It should be administered to out-patients only under close daily monitoring.

Assess physical health, looking for malnutrition, infections and peripheral neuritis, check liver function and test for any signs of an early dementia. Formal psychological memory testing will provide a baseline for the future, and a computerised tomography (CT) or MRI scan indicate degree of brain shrinkage and ventricular dilatation.

Any persisting psychiatric illness must be treated, for instance depression, paranoid or anxiety states. Some persisting paranoid psychoses respond like schizophrenia to antipsychotic drugs, but in some the ingestion of alcohol causes acute deterioration despite antipsychotic medication.

Prevention of drinking

If detoxification is needed for the heavily dependent, psychological help should begin as soon as the person is accessible. Residential units run by voluntary groups provide care for many months to serious problem drinkers to establish abstinence, a process of self-awareness, re-education and peer support.

For the less urgent and severe, most districts have set up alcohol advisory centres, open to referrals from any agency or to individuals themselves. Thus, a problem drinker picked up early (by GP, accident and emergency, screening, out-patients, family or friends) can be offered help before the pattern becomes entrenched. The centres provide a range of information, including contacts for counselling or support, Alcoholics Anonymous (AA) and other self-help groups. These provide the basis for long-term management.

For any treatment to be successful, the person has to admit to him-/ herself that alcohol is getting the better of him/her. He/she must want to regain self-control. He/she can be helped by recognition of the situations that particularly provoke drinking, and by understanding the harmful results to him-/herself. Some people live in particularly predisposing situations; for example, he/she may have a job that favours frequenting pubs and bars. Social or sexual timidity may be relieved by alcohol. Lack of leisure interests, loneliness at home or bereavement may lead to drinking. Identification of the pattern, and of provoking factors (for example, writing down a balance sheet of the pros and cons of continuing, reducing or stopping drinking) may lead to helpful changes in lifestyle. For most, complete abstinence from alcohol in any form must be the target; for a few, very limited moderate drinking may be achievable. Regular contacts over a lengthy period with a doctor, nurse, psychologist or counsellor who will be accepting, encouraging and non-judgemental are likely to aid the patient in achieving rehabilitation. Short admissions to hospital at difficult times can be useful during relapses, but most longer-term treatment is now outside hospital.

Apart from solving the problem of homelessness, a hostel may give valuable support and produce change. Much social help over finance, employment, marriage, loneliness and isolation, and development of new interests may be needed. Special attention must be given to the family. The therapist must be prepared for long-term supervision and for repeated setbacks in some cases. The support of fellow sufferers in therapeutic groups can be crucial.

Drugs in prevention

Prescription of thiamine 25 mg daily should help avoid deficiency and Wernicke's encephalopathy.

Some patients with chronic depressive features do well with lithium or an antidepressant if they take them regularly. It is also claimed that lithium carbonate may help abstinence, even in the absence of depression.

One marginally useful method of drug treatment involves disulfiram ('Antabuse'). The patient, who must be in good health, takes this regularly every morning, possibly under some supervision, for a long period (see chapter 35).

DRUG TREATMENT

Table 20.1 Nalmefene treatment of recently abstinent volunteers with alcohol dependence

Treatment (n)	Duration (weeks)	Criterion of improvement	Drop-outs	Response (%)	ARR (%)	NNT (95% CI)
Nalmefene + CBT (70)	12	No relapse to heavy drinking	36	63	32	4 (2–8)
Placebo + CBT (35)			34	31		

ARR, absolute risk reduction; NNT, number needed to treat; CBT, cognitive–behavioural therapy.

Drugs to reduce craving

The growing understanding of the neurobiology of substance dependence (see p. 211) has raised hope that substances that reduce the euphoriant effects of drugs or alcohol may interrupt the process of conditioning and cue-related craving.

Acamprosate (calcium acetyl homotaurinate) is a new treatment that is intended to reduce craving (see chapter 35). It can be useful as an adjunct for preventing relapse in some heavy drinkers, but the characteristics of those likely to respond have yet to be identified.

The opiate antagonists naltrexone and nalmefene (see Table 20.1) can also reduce relapse in a proportion of heavy drinkers, but are not licensed for this indication (see p. 372). Nalmefene has fewer side-effects.

USEFUL CONTACTS

The Medical Council on Alcoholism, 3 St Andrew's Place, Regent's Park, London NW1 4LB; tel: 020 7487 4445; website: http://www.medicouncilalcol.demon.co.uk.
Alcohol Concern, Waterbridge House, 32–36 Loman Street, London SE1 0EE; tel: 020 7928 7377; website: http://www.alcoholconcern.org.uk.
Al-Anon Family Groups, 61 Great Dover Street, London SE1 6YF; tel: 020 7403 0888.

FURTHER READING

Chick, J. & Cantwell, R. (eds) (1994) *Seminars in Alcohol and Drug Misuse*. London: Gaskell.
Hore, B. D. & Ritson, E. B. (1989) *Alcohol and Health. A Handbook for Medical Students*. London: The Medical Council on Alcoholism.
Mason, B. J., Salvato, F. R., Williams, L. D., *et al* (1999) A double-blind placebo-controlled study of oral nalmefene for alcohol dependence. *Archives of General Psychiatry*, **56**, 719–724.
Nutt, D. (1999) Alcohol and the brain. Pharmacological insights for psychiatrists. *British Journal of Psychiatry*, **175**, 114–119.

The term 'drug abuse' is used in international legislation and in DSM–IV, but 'drug misuse' has been used in recent official publications in the UK about its management. The drugs currently posing the greatest challenges are the opiates and psychostimulants, especially cocaine. Misuse has particularly serious consequences for people already suffering from or predisposed to a mental disorder, and leads to the problem of comorbid drug misuse or dual diagnosis (although this term is used also in other contexts). Dependence on drugs can be categorised broadly according to the extent to which it is associated with psychological or physical withdrawal problems.

THE NEUROCHEMISTRY OF WITHDRAWAL PROBLEMS

Both psychological and physical withdrawal problems have neurochemical counterparts, which differ from one drug to another.

The nucleus accumbens, the central nucleus of the amygdala and the bed nucleus of the stria terminalis form part of the extended amygdala that is thought to be the substrate for the reinforcing actions of all major drugs of misuse.

Psychological dependence (with its intense cue-driven craving) may be mediated by the interaction of drugs, including opiates and stimulants, with the mesolimbic dopamine pathway, terminating in the nucleus accumbens of the ventral striatum (see chapter 7), that subserves drive-oriented behaviour, or the amygdala. Craving becomes strongly cued to environmental triggers; it is thought that the amygdala mediates the environmental influences and regulates their impact upon the nucleus accumbens, which itself provides an interface between affect and action. A further component of stimulant withdrawal is clinical depression, thought to be the result of depletion of catecholamines (noradrenalin and dopamine). The euphoric effects of cocaine can be blocked by dopamine antagonists, including the D_1/D_5 antagonist ecopipam. Drugs of this type may be developed for their ability to reduce craving.

Physical withdrawal symptoms from opiates arise in part from disinhibition of noradrenergic neurons in the locus coeruleus (see p. 71), and of other neurons peripherally, including cholinergic neurons in the gut. Endogenous opiates (enkephalins and endorphins) normally exert inhibitory effects on these neurons.

THE DRUG SCENE

The pattern of drug misuse changes over time. Surveys have shown that high proportions of teenagers use cannabis on at least one occasion, usually as part of a peer group activity. Stimulants and psychotomimetics are used widely in the 'club' scene, especially by the young who are interested in the experiences they induce. Only a minority continues taking such drugs regularly and even fewer become addicted. However, the illicit nature of such drug use places users in a vulnerable situation, and open to exploitation; furthermore the deleterious effects of drug use upon their self-esteem, their academic performance and their social integration means that the boundary between recreational drug taking and drug misuse requiring treatment is unclear.

Unstable opiate addicts

The more serious problems presenting to casualty medical and psychiatric services arise in the unstable opiate addicts. These people are usually young, often with serious difficulties in maintaining relationships and work, and consequently with formidable social problems. Their addiction history is of increasing the amounts taken until they have to support an expensive daily habit. This may involve significant criminal activity, which is both costly and damaging to the individual and wider society. The young addict may have dabbled with many drugs, having begun with the less toxic. Later he/she experiments with opiates, for example heroin or methadone. He/she begins by taking the drug orally, or by inhalation and later learns to use intravenous injections. Veins become thrombosed, and a source of systemic infection. When other veins are occluded he/she may resort to injecting into the femoral vein. Stimulants and barbiturates are sometimes added to enhance the effect, increasing the risk of a fatal outcome. Drugs obtained illicitly vary widely in their potency, and may be contaminated or 'cut' with other substances, increasing the risk of adverse outcomes.

A drug subculture might provide a reasonably stable and satisfying lifestyle, but, even so, there may be accidental or deliberate overdoses, intoxication, infection including hepatitis and HIV, abstinence symptoms, acute toxic states and social problems such as domestic crises, homelessness, unemployment or conflict with the law. Alcohol and cannabis use are common in opiate users, and contribute to their problems, and there may be polydrug use.

Addicts who present themselves unexpectedly at hospital may wish to obtain drugs from the hospital, so the histories they give may be unreliable. On the other hand, they may be suffering from the unwanted effects of serious addiction, especially infections, that must be looked for and treated.

Illicit drug taking is sometimes one symptom of a disturbed personality. A healthy scepticism in the face of an apparent sudden desire to cease drug taking may be appropriate. There may be new pressures, such as court proceedings or threats of separation from relatives. These are opportunities when the patient is motivated to make important changes, but they may be half-hearted; the drug may be the only aid the patient now has to maintain a semblance of feeling normal. Nevertheless, it may be possible for a case worker to increase the patient's motivation. With encouragement and practical help the patient may gain in confidence. Such opportunities to promote change should be taken, and the patient should be put in contact with the relevant services.

MANAGEMENT OF DRUG MISUSE

All doctors must expect to see drug misusers presenting for care, and have a responsibility to attend to both their general health needs and their drug-related problems. A doctor who treats a patient for his/her drug problem should complete a regional drug misuse database form, when the patient first presents or if they return after an interval of more than 6 months. This form is now the only national source of epidemiological information on drug misuse, since the Home Office registration scheme was ended. Unlike the latter, the regional databases are anonymous and therefore cannot be used to avoid double prescribing.

The high morbidity and mortality associated with the use of opiates means that users should be in contact with treatment services. The strategy of treatment services is to enable people with drug problems to overcome them and to lead healthy and crime-free lives. Drug users should have rapid access to support from appropriate services, including primary care (general practice). There is evidence that treatment reduces drug-related mortality, infectious disease and crime.

The organisation of services is based upon collaboration between hospital, general practice and voluntary agencies. Each health district should have a drugs action team with multi-disciplinary representation. Most districts now have a community drug team that is usually street-based and works closely with GPs, with some advice from a specialist psychiatrist. More specialist care is available for out-patients from the specialist drugs or drugs and alcohol service. Most clinics aim to provide services for those in a defined catchment area, and are likely to require proof of residence. But there is also the need to provide services for homeless drug users.

Specialist (hospital) services are more likely to be needed for those with serious associated problems such as a serious forensic history, complex social problems, polydrug use or schizophrenia and for any in whom a prescription for injectable drugs is being considered.

PRINCIPLES OF MANAGEMENT OF OPIATE PROBLEMS

Patients seeking help because of opiate addiction may have found their lives dominated by the strength of their drug habit. The three main steps in treatment are:

- assessment
- management of dependence and withdrawal (detoxification)
- preventing relapse.

The ultimate aim should be total abstinence, but, while this is being achieved, harm minimisation, particularly in relation to injectable drugs and the risk of hepatitis and HIV infection, is important. This means that hepatitis testing, immunisation for hepatitis B and treatment (with interferon) for hepatitis C are arranged; and

DRUG TREATMENT

information on safer injecting and HIV risk-reduction strategies should be provided, along with clean syringes and needles, to those who continue illicit intravenous use. Needle and syringe exchanges exist in many places where there are large numbers of addicts.

Management starts with assessment of the extent of the drug problem, and is followed by steps to avoid the need for illicit sources and crime and help to stop intravenous use. A prescription for an oral substitute will be offered when it is established that a daily habit exists. A plan should be agreed on how to achieve detoxification.

Assessment

Establish the reasons why the patient is seeking help, the recent pattern of drug use and the history of substance misuse. Does he/she have a problem with alcohol, benzodiazepines or other substances in addition to opiates? Many addicts use cannabis. Cocaine is increasingly available in a cheaper freebase form, 'crack', that is smoked. Ask about the social situation, any legal problems and his/her finances. How much is he/she spending on drugs? How does he/she obtain them and is a doctor already prescribing? Try to determine whether he/she is dependent, by his/her description of withdrawal symptoms for the various drug groups. Is there any history to suggest underlying mental illness or drug-induced psychosis? Clarify the prescribing by contacting the previous prescriber.

Look for current opiate withdrawal symptoms (see Box 21.1). Examine the pupils, which are tiny after opiate use and dilated after stimulant drug use. The conjunctivae may be reddened by cannabis. Check the pulse and blood pressure, which may be raised by stimulants and by opiate withdrawal. If the patient is irritable or hostile, he/she may be intoxicated with alcohol; if paranoid, suspect stimulant misuse, amphetamine or cocaine. Examine the upper limbs for needle marks and thrombosed veins. If in doubt examine also the lower limbs and groin.

The assessment process should encourage the patient's motivation to change, and he/she should not feel rejected. Techniques of motivational interviewing can help, and may at first identify aspects of the user's life for which change is most desired. The patient should be aware that withdrawing is difficult and that he/she will experience withdrawal symptoms.

Box 21.1 Features of opiate withdrawl

Sweating
Running eyes and nose
Yawning
Feeling hot and cold
Abdominal cramps
Nausea, vomiting and diarrhoea
Tremor, insomnia and restlessness
Generalised aches and pains
Fast pulse and raised blood pressure
Goose bumps
Dilated pupils

Table 21.1 Duration of time drugs can be detected in the urine

Drug	Time
Heroin (as metabolite morphine)	48 hours
Methadone	7 days
Amphetamines	24 hours
Cocaine as metabolites	2 days
Cannabis (single use)	3 days
Cannabis (daily use)	10–30 days
Diazepam	7 days and more

A specimen of urine should be taken for analysis. This may confirm the patient's account of what he/she is using, identify additional drugs that he/she has denied or not mentioned, or may contradict the patient's claim to be using a drug regularly. For assessing the longer history of drug use over previous weeks hair analysis may be useful, but is available only commercially; drugs such as opiates and cocaine are easily detected, cannabis is more difficult.

Table 21.1 shows for how long the drugs remain detectable in urine using the sensitive and highly specific method of gas chromatography and mass spectrometry.

If a person has a daily habit, then every specimen should contain the relevant drug unless he/she is obviously withdrawing at the time it is given. It is usual to require 2–3 specimens of urine provided on separate days to be positive for the opiate before a prescription is issued for substitution therapy with oral methadone. There should also be evidence that he/she experiences withdrawal symptoms when he/she does not take the drug.

Blood tests might include blood count, renal and liver function tests and tests for hepatitis B and C and HIV, but these require special attention to informed consent, which usually involves counselling about the consequences of a positive test result.

Management of dependence and withdrawal

Once it has been established that the person is dependent upon opiates, a prescription can be agreed for oral substitution, usually with methadone. The intention is to provide him/her with a secure supply of an opiate in a less harmful form so that it is not necessary for him/her to inject him-/herself or to break the law to obtain drugs. All prescribers should be aware of the need to minimise the risk that prescribed drugs are diverted onto the illegal drug market.

A patient presenting for the first time, for instance in casualty, should not be given a prescription for an opiate, but should be referred to the local drug service for assessment and treatment. However, if a patient is admitted to hospital or detained in a police cell, then assessment and treatment should be carried out.

Dose initiation

Only one person should provide each patient's prescription for a drug of dependence and the dose should be kept to the minimum required.

The maximum dose of methadone for initial prescription is 30 mg. With doses higher than this there is a risk of fatal overdose in drug-naive people, especially in combination with a benzodiazepine.

Treatment should be planned in the form of a contract between the doctor or clinic and the patient. The details will vary depending on the patient, the clinic's facilities and the approach, which should be consistent for all addicts. The contract will include conditions about the plan for reducing the dose and the total length of treatment, which may range from 3 to 6 months, and will require the patient to attend regularly and provide urine specimens on request. The consequence of a patient breaking the contract may be that his/her course of treatment is temporarily suspended.

Having agreed the starting dose of methadone, the prescription will be written for a named pharmacist identified by the patient and contacted by the clinic. The pharmacist will supply the drug daily but will not supply more drugs or replace them if they are lost. The patient is then seen every week or so for counselling and support, and encouraged to reduce the dose of the drug.

For some patients, supervised consumption in either the clinic or the community pharmacy is recommended. Further urine tests are used, to confirm that they are taking the drug prescribed and no others. The dose is adjusted over the following days to be sufficient to prevent withdrawal symptoms.

Alternatives to methadone

In a few patients oral methadone induces vomiting. For these, and for some others, including patients who have become addicted through therapeutic prescription of opiates, an alternative drug is dihydrocodeine or buprenorphine (see p. 370).

Stabilisation

During the period of stabilisation the patient's use of alcohol and tranquillisers should also be addressed. Ideally there should be a policy about prescribing benzodiazepines to addicts, agreed between the drug services and local GPs, to ensure that patients receive prescriptions from only one doctor, and that benzodiazepines are not prescribed other than for patients with confirmed dependence who are receiving counselling to withdraw from them.

Most clinics do not find it necessary to prescribe more than 60–80 mg of methadone daily, though doses up to 120 mg are occasionally used. For some patients single daily doses are less helpful than divided doses, because withdrawal symptoms emerge before the next dose is due in 24 hours.

Patients who have been using large quantities of drugs or combinations with alcohol and benzodiazepines may need to be admitted for stabilisation. During the admission they are given a prescription for methadone up to 80 mg daily, while alcohol withdrawal symptoms are treated and their benzodiazepine dose is assessed.

Prescriptions for injectable drugs are rarely appropriate, other than to a small number of addicts, including those who have been receiving such prescriptions since the 1970s when that approach was tried.

Maintenance prescribing

Some patients require the support of prescribed drugs for many months or years. The bulk of treatment evaluation suggests that the greatest amount of gain to health and society can be achieved by prescribing oral methadone or another opiate agonist. The maintenance dose is generally between 60 and 120 mg daily.

Supervised consumption remains an important option during the period of stable prescribing. Random urine checks, for instance twice a year, may be helpful, and at other times when suspicion is raised.

Detoxification

Withdrawal symptoms from heroin reach a peak at 36–48 hours and last for about 5 days. Methadone withdrawal symptoms last longer, peaking at about 5 days and subsiding slowly for 12 days and longer. The withdrawal symptoms (but not the cue-related craving) can be reduced by drugs, such as the noradrenalin α2 agonist lofexidine, which decreases firing of noradrenalin neurons. An alternative to lofexidine is clonidine, but it is not licensed for this use and produces more hypotension. Other drugs that are used for symptomatic treatment of individual withdrawal symptoms are: loperamide (for diarrhoea), metoclopramide (for nausea, vomiting) and aspirin or ibuprofen (for aches and pains).

For some patients, especially those with a short history and low level of tolerance, an early discontinuation of opiates may be possible, and a prescription for lofexidine or clonidine may assist the withdrawal. Many patients find it possible to gradually reduce their dependence on methadone over the course of 3–6 months and discontinue it. Others find each step in the reduction difficult and are liable to supplement the prescription with illicit drugs, including heroin, that are then detected in the urine. If the patient is unable to reduce as an out-patient or wants to discontinue methadone more quickly, then in-patient detoxification should be arranged. This may be done by stepwise reduction of methadone at the rate of 5–10 mg a day over the course of 10 days as an in-patient on a psychiatric ward. This is often unsuccessful because patients experience withdrawal symptoms lasting weeks, and their interactions with other patients and the staff can be difficult to manage.

Accelerated detoxification

An alternative method of detoxification can be used, in which the withdrawal is speeded up by the use of the opiate antagonist naltrexone. However, it must be explained to the patient that this can be an unpleasant procedure, and he/she must be motivated to take part voluntarily. The patient is admitted to hospital and observed for 24 hours without drugs. Treatment of the withdrawal symptoms is started with lofexidine to make sure that this drug is tolerated, pulse and blood pressure being monitored (see p. 371). If it is, and if the withdrawal symptoms are not severe, then oral naltrexone is given, leading to the development of acute withdrawal symptoms. These are of maximum intensity at the start but decline in severity over the course of 2–3 days. During this time the patient is treated with further doses of lofexidine, is under expert nursing observation and is given much reassurance; a benzodiazepine can be prescribed briefly to reduce restlessness. He/she should be able to leave hospital, no longer experiencing withdrawal symptoms, about 6 days after admission. This regimen can be successful on a general psychiatric ward if the staff are familiar with it and have a bed reserved for the purpose. Special care is also required with those who have alcohol problems that should be dealt with before the opiate detoxification. Patients with grossly antisocial personalities may not be suitable, especially if they are HIV positive and might pose a deliberate risk to others.

More problematic addicts need longer periods of in-patient treatment, which is best provided by specialist units.

Rehabilitation and relapse prevention

One of the great challenges for services is to maintain abstinence after it has been achieved in patients. Detoxification is only the first step in a lengthy period of rehabilitation. Here, voluntary agencies play a very large part, especially if the patient is sensitive to environmental cues and factors that produce craving. Placement (voluntarily) in a different setting and away from sources of supply may be a necessary step. Residential facilities ranging from Minnesota Model, Concept House or Christian Therapeutic Communities are of considerable help to many people. Self-help groups run by Narcotics Anonymous operate along the same lines as AA. Individual, family and group psychotherapy may be needed and for some patients attendance at a day centre is helpful.

During this phase there is an emphasis on avoiding reliance on all substances of dependence. It has been suggested that naltrexone taken regularly may encourage the avoidance of opiates, by blunting any effects they would have. However, this has not been found superior to a placebo treatment.

A specialised type of relapse prevention counselling has been developed.

BARBITURATES

Barbiturates are sedative and anticonvulsant. They are seldom prescribed nowadays following a voluntary agreement among GPs not to do so 30 years ago. Their use was associated with tolerance and physical dependence. Overdoses produced respiratory and cardiovascular depression, and death. A dangerous feature was that patients would take their night-time dose repeatedly, after becoming drowsy and forgetting that they had already taken it. Withdrawal is associated with anxiety, insomnia, tremor, convulsions and a confusional state, and other symptoms similar to alcohol withdrawal. A tiny number of addicts still obtain barbiturates. Withdrawal from them can be managed by switching to chlormethiazole (as an in-patient) and reducing the dose as in the treatment of alcoholism; the adjustment may take longer, for instance 3–6 weeks. Irritability and sleeplessness may continue for up to 3 months: the patient should be warned of this and encouraged to tolerate it rather than seek relief from other drugs.

STIMULANTS

Amphetamines are no longer widely available on prescription because of a voluntary ban on their use other than for narcolepsy and ADHD. A few diet clinics prescribe these drugs although there is no medical justification for doing so. Patients become psychologically dependent and ask for private prescriptions for drugs such as phentermine, claiming to want help to reduce weight. However, amphetamines are easily synthesised and readily available from illicit sources. They are mainly inhaled or ingested but can be injected subcutaneously or intravenously for greater effect. Their use in small doses produces symptoms of elation, racing thoughts, pressure of speech and overactivity resembling mania but of short duration. Appetite, however, is suppressed. Larger doses produce paranoid symptoms and a state resembling paranoid schizophrenia. This requires hospital admission and can usually be suppressed with haloperidol or chlorpromazine. Sometimes a longer episode of mania is precipitated in a bipolar patient, and schizophrenia may be exacerbated. Spontaneous recurrences of psychosis may occur later at times of stress.

The abstinence or crash syndrome is manifested by lethargy, dullness and depression; psychological support may be required for a short period and occasionally antidepressant treatment is needed. There is no evidence-based medical justification for prescribing amphetamines to addicts; attempts to do so tend to exacerbate the problems of paranoid psychosis, disinhibited behaviour and manic states.

Cocaine produces mental changes similar to amphetamines. When used as the freebase (crack) its onset when inhaled is similar to intravenous use, and it is more dependence-inducing. Treatment with antidepressants such as fluoxetine reduces the depression but has not been found to improve the outcome as judged by urine analysis.

Some amphetamine derivatives are metabolised in the body to produce neurotoxic compounds. These can damage particular neurons in animals. It is suspected that Ecstasy (methylene-dioxy-methamphetamine; MDMA) or its metabolites may damage the fine axons of serotonin neurons, causing persistent neuropsychiatric problems – panic, obsessionality and depression. Parkinson's disease can also result from neurotoxic effects of drug metabolites (see p. 283). Ecstasy works mainly by serotonin mechanisms and can cause serious hyperthermia, secretion of inappropriate ADH (SIADH) with hyponatraemia and serotonin syndrome (see p. 87). There have been several deaths through its use in the UK.

PSYCHOTOMINETICS

Lysergic acid diethylamide (LSD25) is no longer prescribed but is used illicitly to enlarge perceptual experience. Emergency treatment may be required during a so-called bad trip, which may cause acute distress or result in the person harming him-/herself or others while under the influence of delusions. Management by friends is usually sufficient, but sometimes it is necessary to terminate the acute psychosis, in which case chlorpromazine 50–100 mg intramuscularly or diazepam 10–20 mg intravenously is effective. Sometimes the experience is vividly relived later in the so-called flashback associated with bouts of anxiety and derealisation. Drugs are rarely needed unless the flashbacks are severe, or frequent. Phenothiazines, in small amounts, given for a few weeks or months may help. More rarely, a chronic paranoid psychosis resembling schizophrenia occurs, and should be treated with antipsychotics. This may be a schizophrenic illness that could have occurred anyway. There are no abstinence phenomena.

Cannabis and cannabinoids

Cannabis (marijuana) can, in large quantities, produce a short-lived schizophrenia-like state, and even in small quantities can cause relapses or exacerbations of paranoid psychosis, schizophrenia and mania.

The active ingredients are cannabinoids, such as tetrahydrocannabinol. Two binding sites for these (CB-1 and CB-2 receptors) occur in the hippocampus, globus pallidum, substantia nigra and the cerebellum. CB-1 receptors in the periaqueductal grey matter are involved in pain control. The receptors exert inhibitory effects on neurons, reducing release of transmitters including dopamine and glutamate. An endogenous ligand, anandamide (an eicosonoid), has been isolated. Pharmaceutical drugs are being developed that are agonists or antagonists or that inhibit the breakdown of anandamide.

Cannabinoids impair memory in animals (and man), reducing encoding rather than retrieval. Tolerance develops over time, but there is some evidence of long-term residual effects on memory.

Cannabis is excreted in two phases, the first with a half-life of 36 hours, the second much slower. Symptoms of withdrawal from cannabis reach a peak 3 days after stopping, and decline over the next week. They are anxiety, irritability, reduced appetite, vivid dreams and waking in sweats.

DUAL DIAGNOSIS

Patients with schizophrenia or bipolar disorder are increasingly found to use drugs of misuse. This represents not just the occurrence of a habit that is common in the community, but an increased association beyond that. Box 21.2 shows the odds ratios for substance misuse in schizophrenia in two large epidemiological surveys. The drugs involved are cannabis, stimulants, especially cocaine, and to a lesser extent, opiates. Similar associations apply with bipolar disorder (see p. 119).

Box 21.2 Lifetime comorbidity of schizophrenia and drug-misuse disorders

Epidemiological Catchment Area (Regier et al, 1990)	National Comorbidity Study (Kessler et al, 1994)
6.2	2.7

Nature of the association

The reasons for the association are complex. In some patients the psychosis appears to be induced or precipitated by the drug (cannabis, stimulants). In others their isolated life in deprived urban areas puts them at risk of exploitation. Some are drawn to drugs that, they feel, dull their positive psychotic symptoms (opiates), counteract their negative symptoms (stimulants) or reduce their anxiety at least transiently (cannabis). The side-effects of classical antipsychotics include lethargy and poor concentration, as well as Parkinsonism, and some feel that a stimulant drug or cannabis helps these. These patients are also often lacking the insight and motivation that are so important to overcoming drug dependence. The relative lack of EPS and cognitive side-effects in the atypical antipsychotics means that these drugs may offer an advantage for patients with dual diagnosis; unfortunately none is yet available as a depot injection.

Complications of drug misuse in psychosis

The complications in these patients include the familiar ones of drug misuse, debts, criminality, violence, suicide and sudden death, physical ill health, self-neglect and a chaotic lifestyle. In the case of cannabis and stimulants there is also evidence that the psychosis itself is worsened, having an earlier onset, more mood swings of depression or mania, atypical symptoms and more frequent relapses. The patients tend to be more difficult to engage and have poorer compliance with medication, and they are more resistant to benefit from standard treatments.

Role of drug services in dual diagnosis

Opiates

The specialist drug services have expertise in the management of opiate problems that are not easily replicated in a general adult psychiatric service, and they should therefore be involved as the main advisers on that part of the patient's care; the general psychiatric service continues to treat the patient's psychosis.

Psychotomimetics and psychostimulants

All psychiatrists now should be familiar with the problems of cannabis in their patients, and in future may be able to intervene more effectively if a cannabinoid antagonist becomes available. However, the most serious immediate challenge is from crack cocaine, which is short acting and highly addictive, and destabilises both psychosis and social structure, dramatically. In urban areas with heavy trade in this substance, it is linked to violent gangs, and patients put their health and safety at risk. A dual-diagnosis service run by a psychiatrist with special interest in drug dependency may be needed to address the complex psychiatric, medical and legal problems that arise; a specialised ward area must have security sufficient to exclude dealers and to treat the patients in a state free of harmful substances.

DRUG TREATMENT

LEGAL ASPECTS

The Misuse of Drugs Act (1971) was the first step to provide better control over misuse of drugs of all kinds and laid down rules for supply and possession. Controlled drugs are classified in three grades, depending on harmfulness when misused (Box 21.3). Penalties for offences are graded similarly.

All doctors can prescribe drugs such as methadone for addicts. Those who do so regularly can apply for a handwriting dispensation (see below). All doctors can prescribe heroin for the relief of severe pain in addicts. Heroin, cocaine and dipipanone can otherwise only be prescribed to addicts by doctors who hold a special licence from the Home Secretary. Licences are usually granted only to doctors working in NHS drug treatment centres.

Special prescription pads, FP10 (HP)(ad) are used in hospital to request community pharmacists to issue drugs on a daily basis. Similar prescriptions FP10 (MDA) are used by GPs to prescribe for daily dispensation.

Special conditions apply to writing a prescription for a controlled drug. It is to be written in the prescriber's own handwriting, in ink, and include the name and address of the patient, the form and strength of the preparation, the dose, the total quantity of the drug, in words and figures, and be signed and dated. Exemption from the handwriting requirement can be obtained for doctors working with large numbers of drug users.

A regional drug misuse database form should be completed when the patient first presents (see above). The *BNF* should be consulted for up-to-date information on controlled drugs for which a licence is required.

USEFUL CONTACTS

Drug Prevention Advisory Service, Home Office, Horseferry House, Dean Ryle Street, London SW1P 2AW; tel: 0207 217 8631.
Drugscope (previously ISSD), Waterbridge House, 32–36 Loman Street, London SE1 0EE; tel: 0207 803 4720; website: http://www.drugscope.org.uk.

Box 21.3 Classes of drugs

Class A

Cocaine, diamorphine (heroin), dipipanone, LSD, methadone, morphine, opium, pethidine, phencyclidine and Class B drugs when injected.

Class B

Oral amphetamines, barbiturates, cannabis, codeine, glutethimide, pentazocine and phenmetrazine.

Class C

Meprobamate, certain drugs related to amphetamines such as benzphetamine and most benzodiazepines.

UK Anti-Drugs Coordination Unit, tel: 0207 270 6057; e-mail: ukadcu@gtnet.gov.uk.

FURTHER READING

Drug misuse

Department of Health (1996) *The Task Force to Review Services for Drug Misusers. Report of an Independent Survey of Drug Treatment Services in England*. London: Department of Health.

——, Scottish Office Department of Health, Welsh Office, *et al* (1999) *Drug Misuse and Dependence – Guidelines on Clinical Management*. Norwich: Stationery Office.

Ghodse, H. (1995) *Drugs and Addictive Behaviour: A Guide to Treatment*. Oxford: Blackwell Science.

Seivewright, N. (2000) *Community Treatment of Drug Misuse: More than Methadone*. Cambridge: Cambridge University Press.

Welch, S. & Strang, J. (1999) Pharmacotherapy in the treatment of drug dependence: options to strengthen effectiveness. *Advances in Psychiatric Treatment*, **5**, 427–434.

Wolff, K., Welch, S. & Strang, J. (1999) Specific laboratory investigations for assessments and management of drug problems. *Advances in Psychiatric Treatment*, **5**, 180–191.

Dual diagnosis

Mueser, K. & Lewis, S. (2000) Treatment of substance misuse in schizophrenia. In *Schizophrenia and Mood Disorders: The New Drug Therapies in Clinical Practice* (eds P. F. Buckley & J. Waddington), pp. 286–296. Oxford: Butterworth Heinemann.

Seivewright, N. & McMahon, C. (1996) Misuse of amphetamines and related drugs. *Advances in Psychiatric Treatment*, **2**, 211–218.

Ziedonis, D. M. & D'Avanzo, K. (1998) Schizophrenia and substance abuse. In *Dual Diagnosis and Treatment* (eds H. R. Kranzler & B. J. Rounsaville), pp. 427–466. New York: Marcel Dekker.

Stimulants

Bruce, M. (2000) Managing amphetamine dependence. *Advances in Psychiatric Treatment*, **6**, 33–39.

Croft, R. J., Klugman, A., Baldeweg, T., *et al* (2001) Electrophysiological evidence of serotonergic impairment in long-term MDMA ("ecstasy") users. *American Journal of Psychiatry*, **158**, 1687–1692.

Pope, H. G., Gruber, A. J., Hudson, J. I., *et al* (2001) Neuropsychological performance in long-term cannabis users. *Archives of General Psychiatry*, **58**, 909–915.

Reneman, L., Lavalaye, J., Schmand, B. *et al* (2001) Cortical serotonin transporter density and verbal memory in individuals who stopped using 3,4-methylenedioxymethamphetamine (MDMA or "ecstasy"): preliminary findings. *Archives of General Psychiatry*, **58**, 901–906.

Romach, M. M. K., Glue, P., Kampman, K., *et al* (1999) Attenuation of the euphoric effects of cocaine by the dopamine D1/D5 antagonist ecopipam (SCH 39166). *Archives of General Psychiatry*, **56**, 1101–1106.

Yui, K., Ishiguro, T., Goto, K., *et al* (1998) Factors affecting the development of spontaneous recurrence of methamphetamine psychosis. *Acta Psychiatrica Scandinavica*, **97**, 220–227.

Studies quoted

Kessler, R. C., McGonagle, K. A., Zhao, S., *et al* (1994) Lifetime and 12-month prevalence of DSM–III–R psychiatric disorders in the United States. Results from the National Comorbidity Survey. *Archives of General Psychiatry*, **51**, 8–19.

Regier, D. A., Farmer, M. E., Rae, D. S., *et al* (1990) Comorbidity of mental disorders with alcohol and drug abuse. Results from the Epidemiology Catchment Area (ECA) Study. *JAMA*, **264**, 2511–2518.

DRUG TREATMENT

Symptoms of sexual dysfunction are often overlooked if the doctor does not make direct enquiries in a sensitive manner. However, there is increasing interest and expectation among patients about sexual function; and there is increasing knowledge of its physiology and of how drugs affect it, for the worse or for the better.

SEXUAL FUNCTION

Sexuality can be separated into gender identity, sexual orientation or preference; libido or drive; responsiveness with arousal (including erection in males and lubrication in females); and orgasm (and ejaculation).

SEX HORMONES, GENDER IDENTITY AND LIBIDO

Androgens

The male sex hormones, androgens, are testosterone, formed mainly in the testis (and in the adrenal cortex in females), and dihydrotestosterone. The latter is produced in the target tissues by the action of the enzyme testosterone 5-α-reductase. Receptors for androgens are present in the CNS as well as in the genitalia, and are important from before birth – when testosterone masculinises the brain and internal genitalia, whereas dihydrotestosterone masculinises the external genitalia.

In people with a deficiency of testosterone 5-α-reductase, dihydrotestosterone is not produced, and the external genitalia of the male at birth appear female. At puberty such individuals undergo a striking virilisation, the most surprising part of which is that their gender identity and psychosexual orientation are those of heterosexual males, despite having been reared as females – the Imperato-McGinley syndrome.

Oestrogens

Oestrogens (oestradiol, oestrone, oestriol) are produced mainly in the ovaries; but the aromatase enzyme that converts androgens to oestrogens is also present in adipose tissue, where it produces most of the oestrogen after the menopause, and leads to higher oestrogen levels in obese men and women. The interactions of oestrogens and progestagens with neurotransmitter systems are discussed in chapter 7.

Sexual drive

Androgens support the sex drive and responsiveness in men and in women. Circulating levels of androgens in men decline with age from about 40. However, this is not the only factor affecting decreasing sexual drive and responsiveness in older males. If testosterone levels are found to be below the normal range, the person should be referred to an endocrinologist for assessment. The notion of male menopause requiring replacement therapy is not valid. Healthy premenopausal women show increased sexual responsiveness after receiving testosterone. A minority of men given high doses of testosterone for several weeks become hypomanic and aggressive.

AROUSAL AND ERECTILE FUNCTION

Sexual arousal results from psychological and tactile stimulation. Penile erection also occurs during sleep, mainly in the early morning during REM sleep.

Autonomic innervation is from the hypogastric (sympathetic) and sacral (parasympathetic) nerves. The former is anti-erectile. It is now known that penile erection is totally dependent on the generation of nitric oxide (NO) by nitrergic nerve fibres terminating around blood vessels in the corpus cavernosum. This causes arteriolar vasodilatation that fills the lacunar spaces with blood and thereby (because of the inelasticity of the tunica albuginea) compresses the veins and restricts the outflow of blood, so that intracavernosal pressure rises and engorgement develops. Similar, less well-documented mechanisms occur in females.

Other factors that cause vasodilatation in the territory of the pudendal artery, and can contribute to erection, are parasympathetic tone or cholinergic drugs, prostaglandins and drugs blocking noradrenalin α-receptors or stimulating histamine (H-2) receptors.

Detumescence results from the return of sympathetic noradrenergic (α-1) tone, with contraction of smooth muscle in the corpus cavernosum. Other factors contracting the corpus cavernosum and opposing erection are 5-HT receptor activation and histamine (H-1) receptors.

ORGASMIC FUNCTION

This involves a spinal reflex and is sensitive to serotonergic influence. Coordinated contractions of the vas deferens, and the bulbocavernosus smooth muscle surrounding the urethra, result in ejaculation and are mediated through noradrenergic sympathetic nerves. Retrograde ejaculation (into the bladder) results if the internal urethral sphincter does not close (if noradrenergic input is blocked). The corresponding mechanisms in females are less clear, but may involve periurethral glands.

CAUSES OF SEXUAL DYSFUNCTION

Sexual dysfunction may result from physical or psychiatric illness, or in the course of drug treatment; it may also present as isolated symptoms. It may be associated with personality or marital problems. The most common complaint is of erectile dysfunction or failure, formerly known as impotence, and this has many causes (see Box 22.1).

Box 22.1 Causes of erectile dysfunction

Risk factors	Ageing, smoking, hypertension, hyperlipidaemia
Neurological	Neuropathy, spinal cord injury, multiple sclerosis
Endocrine	Diabetes, hyperprolactinaemia, hypogonadism, thyroid disease
Vascular disease	Atherosclerosis, Leriche's syndrome
Drugs	Thiazides, antihypertensives, antidepressants, sedatives, alcohol, opiates, antipsychotics, atropinics, cimetidine
Psychiatric illness	Depression, anxiety
Systemic physical illness	e.g. Renal failure

The prevalence of erectile dysfunction increases with age from 40 to 70. The diagnosis requires investigation of the psychological state, drug and alcohol history, and of physical health, particularly endocrine aspects (blood sugar, prolactin, testosterone and luteinizing hormone (LH), and vascular and neurological function. The occurrence of nocturnal erections provides evidence of functional integrity, but these can be also lost as a result of depression or drug treatment.

DRUG SIDE-EFFECTS

Some drug effects are predictable from the pharmacology, affecting either the autonomic nerves or the central reflexes and higher integrative functions. The drugs used to treat psychiatric illness often affect sexual function in an unwanted way. Thus, some antidepressants (e.g. clomipramine and the SSRIs) have marked inhibitory effects on orgasm and ejaculation through 5-HT. This is less apparent with citalopram and fluvoxamine than with fluoxetine, sertraline or paroxetine. It may be reversed by a drug that blocks 5-HT-2 receptors, such as cyproheptadine; nefazodone, mirtazapine and certain atypical antipsychotics with serotonin antagonist properties can also act in this way. The SSRIs also reduce libido and responsiveness (see chapter 25). When tolerance to the drug develops, or the drug is stopped, sexual function usually returns to normal. Conversely fluoxetine and clomipramine occasionally produce spontaneous orgasmic sensations in women, sometimes combined with yawning. Antidepressants with noradrenergic effects tend to oppose erection, as to a small extent do anticholinergic effects. Trazodone can cause persistent erections or priapism.

Some antipsychotics cause hyperprolactinaemia (see p. 286) that may reduce libido; some block noradrenalin α-1 receptors and interfere with ejaculation, for example the antipsychotics thioridazine risperidone and sertindole.

Sedatives, alcohol and opiates impair libido and the central integration of sexual responses.

Sexual symptoms in psychiatric disorders

Depression lowers sexual drive and performance, leading to indifference, erectile failure or frigidity. In a previously well-adjusted couple, a serious misunderstanding can result. Explanation of the biological nature of the change, and the effects of antidepressants, and reassurance that normal sexual response will return on recovery from depression usually enables a couple to accept the situation.

Mania, in contrast, heightens sexual drive and sexual enjoyment, the only mental illness to do so. Increased sexual demand in marriage may become a problem for the spouse of a patient with mania, and so may promiscuity or sexual deviations as a result of disinhibition.

Schizophrenia is associated with low sexual drive that, with deficits in emotional responses, limits sexual activity. With early onset, marriage is infrequent and fertility is low, especially in males. Sexually embarrassing or deviant behaviour occurs sometimes in chronic schizophrenia and presents potential problems for the community.

Erectile impotence places strains on a relationship and the dangerous condition of morbid jealousy, with paranoia, may develop in some individuals.

In people with learning disabilities lack of sexual experience and poorly controlled impulses can lead to inappropriate sexual behaviour. Recognition of the problems and guidance by a therapist should be of help.

Sexual dysfunction arising in these ways usually needs no treatment other than of the primary psychiatric illness. Embarrassing or potentially criminal sexual conduct occurring in schizophrenia or mental handicap when related to high sexual drive may respond to drugs that reduce the drive (see below).

Sexual disorders

Sexual dysfunction presenting in the absence of any causal illness or relationship difficulties requires treatment of sexual performance itself. The treatment of such primary dysfunctions generally involves a behavioural approach directed to improving the sexual response of a couple to each other. Success depends on motivated, cooperative, sexual partners and a therapist with special skills. The partner may him-/herself have sexual problems that need to be addressed. After a few sessions of couple therapy a drug treatment may be introduced, for a defined period of, for instance, 3 months.

Certain SSRIs such as paroxetine, sertraline and fluoxetine are sometimes helpful as adjuncts in the treatment of premature ejaculation.

Treatment of erectile dysfunction

Sedative drugs may have a small part to play when anxiety and erectile impotence are linked, especially in the uncertain young man or the overconsciously ageing one. If taken shortly before intercourse, sedative drugs can sometimes improve performance.

DRUG TREATMENT

The discovery of the role of NO and of the drug sildenafil, which potentiates it and improves erectile function, has transformed the management of erectile failure (see p. 387).

Other oral treatments under investigation include yohimbine (an α-2 antagonist), apomorphine (dopamine agonist) and trazodone.

Previous treatments included the injection into the corpus cavernosum of drugs such as papaverine, or alpha adrenoceptor antagonists such as thymoxamine. For insulin-dependent diabetics, the use of such injections is not the threat that it might be to others. Alternatively, a pellet of prostaglandin E1 (alprostadil, 'Caverject') could be introduced into the urethra. These are effective for all causes of erectile dysfunction, but carry the risk of causing priapism and cavernosal fibrosis.

SEXUAL PROBLEMS IN WOMEN

The most common problems are reduced libido, dyspareunia and orgasmic dysfunction. Their management involves a combination of medical and counselling interventions, including treatment of underlying medical and psychiatric conditions and marital therapy. There are reports of sildenafil being useful in dysfunction of female arousal and orgasm, induced by antidepressants, and unconfirmed reports of its usefulness in other types of dysfunction in females.

DRUGS TO REDUCE LIBIDO

A high level of sexual activity, especially if associated with personality disorder or sexual deviance, can be a serious problem in men and may result in crime and loss of liberty. Treatments that reduce sexual drive may reduce undesirable conduct. Cyproterone acetate, an antiandrogen that also lowers testosterone levels, and reduces sexual drive, can be effective (see chapter 39). Medroxy-progesterone acetate ('Depo-Provera') by intramuscular injection or goserelin, a long-acting analogue of LH are also used to lower androgen levels (see p. 385). In some patients the benefits from these drug treatments are transient despite continuing low levels of testosterone; then consideration should be given to physical castration, which some patients request.

When the unwanted behaviour is not sex-drive dependent, as in the older male or the person with an aggressive psychopathic personality, drugs that reduce sex drive are less likely to work.

The butyrophenone benperidol has been recommended for the reduction of deviant antisocial sexual behaviour but is not of proven value.

Drugs should be combined with psychological treatment aimed at increasing the patient's motivation to alter behaviour and improve self-control.

FURTHER READING

Eardley, I. (1998) New oral therapies for the treatment of erectile dysfunction. *British Journal of Urology*, **81**, 122–127.

Hermann, N. (2000) Sex and drugs for the senior citizen. *Old Age Psychiatry*, **16**, 6.

Imperato-McGinley, J., Peterson, R. E., Gautier, T., *et al* (1979) Androgens and the evolution of male-gender identity among male pseudo-hermaphrodites with 5-alpha-reductase deficiency. *New England Journal of Medicine*, **300**, 1233–1237.

Pope, H. G., Kouri, E. M. & Hudson, J. I. (2000) Effects of supraphysiological doses of testosterone on mood and aggression in normal men: a randomised controlled trial. *Archives of General Psychiatry*, **57**, 133–140.

Stein, J. D. & Hollander, E. (1997) Sexual dysfunction associated with the drug treatment of psychiatric disorders. *CNS Drugs*, **2**, 78–86.

Sternbach, H. (1998) Age-associated testosterone decline in men: clinical issues for psychiatry. *American Journal of Psychiatry*, **155**, 1310–1318.

Tuiten, A., van Honk, J., Koppeschaar, H., *et al* (2000) Timecourse of effects of testosterone administration on sexual arousal in women. *Archives of General Psychiatry*, **57**, 149–153.

Wylie, K. R. (1998) Physical treatments for sexual dysfunctions. In *Seminars in Psychosexual Disorders* (eds H. Freeman, I. Pullen, G. Stein, *et al*), pp. 84–100. London: Gaskell.

Yates, W. R. (2000) Testosterone in psychiatry: risks and benefits. *Archives of General Psychiatry*, **57**, 155–156.

DRUG TREATMENT

23. WEIGHT CHANGES AND EATING DISORDERS

UNDERWEIGHT

Loss of weight is a common non-specific symptom of much serious mental and physical disease, normally one symptom among many. There is, however, one group of conditions collectively called eating disorders in which weight change is the focus of concern.

Anorexia nervosa

The most extreme form is anorexia nervosa, in which loss of weight results from self-starvation. The patient refuses to eat, even if hungry, or eats only a little protein food but avoids carbohydrate and fat, secretly vomits after eating, takes laxatives and diuretics or exercises to excess in an attempt to lose weight. Such patients have fears of being too fat, of gaining weight or of developing a normal sexually mature figure and may be determined to be thin to the point of endangering their lives. The psychological background is varied and complex, and not within the scope of this book. However, difficulty in engaging in a therapeutic relationship is often a feature of eating disorders. There is frequently a disturbed relationship with a family member, usually a parent. The patient may have a distorted body image, tending to overestimate his/her size. The patient with anorexia nervosa is liable to give false reports of weight gain and to mislead the doctor about him-/herself in order to allay concern about his/her condition. In adolescent girls and young women anorexia nervosa is accompanied by amenorrhoea and other somatic effects of starvation. But anorexia with refusal to eat an adequate amount of food does also occur, though much less often, in adolescent boys and in older women and men. Refusal to eat may be used to achieve a sense of control, punish another or to attract special concern.

Because extreme weight loss predisposes the patient to pneumonia, to gastric dilation and to dying of self-starvation, re-feeding may become urgent. It must be carried out away from family pressures, in hospital, and is likely to entail strict supervision, in bed if necessary, and no home leave. Nurses who are firm, friendly and aware of the ways of such patients can produce weight gain with the help of food supplements alone. Sometimes drugs are necessary to assist psychological treatment. Chlorpromazine (150–300 mg daily) stimulates appetite and causes weight gain, although it is used less often now; olanzapine has also been used. Amitriptyline is occasionally prescribed in the belief that there is an atypical depressive illness to be treated; amitriptyline, like chlorpromazine, has appetite-stimulating and weight-gaining effects over a period. SSRIs are not considered helpful in acute anorexia nervosa but may have a place in preventing relapse of the condition in recovered patients.

Bulimia nervosa and binge eating disorder

Bulimia nervosa, with a morbid fear of becoming fat, is characterised by an urge to overeat, followed by self-induced vomiting, purging, exercising and other measures aimed at alleviating the morbid fear. It is almost exclusively a disorder of women. More so than anorexia nervosa, bulimia may affect older women and some who are married with children. It is commonly accompanied by depression. Often the sufferers have concerns about the control of their lives and impulses on a broad basis.

Fluoxetine has been used in doses of up to 60 mg daily, and was beneficial even in those who were not depressed. However, the number experiencing a complete abolition of binges within 6 weeks is very low (see Table 23.1). Another SSRI found to be effective is fluvoxamine. Phenelzine has also been shown to be of benefit but is less safe because of interactions with tyramine in foods. The SSRIs have not been shown to be superior to less-specific drugs such as TCAs. Unfortunately these modest improvements from drugs do not generally last; almost one-third of those who benefit in the first 3 months relapse over the following 3 months.

CBT is the best-established treatment. IPT is also of proven effectiveness, and the gains may be more enduring.

Drug treatment with antidepressants, including the SSRIs, may be helpful in combination with CBT, at least in the first few months. As yet no long-term benefit of combining drug treatment with this has been shown.

Binge eating disorder is associated with episodic bingeing in the absence of purging behaviour and is usually associated with obesity. Fluvoxamine reduces the frequency of binge eating, to a modest extent.

Pathophysiology

Human appetite involves the transmitters noradrenalin and dopamine, and satiety is thought to involve 5-HT. Receptor and neurotransmitter functions are poorly understood, but there is evidence of abnormal cerebral 5-HT function in the eating disorders.

In animals noradrenalin acts at α-1 receptors in the paraventricular nucleus to reduce feeding, and at α-2 to increase it. Phenylpropanolamine acts as an appetite suppressant via α-1. Amphetamine also releases dopamine to act in the parafornical hypothalamus to reduce food intake. α-1 blockade (phenoxybenzamine) can increase body weight in anorexia nervosa.

Adipose tissue secretes a hormone, leptin, that signals the size of the adipose tissue to the brain. Leptin levels are low in anorexia nervosa and rise as body mass returns.

In bulimia nervosa there is reduced turnover of 5-HT and dopamine, as judged by CSF levels of their metabolites. There are also blunted prolactin responses to fenfluramine, which releases 5-HT, and to the 5-HT receptor agonist m-chlorophenylpiperazine. Furthermore, acute depletion of brain 5-HT, in recovered patients with bulimia, by ingestion of a tryptophan-free amino acid mixture, leads to lowering of mood, increased concern about body image and a sense of loss of control of eating. In people who lose weight, there are increased neuroendocrine responses to L-tryptophan, and 5-HT-2C receptor supersensitivity.

Table 23.1 Efficacy of fluoxetine in bulimia nervosa

Treatment (n)	Duration	Drop-outs (%)	Criterion of improvement	Response (%)	ARR (%)	NNT (95% CI)
Fluoxetine (296)	16 weeks	41	100% reduction in vomiting	18.3	6.3	NSD
Placebo (102)		52		12		
Fluoxetine (296)	16 weeks	41	50% reduction in binges	51.4	15.4	7 (4–23)
Placebo (102)		52		36		

ARR, absolute risk reduction; NNT, number needed to treat; NSD, not statistically significant.
Adapted from Goldstein et al. 1995.

This evidence points to a role for lowered brain 5-HT function (to which dieting might also contribute) in the development of eating disorders in predisposed individuals.

Special weighing

It is worth knowing that total starvation will not produce a daily weight loss of more than 500 gm in a sedentary person receiving water only; and that excessive feeding will not add more than a maximum of 200 gm a day to the body's fat and flesh weight. Larger changes over 24 hours are owing to losses or gains of body fluid (losses through urine, sweat or diarrhoea, perhaps). Emptying the bladder of overnight urine, volume 600 ml, means a weight loss of 600 gm. Eating dinner will immediately add 500 gm to body weight, drinks apart (these are rough values). When dieting, initial weight loss involves depletion of glycogen stores and water, and this is difficult to sustain.

Accurate weighing is important in certain clinical conditions and in medical research. The instrument must be reliable, and cantilever scales are required. Weighing someone several times a day can be a check on whether a patient with anorexia or bulimia has been eating normally or not. In patients prone to excessive water drinking (polydipsia, leading to water intoxication) comparison of the body weight at midday and 4 p.m. with that at 8 a.m. may reveal the extent of overdrinking and the approach to the danger zone of hyponatraemia (below 120 mmol/l). A weight gain of 7% on the early morning body weight is the permitted maximum. In the rare Prader-Willi syndrome (obesity, poor growth, failure of sexual maturation and mental retardation), where the child or adolescent will ransack refrigerators and break down doors to get excessive food, frequent weighing can be used to detect the food intake and monitor the effect of treatment.

OVERWEIGHT

The psychiatrist encounters increased body weight as a result of long-term medication with phenothiazines, depot antipsychotics, atypical antipsychotics, certain antidepressants and lithium. With these drugs it is thought that blockade of 5-HT-2C receptors is important in producing increased food intake. Histamine H_1-receptor blockade may also contribute to weight gain, by producing sedation and inactivity. All antipsychotics cause weight gain to some extent, even specific D_2/D_3 antagonists, such as the benzamides, so dopamine receptor blockade is also important. Weight gain on antipsychotics develops to a plateau over the course of about 9–18 months.

Occasionally, an affective illness results in weight gain instead of loss, and an anxiety state causes comfort overeating. Rarely, refractory obesity, thought to be psychological after defying medical and surgical efforts, is referred to the psychiatrist.

Obesity resulting from a depressive illness almost always disappears after successful treatment.

The treatment of gross obesity with a suspected psychological cause should be approached by investigating for evidence of overeating induced by anxiety, depression or disturbed interpersonal relations.

Treatment directed at these conditions, including the appropriate psychotropic drugs, sometimes reduces weight.

A behavioural approach or a group like Weight Watchers, which encourages reducing food intake and increasing energy output over the long term, can be successful.

Drugs to reduce weight

The appetite-suppressing drugs, phentermine and mazindol, that are central stimulants related to amphetamine, are potentially addictive and should not be prescribed.

dl-Fenfluramine ('Ponderax'), a serotonin releaser with a sedative action and which is less addictive, used to be prescribed in severe obesity but not for longer than 3 months. D-Fenfluramine is the active isomer and was available as 'Adifax', but has been withdrawn in most countries because of fibrosis in the heart. Centrally acting drugs have at present no place in the long-term treatment of chronic obesity.

A new drug, orlistat ('Xenical'), which reduces lipid absorption by blocking pancreatic lipase, may be required in severe obesity, but unpleasant gastrointestinal adverse effects are common. The National Institute for Clinical Excellence has recommended its use in people with a body mass index (BMI) of over 30 and who demonstrate motivation by losing some weight first.

Sibutramine, a sympathomimetic and 5-HT agonist is also effective (see p. 382).

Drug-induced weight gain

Antidepressants are frequently associated with weight increases of up to 5 kg over several months. Amitriptyline is most often implicated, but some newer antidepressants such as mirtazapine do this too. With amitriptyline a reduction in metabolic rate has been reported, perhaps related to sedation. Amitriptyline can also produce a craving for sweet foods such as chocolate, which has a high fat and carbohydrate content. Antagonism of central 5-HT and H_1 receptors is the suggested mechanism. The SSRIs, NRIs and SNRIs should not block receptors or stimulate food intake. Weight changes are in fact at placebo levels with SSRIs, nefazodone, venlafaxine and reboxetine, and fluoxetine may even lead to short-term loss of weight. The NaSSA mirtazapine blocks 5-HT-2C and H_1 receptors, and weight gain is a prominent side-effect.

Lithium and valproate can also cause weight gain. The mechanisms involved are unclear. With lithium, polydipsia may provoke a high intake of sugary drinks, but many patients gain weight without this. Weight gain is greater with blood levels above 0.8 mmol/L. Carbamazepine may be an appropriate substitute in cases of severe weight gain. The anticonvulsant topiramate is interesting because it is associated with weight loss.

Among antipsychotics, butyrophenones and substituted benzamides are associated with the least weight gain (around 1–2 kg over 10 weeks). The low-potency phenothiazines, such as chlorpromazine, cause more weight gain. Antagonism of dopamine D-2/3 and 5-HT-2C is thought to be causative; blockade of histamine H_1 receptors may contribute by causing sedation and inactivity. Clozapine and olanzapine are usually associated with substantial weight gain, often 5 kg or more; quetiapine less so. Risperidone and zotepine cause moderate weight increases (around 2 kg on average over 10 weeks) and ziprasidone appears not to alter weight. The lack of any effect with ziprasidone is surprising, considering its moderately potent antagonism of H_1, 5-HT-2C and D_2 receptors.

Levels of the hormone leptin increase during treatment with clozapine and olanzapine, as body weight increases.

For the most part, patients gain weight because of an increase in appetite, which causes an increase in food intake. Some atypical antipsychotics such as clozapine and olanzapine are clearly associated with binge eating. In some there is also a low level of physical activity that may be worsened as a result of sedation.

Some patients develop impaired glucose tolerance and hyperlipidaemia, and some diabetes. This may arise from a direct effect of drugs, particularly clozapine, upon receptors for insulin or glucose.

BMI and depot antipsychotics

A simple measure of body weight is BMI (the weight in kg divided by the square of the height in metres). If the BMI is over 30, there is Grade II (clinically relevant) obesity; over 40 is Grade III (crippling obesity). In a study of patients in London on long-term depot antipsychotic medication, 30% had Grade II and 5% had Grade III obesity, compared with 5% and zero in the normal working population in the UK. National differences in population figures for obesity are striking, with higher rates in the US, for example, and low rates in developing countries.

The phenothiazine fluphenazine decanoate and the butyrophenone haloperidol decanoate show no difference in their effects on body weight during 1 year of treatment.

Management of drug-induced weight gain

Obesity induced by psychotropic drugs nearly always disappears gradually after the drug is stopped. But stopping the drug may be inadvisable because of the risk of relapse. A reduction in dose or a switch to a drug that does not cause weight increase should be undertaken whenever possible. For lithium, a reduction in the daily dose may be tried, risking relapse for a slimmer figure, or carbamazepine, which does not cause weight gain, may be substituted; valproate has also been associated with weight gain (and polycystic ovary syndrome), but lamotrigine has not. A slimming diet may help, preferably with the advice of a dietician.

Often, however, obesity is the price of drug control of positive symptoms of a psychosis, contributing to the clinical picture of the long-term patient. Clearly, new antipsychotics with less propensity for weight gain are needed.

The best predictor of weight control is the patient's motivation to succeed. In severe cases of weight gain, orlistat may be considered, although its efficacy in drug-induced obesity has not been established.

DRUG TREATMENT

235

FURTHER READING

Bulimia nervosa

American Psychiatric Association (2000)Practice guideline for the treatment of patients with eating disorders (revision). American Psychiatric Association Work Group on Eating Disorders. *American Journal of Psychiatry*,**157**(Suppl.), 1–39.

Fluoxetine Bulimia Nervosa Collaborative Study Group (1992) Fluoxetine in the treatment of bulimia nervosa: a multicentre, placebo-controlled, double-blind trial. *Archives of General Psychiatry*, **49**, 139–147.

Walsh, B. T., Wilson, G. T., Loeb, K. L., *et al* (1997) Medication and psychotherapy in the treatment of bulimia nervosa. *American Journal of Psychaitry*, **154**, 523–531.

Pathophysiology

Cowen, P. J., Clifford, E. M., Walsh, A. D., *et al* (1996) Moderate dieting causes 5-HT2c receptor supersensitivity. *Psychological Medicine*, **26**, 1155–1159.

Goodwin, G. M., Shapiro, C. M., Bennie, J., *et al* (1989) The neuroendocrine responses and psychological effects of infusion of L-tryptophan in anorexia nervosa. *Psychological Medicine*, **19**, 857–864.

Smith, K. A., Fairburn, C. G., Cowen, P. J. (1999) Symptomatic relapse in bulimia nervosa following acute tryptophan depletion. *Archives of General Psychiatry*, **56**, 171–176.

Antipsychotics and weight gain

Allison, D. B., Mentore, J. L., Heo, M., *et al* (1999) Antipsychotic-induced weight gain: a comprehensive research synthesis. *American Journal of Psychiatry*, **156**, 1686–1696.

Baptista, T. (1999) Body weight gain induced by antipsychotic drugs: mechanisms and management. *Acta Psychiatrica Scandinavica*, **100**, 3–16.

Kinon, B. J., Basson, B. R., Gilmore, J. A., *et al* (2001) Long-term olanzapine treatment: weight change and weight-related health factors in schizophrenia. *Journal of Clinical Psychiatry*, **62**, 92–100.

Kraus, T., Kaack, M., Schuld, A., *et al* (1999) Body weight and leptin plasma levels during treatment with antipsychotic drugs. *American Journal of Psychiatry*, **156**, 312–314.

Mir, S. & Taylor, D. (2001) Atypical antipsychotics and hyperglycaemia. *International Clinical Psychopharmacology*, **16**, 63–74.

Silverstone, T., Smith, G., Goodall, E. (1988) The prevalence of obesity in patients receiving depot antipsychotics. *British Journal of Psychiatry*, **153**, 214–217.

Antidepressants and weight

Finkel, S. I., Richter, E. M., Clary, C. M., *et al* (1999) Comparative efficacy of sertraline vs. fluoxetine in patients age 70 or over with major depression. *American Journal of Geriatric Psychiatry*, **7**, 221–227.

Michelson, D., Amsterdam, J. D., Quitkin, F. M., *et al* (1999) Changes in weight during a 1 year trial of fluoxetine. *American Journal of Psychiatry*, **156**, 1170–1176.

Paykel, E. S., Mueller, P. S. & De la Vergne, P. M. (1973) Amitriptyline, weight gain and carbohydrate craving: a side effect. *British Journal of Psychiatry*, **123**, 501–507.

Studies quoted

Goldstein, D. J., Wilson, M. G., Thompson, V. L., *et al* (1995) Long-term fluoxetine treatment of bulimia nervosa. *British Journal of Psychiatry*, **166**, 660–666.

Amitriptyline and imipramine, introduced in 1957, are two of the oldest and best known drugs for treating depressive illness. Their chemical structure, three joined rings of atoms with a centrally attached tail or side-chain, is termed 'tricyclic' (Figure 24.1). The central ring has seven atoms, not six as in phenothiazines, a structure that makes the molecule V-shaped and unable to lie flat. The side-chain influences potency and sedative action. Other drugs with tricyclic molecules that are not antidepressants include cyproheptadine, which blocks 5-HT and histamine and is used as an appetite stimulant, and carbamazepine, an anticonvulsant.

The wide range of TCAs that are marketed results from minor structural modifications of the fundamental molecule. If a fourth ring is added, as in maprotiline, then the compound is called tetracyclic. Other new antidepressants such as the SSRIs have different structures without tricyclic rings. The TCAs have in common the ability to increase the concentration of noradrenalin, 5-HT, or dopamine in the synaptic cleft, and achieve this mainly by binding to the transporters (chapter 7) and thereby blocking the reuptake process. They are therefore known collectively as MARIs.

Reuptake inhibition

The older TCAs, imipramine and amitriptyline, block both 5-HT and noradrenalin reuptake; their demethylated metabolites, desipramine and nortriptyline, are more specific noradrenalin reuptake inhibitors (see Table 24.1). Clomipramine is the most specific of the older drugs for blockade of the reuptake of 5-HT, as opposed to noradrenalin or dopamine. It should be noted, however, that the range of pharmacological activities is not necessarily the same as the mode of action for the antidepressant effect (see below).

Newer antidepressants

Subsequently other (non-tricyclic) MARIs have been developed and these are classified further, according to their main pharmacological actions, into SSRIs, SNRIs, NRIs and NaSSAs. The naming of these classes owes as much to marketing considerations as to pharmacology.

Mechanism of antidepressant effect

The MARIs act primarily by binding to the transporter proteins (NAT and SERT, see chapter 7, p. 75) and thereby blocking the reuptake of noradrenalin, 5-HT and to some extent dopamine. This increases the concentration of the transmitters at their receptors, which are both pre- and post-synaptic in the synaptic cleft, and on the cell bodies (autoreceptors). Some may achieve this also by blocking pre-synaptic noradrenalin α-2 autoreceptors, thereby increasing the release of

Figure 24.1 Tricyclic drug structures

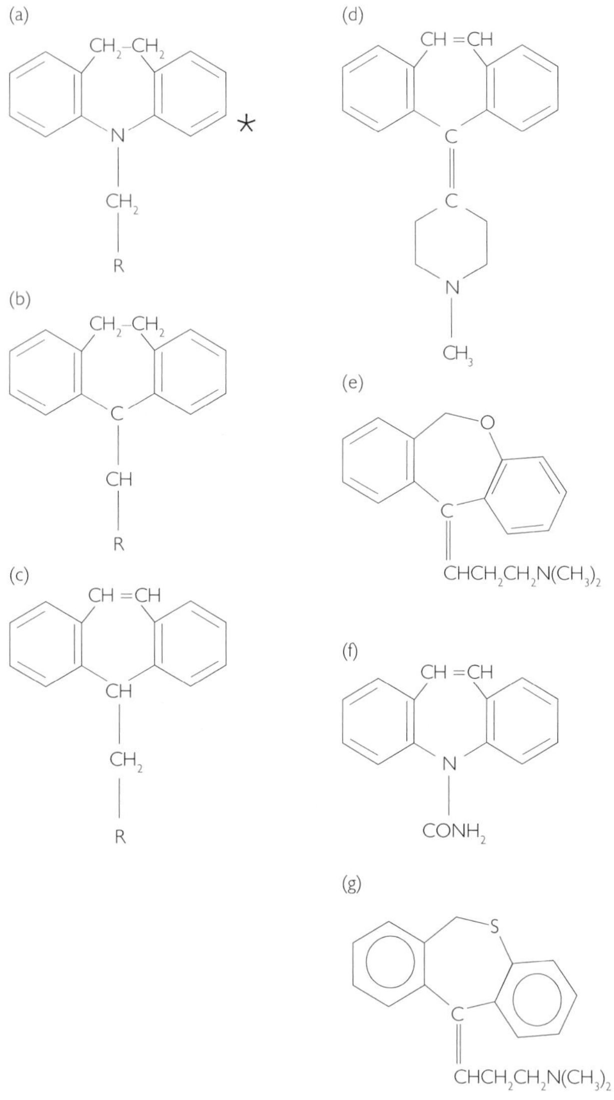

(a) For imipramine R is $CH_2CH_2N(CH_3)_2$; for desipramine R is $-CH_2CH_2N(CH_3)H$; for trimipramine R is $-CH(CH_3)-CH_2N(CH_3)_2$; when a chlorine atom instead of a hydrogen atom is attached to the carbon marked $*$ in the imipramine structure, clomipramine is formed. (b) For amitriptyline R is as for imipramine; for nortriptyline R is as for desipramine. (c) For protriptyline R is as for desipramine. (d) Cyproheptadine, (e) doxepin, (f) carbamazepine and (g) dothiepin. In (e) and (g) R is as for imipramine.

Table 24.1 Affinities of TCAs for reuptake sites and receptors of human brain

Drug	NRI	SRI	DRI	H-1	ACh M	NA α-1	NA α-2	5-HT-2A
Amitriptyline	2.9	23	0.03	91	6	4	0.1	3
Clomipramine	2.7	362	0.05	3	3	3	0.03	4
Desipramine	120	5.7	0.03	0.9	0.5	0.8	0.01	0.4
Dothiepin	2.2	12	0.02	28	4	0.2	0.04	0.4
Imipramine	2.7	71	0.01	9	1	1	0.03	1.3
Lofepramine	19	1.4	0.005	0.3	1.5	1	0	0.5
Nortriptyline	23	5.4	0.09	10	0.7	1.7	0.04	2.3
Trimipramine	0.04	0.7	0.03	370	2	4	0.2	3

NRI, noradrenalin reuptake inhibition; SRI, serotonin reuptake inhibition; DRI: dopamine reuptake inhibition; H, histamine receptor; AChM, acetylcholine muscarinic receptor; NA, noradrenalin; 5-HT, serotonin.

Affinity is expressed as $1/10^7 \times Kd$, where Kd is equilibrium dissociation constant in molarity. Thus, higher numbers indicate greater strength of that action. Ratios of different figures in the rows show how many times more potent the drug is in the two actions.

Adapted from Leonard & Richelson (2000).

noradrenalin, but this applies mainly to newer antidepressants such as mirtazapine (see chapter 26). The other actions of the TCAs, blocking receptors for acetylcholine, histamine, noradrenalin and serotonin, are thought to influence side-effects but not antidepressant efficacy.

Table 24.1 shows the relative potencies of the TCAs in blocking the transporters for noradrenalin, 5-HT and dopamine, and in blocking receptors for histamine, noradrenalin acetylcholine and 5-HT.

The gradual development of the antidepressant effect suggests that adaptive processes are important in the mechanism of action. One type of adaptive change occurs in the transmitter receptors. Thus noradrenalin β- and α-2 receptors are gradually reduced in number (downregulated) during antidepressant treatment, while noradrenalin α-1 receptors are upregulated. Slow changes occur too in both pre- and post-synaptic serotonin receptors. These are discussed further in relation to serotonin in chapter 25 and to noradrenalin in chapter 26.

Other slow processes that may be set in train include the transport of enzymes from the cell body of the neuron along the axon to the nerve endings. These enzymes are involved in the synthesis of transmitters and the neuropeptide modulators. Although the basis of the antidepressant effect is not fully understood, the available evidence suggests that the overall effect of antidepressants is to increase transmission at noradrenalin or 5-HT synapses.

Disadvantages of TCAs

The TCAs have a number of shortcomings:

- their antidepressant effect develops slowly, from 1–6 weeks
- they are effective in only a proportion of patients

THE DRUGS

- they have many side-effects that are largely predictable from their pharmacological actions, which limit their acceptability to patients, and reduce adherence or lead to early discontinuation in clinical trials
- they are cardiotoxic, and are associated with fatalities in overdose
- they have interactions with other drugs

New antidepressants have been developed in the hope of overcoming these problems. Those so far available are much less toxic in overdose, and have a different pattern of side-effects that are sometimes better tolerated by patients. None has proved more effective in depression than amitriptyline or clomipramine, though some may be more effective in anxiety states. All exert their clinical actions gradually, with little evidence of differences in time course.

Pharmacological side-effects

Pharmacological side-effects are not necessarily a disadvantage in an antidepressant. For instance, night-time sedation is useful for those patients in whom insomnia is a symptom of their illness, and dryness of the mouth can be tolerated and be a useful biological marker of compliance and a guide to the adequacy of dose with amitriptyline or imipramine. However, some side-effects are particularly intolerable and may either cause complications or lead the patient to discontinue treatment; this results in failure to improve and prolongs the illness, with a need for alternative treatment.

In addition to blocking the reuptake of monoamines, the TCAs have other pharmacological actions, including blocking the receptors for particular neurotransmitters (especially acetylcholine-M, histamine H_1, noradrenalin α-1 and α-2, and 5-HT receptors) and interfere with the ionic channels in cell membranes (membrane stabilising or local anaesthetic actions). These differing pharmacological actions can be related to particular patterns of side-effects in the following ways (see Box 24.1).

Anticholinergic effects

Antagonism of acetylcholine muscarinic receptors causes a variety of side-effects through blockade of the parasympathetic nerves, such as the vagus (see Box 24.1). Reduced salivation leads to dry mouth and may exacerbate gum disease and dental caries. The pre-existing constipation of the patient with depression is worsened. In high doses or in the elderly, paralytic ileus may occur. Urinary hesitancy occurs, especially in males, and acute retention may develop if the prostate is enlarged.

Blurred vision, with difficulty in accommodating, is a common but not usually severe side-effect. The precipitation of acute narrow-angle glaucoma is serious but rare.

Cognitive impairment by this mechanism is not uncommon in the elderly, and confusional states may occur. Those with pre-existing cholinergic deficits owing to Alzheimer's disease may be more susceptible to manifest this side-effect.

Tardive dyskinesia tends to be made worse by anticholinergic effects of drugs, though not caused by them. These side-effects are particularly

---

Box 24.1 Pharmacological side-effects of antidepressants

Anti-muscarinic (acetylcholine)

Dry mouth, constipation, urinary retention, blurred vision, cognitive impairment and worsened tardive dyskinesia

Noradrenalin reuptake blockade

Dry mouth, constipation, urinary retention, blurred vision, tachycardia, insomnia and raised blood pressure

Noradrenalin α-1 blockade

Postural hypotension and ejaculatory impotence

Histamine blockade (H_1)

Sedation, cognitive impairment and falls

5-HT reuptake blockade

Diarrhoea, headache and drowsiness

5-HT-1 agonism

Serotonin syndrome

5-HT-2 agonism

Nervousness, insomnia, anorexia, sexual dysfunction, akathisia, Parkinsonism and dystonia

5-HT-3 agonism

Nausea

5-HT blockade

Weight gain

Dopamine reuptake blockade

Nausea, activation, anti-Parkinsonian and psychosis

Complex/unclear

Fine tremor, sweating, myoclonus, secretion of inappropriate antidiuretic hormone, epilepsy and mania/rapid cycling

Membrane-stabilisation

Cardiac dysrhythmia and asystole

---

common with amitriptyline, imipramine and clomipramine, less so with dothiepin, lofepramine and maprotiline. Nortriptyline blocks acetylcholine weakly. The newer drugs – trazodone and the SSRIs (with the exception of paroxetine) – produce little blockade of acetylcholine receptors; sertraline and citalopram also produce dry mouth, probably by a different mechanism. The SNRIs, NRIs and NaSSAs are largely devoid of anticholinergic actions, but some similar though less severe side-effects can still occur, probably through potentiation of the sympathetic nervous system (via increased noradrenergic function).

Noradrenalin reuptake inhibition

Blockade of noradrenalin reuptake tends to produce sympathomimetic effects such as tachycardia, dry mouth, constipation, urinary hesitancy and blurred vision, and therefore to act synergistically with the anticholinergic effects that block the parasympathetic component of the autonomic nervous system. However, this action does not produce cognitive impairment, unlike anti-cholinergic drugs; it is more likely to cause increased arousal. Increased blood pressure can occur, mainly with venlafaxine at high doses.

Histamine H_1 blockade

Histamine H_1 blockade underlies night-time sedation, but also impairs psychomotor coordination during the daytime. It is associated with falls in the elderly and with cognitive slowing, and contributes to road traffic accidents. TCAs such as amitriptyline, clomipramine and dothiepin are sedative. Imipramine and nortriptyline are less so. Lofepramine and desipramine cause little blockade of histamine receptors and are not generally sedative. Among the newer drugs, trazodone, nefazodone and mirtazapine block H_1 receptors and are sedative. Maprotiline, the SNRIs and the NRIs do not block H_1 receptors and are not sedative. The SSRIs do not block H_1 receptors, and do not increase sleep, but some do cause daytime drowsiness, particularly paroxetine (see p. 256).

Noradrenalin α-1 receptor blockade

Noradrenalin α–1 receptor blockade leads to postural hypotension, which may cause dizziness and falls, especially in the elderly; it is also thought to contribute to ejaculatory impotence. This action is strong with amitriptyline, clomipramine and imipramine. It is weak with dothiepin, nortriptyline, lofepramine and maprotiline. It does not occur with the SSRIs, SNRIs, NRIs or with viloxazine. It does occur with nefazodone and mirtazapine and strongly with trazodone. A comparative study of nortriptyline and imipramine in the elderly showed that nortriptyline produced less postural hypotension.

Blockade of 5-HT receptors

Serotonin receptors are now classified into at least three main types and eight subtypes (see chapter 7). 5-HT antagonists such as cyproheptadine tend to increase appetite and body weight. The 5-HT-2C receptor is thought to be especially important in this regard. It is probably by this mechanism that antidepressants such as amitriptyline cause excessive weight gain, which is lost again when the drug is stopped. Carbohydrate craving can occur as a dose-related side-effect of amitriptyline. Blockade of histamine receptors has also been suggested as contributing to weight gain.

Weight gain is not a problem with the SSRIs, the SNRIs or the NRIs, or with trazodone or nefazodone, but does occur with the NaSSA mirtazapine.

Serotonin reuptake inhibition

The development of SSRIs has provided a clearer picture of the side-effects that are attributable to serotonin reuptake inhibition (see Boxes 25.2, p. 259, and 25.3, p. 260). The most common side-effects emerging with these drugs have been nausea, nervousness, insomnia, drowsiness, sexual dysfunction (reduced libido, erectile impotence and ejaculatory/orgasmic failure), fine tremor, diarrhoea, headache, akathisia and increased sweating. Much less common are acute dystonia and Parkinsonism.

These side-effects are believed to arise through stimulation of various 5-HT receptor types, for instance ejaculatory problems from 5-HT-2, anxiety and anorexia from 5-HT-2C, and nausea and vomiting from 5-HT-3.

Anorgasmia and ejaculatory difficulties occur also with clomipramine, which is a strong serotonin reuptake inhibitor. Cyproheptadine, which blocks 5-HT receptors, if taken 2 hours earlier, can counteract this problem.

Serotonin syndrome is a serious toxic reaction to excessive 5-HT in the brain. It is usually the result of an interaction occurring when a drug blocking serotonin reuptake is combined with a drug potentiating 5-HT transmission by another mechanism, particularly an MAOI but also sometimes L-tryptophan, lithium or carbamazepine (see p. 87–88).

Dopamine reuptake inhibition

This property is likely to produce nausea and activating effects, and to risk precipitating psychosis. However, mania is less likely to be triggered. Drugs with this action at high doses include sertraline, clomipramine and amitriptyline.

Side-effects with unclear or complex pharmacology

A fine tremor occurs with the tricyclic drugs and to a similar extent with the SSRIs. Propranolol reduces this side-effect but blocks both noradrenalin β-receptors and 5-HT receptors, and the underlying mechanism of the tremor is uncertain.

Excessive sweating occurs to a greater extent with imipramine and other TCAs than with the SSRIs, indicating that the mechanism is complex.

Secretion of inappropriate antidiuretic hormone with hyponatraemia has been reported with dothiepin, lofepramine, the SSRIs and venlafaxine as well as other TCAs, and may be a possible side-effect with all antidepressants.

Symptomatic hyponatraemia presents as a confusional state with weakness, lethargy, or drowsiness, usually only when serum levels are less than 123 mmol/l. The elderly are predisposed because of renal and endocrine changes associated with ageing. The risk is increased by medical disorders, mental illness and use of drugs, including antidepressants associated with secretion of inappropriate antidiuretic hormone. With SSRIs, people over 70 are particularly vulnerable to develop hyponatraemia, which usually occurs within the first few weeks and resolves within 2–3 weeks of stopping the drug. Sodium levels taken within the first and second weeks after commencing an SSRI should detect the problem. Priapism can occur with trazodone; the mechanism is not certain. Muscular twitching (myoclonus) occurs with the TCAs and SSRIs.

Epileptic fits occur in a dose-dependent manner with the TCAs, up to 1% of patients being affected by higher doses. The mechanism of this effect of antidepressants is not known, but maprotiline, bupropion and amoxapine are particularly liable to cause it. Drugs with less ictogenic potential include viloxazine, the SSRIs and moclobemide. Existing epilepsy is not necessarily worsened by treatment with MARIs. The SSRIs may prolong the duration of seizures during ECT (see chapter 40).

The development of mania or rapid-cycling bipolar disorder during the course of antidepressant treatment is more likely to occur when there is a previous history of mania. This has been reported with both the TCAs and some of the newer drugs, but is less common with bupropion and the SSRIs. It is difficult to know in individual cases whether the switching is spontaneous or a result of treatment, and few controlled trials have involved bipolar depressed patients (see chapter 12).

Membrane-stabilising activity

Many centrally acting drugs have membrane-stabilising or local anaesthetic properties at high doses. This action is responsible for cardiac dysrhythmias associated with overdoses of antidepressants, and can lead to asystole and fatal outcome in suicide attempts. This mechanism of action is unrelated to either the anticholinergic effects or any of the other properties discussed above. It is due to interference with ionic channels for sodium, potassium or calcium currents in Purkinje cells of the myocardium. By blocking sodium conductance channels, the drugs are typed as Class I in the classification of anti-arrhythmic drugs by the pharmacologist Vaughan-Williams (Page *et al*, 1997). Thus, in spite of its low anticholinergic properties, a drug such as dothiepin owes its lethality in overdose to this membrane-stabilising property.

The occurrence of ectopic beats is not a contraindication to use of the tricyclic drugs; the membrane-stabilising activity may in fact reduce the number of ectopics in such patients. However, cardiologists in the Cardiac Arrythmia Suppression Trial (CAST; Ruskin, 1989) discovered to their horror that the use of a Class I anti-arrhythmic drug as prophylaxis (encainide or flecainide) after myocardial infarction, led to higher not lower rates of cardiac-related death. Therefore, for the treatment of depressive illness after a myocardial infarction, an antidepressant free of membrane-stabilising activity should be used.

Antidepressants with weaker membrane-stabilising activity include lofepramine and the newer drugs viloxazine, the SSRIs, venlafaxine (SNRI), reboxetine (NRI), mirtazapine (NaSSA) and nefazodone. These should be used if an antidepressant is required in a patient with cardiac disease, especially one with a conduction defect or after a myocardial infarction. Trazodone and citalopram may produce ECG abnormalities in overdose, and fatal dysrhythmias.

Overdoses

Overdoses of imipramine or amitriptyline lead to unconsciousness in 1–5 hours, with a catastrophic fall in blood pressure, cardiac arrhythmias, epileptic fits and sometimes status epilepticus. Likewise, an overdose of dothiepin leads to cardiac arrhythmias or asystole. Stomach washout, control of fits and maintenance of blood pressure and hence of kidney function must be carried out in a medical ward under specialist advice. Prognosis is good where treatment begins shortly after the overdose.

Fatal toxicity index

The tendency of drugs to be fatal in overdose can be gauged by the number of such incidents reported to coroners as compared with the number of prescriptions issued for individual drugs.

It is therefore possible to calculate a fatal toxicity index (Table 24.2). In this way it has been found that amitriptyline and dothiepin carry the highest risks. There is a small safety margin between the therapeutic level of these drugs (e.g. 150 µg/l for amitriptyline) and the fatal cardiotoxic level (above 500 µg/l).

Antidepressants with the lowest fatal toxicity index include lofepramine, the SSRIs and newer drugs such as venlafaxine, nefazodone, mirtazapine and reboxetine.

Drop-outs from treatment

Most side-effects are dose- and age-related and some, for instance nausea, tend to decrease with continued treatment. The risk of drop-outs may be reduced by starting on a lower dose, especially in the elderly. In research studies of the newer drugs, a smaller proportion of patients discontinued treatment because of side-effects compared with the older TCAs, imipramine or amitriptyline. About 20% discontinued TCA treatment because of new symptoms, compared with 15% on SSRIs and 5% on placebo. Among the TCAs, lofepramine produces less severe side-effects and is much less cardiotoxic.

Toxic and allergic side-effects

Abnormal liver function tests occur occasionally with many antidepressants; most are unpredictable and independent of dose, and their potential severity varies widely. Previous exposure to enzyme-inducing agents may increase the rate of formation of reactive drug metabolites and potentiate hepatotoxicity. Anticonvulsants and chronic

THE DRUGS

Table 24.2 Fatal toxicity index for antidepressants

Drug	Observed deaths	Expected deaths	Deaths per million prescriptions (95% CI)
Dothiepin	801	504	47.7 (44.6–51.2)
Amitriptyline	509	394	38.9 (35.6–42.4)
Imipramine	111	106	31.5 (25.9–37.7)
Clomipramine	26	108	13.9 (9.6–19.0)
Lofepramine	10	125	2.4 (1.1–4.1)
Sertraline	1	5	6.2 (0.0–24.4)
Fluvoxamine	2	13	4.8 (0.4–13.7)
Paroxetine	1	12	2.6 (0.0–10.2)
Fluoxetine	1	46	0.7 (0.0–2.6)

Adapted from Henry (1997).

alcohol ingestion may be important in this respect. With lofepramine, jaundice may develop in the first 8 weeks but is reversible on discontinuing the drug.

These are generally rare and only detected after the drug has been marketed and several thousand patients treated.

Blood dyscrasias have occasionally resulted from TCAs and from mianserin. The elderly are particularly at risk.

Drug interactions

The TCAs interfered with the control of blood pressure by older adrenergic blocking drugs, such as guanethidine, that have to be taken up into nerve endings in order to act. They also potentiate the action of adrenalin in local anaesthetics by preventing adrenalin reuptake, thereby causing a rise in blood pressure. Substances that induce the liver mono-oxygenase P450 enzyme system, for example carbamazepine, barbiturates, phenytoin and hydrocarbons in tobacco smoke or in barbecued food, may lower the plasma concentration of TCAs. Oestrogens inhibit the metabolism of TCAs, leading to higher blood levels or the need for lower doses. Cimetidine also raises the plasma concentration of TCAs. Some phenothiazines, such as chlorpromazine and thioridazine, increase the plasma concentration of TCAs by inhibiting cytochrome hydroxylase enzymes CYP IID6 in the liver. The SSRIs to varying extents also inhibit the same enzymes (see Box 25.4, p. 264).

Discontinuation reactions

Discontinuation reactions after abrupt cessation of TCAs include nausea, vomiting, sweating and insomnia, lasting for a few days. Dependence, with drug-seeking behaviour or craving, is not a problem with the TCAs or other antidepressants, unless they have stimulant properties, for example the MAOI tranylcypromine.

CLINICAL EFFECTIVENESS OF THE TCAs

The tricyclics at doses of 125–150 mg daily or above are effective in the treatment of depressive illness, especially moderate or severe cases. The benefits of these drugs compared with placebo are much less apparent in milder cases (Hamilton Depression Rating Scale score less than 18; Hamilton, 1960). Amitriptyline and imipramine have been studied most extensively, other tricyclics less so. The meta-analyses show that they consistently produce improvements in about 60–70% of patients with depression compared with rates of 20–30% on placebo, in double-blind RCTs. Newer drugs have generally been shown to be superior to placebo before they are marketed. Many, but not all, have been shown to be of equal efficacy to the older drugs in depressive illness, but not necessarily in other diagnostic groups.

TCAs should generally be continued for 6 months after the acute episode has responded, to avoid relapse. Beyond that time they may be continued to prevent recurrences. Amitriptyline and imipramine have been studied extensively, in prophylaxis. Nortriptyline and

dothiepin have been shown effective for this use in the elderly. For maximal effect in preventing relapses or recurrences, the dose should be the same as was effective in the acute episode; lower doses are rather less effective.

Indications

As well as depressive illness, the TCAs are also used to treat anxiety states (e.g. panic disorder), OCD, PTSD, chronic pain, fibromyalgia, premenstrual dysphoria, eating disorders and nocturnal enuresis in children. Clomipramine (the most selective of the TCAs for 5-HT reuptake inhibition) was found especially useful for anxiety states and OCD, as well as for severe depression.

Blood level monitoring

An approximate therapeutic range has been established for amitriptyline, nortriptyline and imipramine. Assays for measuring these are widely available, offering an advantage in cases where there is a poor response, and where a decision is to be taken on whether to increase the dose or to change to a different drug. In the case of nortriptyline, there is evidence of a therapeutic window (50–150 mg/ml), at levels above which the symptoms are liable to worsen.

The most common cause of failure to relieve depressive illness with a drug is to use too small a dose. As long as side-effects are tolerable the dose can be raised. A second cause is impatience: at least 2 weeks' action is needed and the patient must be aware of this.

Choice of drug

The choice of drug for the treatment of depression should be based upon the pattern of symptoms (especially disturbed sleep and weight changes), the patient's physical health and other medication, the likely tolerability of side-effects for the individual patient and whether there is a risk of overdose (see chapter11). In some cases the cost of treatment is also an issue, and cost-effectiveness may need consideration.

AMITRIPTYLINE

Amitriptyline is described in detail as the typical TCA. To avoid tiresome repetition of shared properties, other tricyclics are only briefly described.

Amitriptyline ('Tryptizol', 'Lentizol') may be started in adults with tablets after food, 10 mg or 25 mg twice daily, or simply 25–50 mg at night, since then a separate hypnotic may not be needed. After 2 days the dose can be raised, and raised again as required. A daily dose of 150 mg is quite usual. There will be only little response except improved sleep for about 2 weeks. Some patients will need a dose as high as 250 mg daily to improve (above the *BNF* limit of 150 mg), but compliance should be checked and a blood level measured; an ECG may also be thought advisable.

Individuals differ in their tolerance of side-effects but tolerance usually increases in a few days, which is the reason for starting with

THE DRUGS

low doses and raising by steps. If side-effects continue to be a problem, a different drug should be tried. Where agitation remains poorly controlled, small doses of a phenothiazine such as chlorpromazine may be necessary; alternatively a benzodiazepine may be given during the day, and temazepam or zolpidem at night. However, the benzodiazepine or hypnotic should be withdrawn once the core depressive symptoms begin to respond to the antidepressant; the risk of dependence increases if the first antidepressant fails to lift the depression.

Patients who get indigestion or vomiting with tablets may try syrup instead. Slow-release preparations of amitriptyline have generally no advantage over tablets in similar dose and may be more expensive.

Amitriptyline is a very effective antidepressant. No single drug has been shown superior in efficacy, and several are inferior in severe depression. It may, however, not be as effective as SSRIs in panic disorder or OCD, but it seems to be superior for PTSD and chronic pain.

Antidepressants must be continued for some time after recovery. In general, advise the patient to continue treatment for 6 months after he/she is better. Then reduce the dose in steps. If depressive symptoms begin to return, go back to the original higher dose and try reduction again in another 3 months' time. Do not be in a hurry to stop treatment. After a third attack in 3 years prophylaxis by continuing the TCA is a reasonable line of treatment. Sometimes a lower dose is advised, but this carries a greater risk of recurrence. As an alternative (especially for bipolar disorder) lithium may be given. The decision when to start prophylaxis, and when to stop it, depends on weighing the social consequences of a further depression, its likely severity, the risk of suicide, the side-effects of the drug and the patient's motivation.

A similar approach is used for panic disorder and social phobia. In these it is important to start with a very low dose, as there may be an initial worsening. The dose should be gradually increased to similar levels as for depression.

In children amitriptyline 25 or 50 mg at night reduces the frequency of bedwetting. It is less effective than an electric alarm and should not be used where incontinence has physical illness as its cause (see chapter 18).

Brain damage in children and in adults is no contraindication to tricyclic treatment, and depression after a stroke can respond well to the drugs. Heart damage, however – in particular myocardial infarction – carries some risk of dysrhythmia with a TCA. Another class of drug such as an SSRI may be safer. ECT may also be considered but in most cases is best avoided until at least 12 weeks after the attack. TCAs, in therapeutic dose, are not toxic to the healthy heart, but stabilised treatment for hypertension may be upset.

Side-effects are early (within hours) or delayed (after 2 weeks or more of treatment). The early ones are very common: drowsiness, oversedation, indigestion, dry mouth, constipation, blurring of vision, headache, dizziness, postural hypotension and difficulty in urination. The delayed ones, in order of increasing rarity, are weight gain (lost again when drug is stopped), shaking of limbs (myoclonus), hypomania, grand mal attack, toxic hallucinosis (like that from anticholinergics) and paralytic ileus, which causes acute abdominal pain.

Combined MAOI and TCA therapy for resistant depression is possible, but there is no controlled trial data proving efficacy (see chapter 11). Amitriptyline is available as tablets: 10, 25, 50 mg; capsules: 75 mg; syrup: 10 mg per 5 ml; injection: ampoule of 10 ml contains 10 mg per ml; and sustained-release capsules ('Lentizol'): 25, 50 mg.

NORTRIPTYLINE

The clinical effects are like those of amitriptyline except that nortriptyline ('Allegron', 'Aventyl') has little sedative or hypnotic action and produces less postural hypotension. In fact, amitriptyline is rapidly metabolised in the body to nortriptyline, so it is not surprising if the two seem similar. Doses can be a little lower; 75 mg daily may be enough, producing a plasma concentration of 50–150 mg/ml or about 200–600 mmol/l. It has slight anticholinergic effects.

IMIPRAMINE, DESIPRAMINE AND TRIMIPRAMINE

These are very like amitriptyline. Imipramine ('Tofranil') is less sedative but can otherwise be used in the same way, in the same doses, up to 200 mg daily. Doses up to 300 mg daily are used in the US. Desipramine is the metabolite of imipramine and is less sedative still; it is no longer marketed in the UK. Trimipramine is very sedative, but otherwise has similar properties.

DOTHIEPIN

Dothiepin ('Prothiaden') has only one atom different from amitriptyline (a sulphur bridge in the central ring). It resembles amitriptyline in its sedative and antidepressant effect, but is slightly less potent, so that a minimum of 125 mg daily must be given to have more than a placebo effect in acute depression. It has slightly less anticholinergic side-effects and has been much used for the elderly. However, in overdose it is one of the most cardiotoxic of the TCAs, and is tolerated only a little better than amitriptyline.

CLOMIPRAMINE

Clomipramine ('Anafranil') is the most selective of the TCAs for blocking 5-HT rather than noradrenalin reuptake. It is also anticholinergic, sedative and produces postural hypotension. It is slightly more potent than amitriptyline and the doses should be correspondingly lower, being built up from 10 mg to 75–150 mg daily (elderly 75 mg).

It has been recommended for depression resistant to treatment, and may then also be combined with lithium in a plasma level of 0.5–0.8 mmol/l. Formerly L-tryptophan was included in the combination, but this was temporarily withdrawn because of eosinophilia – myalgia syndrome – and is now available only on a named patient basis. Clomipramine must not be combined with or used within 3 weeks of MAOIs because this would very likely cause a serotonin syndrome.

Clomipramine is available by intramuscular injection and also by intravenous infusion, which should be given only to patients who are unable to take the drug orally.

Clomipramine has also been used with good effect in OCD, and phobic illness, even without accompanying depression. The dose is generally higher than that used in depression, being built up to 100–150 mg daily (maximum 250 mg) over the course of 2 weeks. Many patients with panic disorder tend to experience intensified anxiety during the first few days of treatment, and the dose should therefore be introduced very gradually.

Some experts consider clomipramine to be still the most effective drug for OCD, although for most uses SSRIs have superseded it.

Clomipramine may, particularly at night, provoke a drug-induced delirious psychosis, which disappears within a few days of stopping the drug.

Clomipramine, like other TCAs, is not very suitable for patients with liver damage or cardiac conditions.

LOFEPRAMINE

Lofepramine ('Gamanil') is a TCA that is non-sedative and has less anticholinergic side-effects and less cardiotoxicity than other TCAs. It is metabolised to desipramine. It can produce hypotension, constipation and tachycardia. Among the tricyclics this is the safest in overdose. Jaundice may develop in the first 8 weeks but is reversible on discontinuing the drug.

The usual dose starts with 70 mg, increasing to 210 mg daily depending upon response. It is available as tablets, 70 mg.

Other related drugs are protriptyline ('Concordin'); doxepin ('Sinequan'); iprindole ('Prondol'); viloxazine ('Vivalan'); and amoxapine ('Asendis').

Drug combinations

These proprietary preparations are listed for information only – we do not recommend them.

Motival: nortriptyline 10 mg plus fluphenazine 0.5mg (Motipress is similar, three times stronger); triptafen DA: amitriptyline 25 mg plus perphenazine 2 mg; and triptafen-M(inor): amitriptyline 10 mg plus perphenazine 2 mg.

FURTHER READING

Cardiac Arrhythmia Suppression Trial (CAST) Investigators (1989) Preliminary report: effect of encainide and flecainide on mortality in a randomized trial of arrhythmia suppression after myocardial infarction. *New England Journal of Medicine*, **321**, 406–412.

Hamilton, M. (1960) A rating scale for depression. *Journal of Neurology, Neurosurgery and Psychiatry*, **23**, 56–62.

Henry, J. (1997) Fatal toxicity index. *Drug Safety*, **16**, 374–390.

Leonard, B. & Richelson, E. (2000) Synaptic effects of antidepressants: relationship to their therapeutic and adverse effects. In *Schizophrenia and Mood Disorders: The New Drug Therapies in Clinical Practice*, pp. 67–84. Oxford: Butterworth Heinemann.

Lipsey, J. R., Robinson, R. G., Pearlson, G. D., *et al* (1984) Nortriptyline treatment of post-stroke depression: a double-blind study. *Lancet*, **i**, 297–300.

Page, C. P., Curtis, M. J., Sutter, M. C., *et al* (1997) *Integrated Pharmacology*. London: Mosby.

Ruskin, J. (1989) The cardiac arrhythmia suppression trial (CAST). *New England Journal of Medicine*, **321**, 386–388.

Task Force of the Working Group on Arrhythmias of the European Society of Cardiology. The Sicilian gambit: A new approach to the classification of antiarrhythmic drugs based on their actions on arrhythmogenic mechanisms. *Circulation*, **84**, 1831–1851.

Virchner, V., Silver, L. F. & Kelly, C. A. (1998) SIADH. *Journal of Psychopharmacology*, **12**, 396–400.

THE DRUGS

The five drugs available are fluvoxamine ('Faverin'), fluoxetine ('Prozac'), paroxetine ('Seroxat'), sertraline ('Lustral'), and citalopram ('Cipramil'). They are called selective serotonin reuptake inhibitors because their most potent pharmacological action is inhibition of the reuptake of serotonin and this action occurs at concentrations much lower than those that inhibit the reuptake of the other transmitters noradrenalin and dopamine, and because they are relatively lacking in blocking activity at the receptors for neurotransmitters. Table 25.1 lists the reuptake inhibitors according to their selectivity for 5-HT in comparison to noradrenalin and dopamine, and in binding the transmitter receptors in biochemical tests in human tissue *in vitro*; the TCA clomipramine is included for comparison.

Fluoxetine is known to have a metabolite that is active as a reuptake inhibitor, norfluoxetine, and this has selectivity and probably antidepressant activity similar to fluoxetine itself. Citalopram has two active metabolites, both selective for serotonin. Citalopram is the most selective of the SSRIs, and fluoxetine the least. Sertraline is unusual in having a lower selectivity than the others for serotonin in comparison to dopamine reuptake, raising the possibility of clinically significant dopamine reuptake inhibition, especially at higher doses.

Pharmacokinetics

The drugs differ in their pharmacokinetics (see Box 25.1). Fluoxetine has the longest elimination half-life (2–3 days) and its active metabolite

Table 25.1 Affinities of SSRIs for reuptake sites and receptors of human brain (clomipramine for comparison)

Drug	NRI	SRI	DRI	H-1	ACh-M	NA α-1	NA α-2	5-HT-2A
Clomipramine	3	360	0.05	3	3	3	0.03	4
Citalopram	0.03	86	0.004	0.2	0.05	0.05	0.007	0.04
Fluoxetine	0.4	120	0.03	0.02	0.05	0.02	0.008	0.5
Fluvoxamine	0.08	45	0.01	0.0009	0.0004	0.01	0.007	0.02
Paroxetine	2.5	800	0.2	0.005	0.9	0	0.006	0.005
Sertraline	0.2	340	4	0.004	0.2	0.3	0.03	0.01

NRI, noradrenalin reuptake inhibition; SRI, serotonin reuptake inhibition; DRI, dopamine reuptake inhibition; H$_1$, histamine receptor; ACh-M, acetylcholine muscarinic receptor; NA α-1, noradrenalin α-1; NA α-2, noradrenalin α-2, 5-HT-2A, serotonin 2A.

Affinity is expressed as $1/10^7 \times Kd$, where Kd is equilibrium dissociation constant in molarity. Thus, higher numbers indicate greater strength of that action. Ratios of different figures in the rows show how many times more potent the drug is in the two actions.

Adapted from Leonard & Richelson (2000).

Box 25.1 Selective serotonin reuptake inhibitor half-lives

Drug	Half-life
Fluoxetine	5 days
Norfluoxetine	15 days (longer in elderly)
Citalopram	33 hours (longer in elderly)
Sertraline	26 hours
Paroxetine	10 hours acute; 21 hours chronic
Fluvoxamine	10 hours acute; 16 hours chronic

---

norfluoxetine has a half-life of 7–9 days. The elimination half-lives of fluvoxamine, paroxetine and sertraline range from 15 to 30 hours. Thus steady-state plasma levels are reached after about 5–7 days with them, but only after 4–6 weeks with fluoxetine.

Other pharmacological actions

These drugs are largely devoid of receptor blocking actions. However, paroxetine does have weak anticholinergic properties (at the M_3 receptor in glandular tissue, smooth muscle and brain), and both sertraline and citalopram have anticholinergic side-effects (mainly dry mouth) clinically, though the mechanism is unknown.

Fluoxetine has direct agonist activity at 5-HT-2C receptors that may be relevant to its effects causing anxiety and lowering appetite.

NO synthetase is inhibited by paroxetine, an action that might contribute to erectile dysfunction (see chapter 22).

Prolactin levels are slightly raised by paroxetine and citalopram, but not by sertraline.

MODE OF ACTION

By binding to the serotonin transporter (SERT, see p. 75) these drugs block the reuptake of released 5-HT, and thus tend to increase the concentration of 5-HT at its receptors, which are both post-synaptic and presynaptic. The receptors are of several types (see chapter 7). The antidepressant and anxiolytic activity is thought to be mediated mainly by subtypes of the 5-HT-1 receptor, but side-effects arise from stimulation of 5-HT-2 (insomnia, agitation and sexual dysfunction) and 5-HT-3 (nausea, headaches). Initially the increased levels of 5-HT act on presynaptic autoreceptors. This action on 5-HT-1A autoreceptors on the cell body and dendrites reduces the electrical firing of the cells; the action on 5-HT-1D autoreceptors at the nerve terminals reduces the release of the transmitter. However, over time adaptive processes occur, which restore the cell firing. These include desensitisation and downregulation of the somato-dendritic 5-HT-1A receptors and possibly of the terminal 5-HT-1D receptors. This leads to a recovery of the release of 5-HT and a further increase in extracellular concentrations of 5-HT. Thus, soon after commencing SSRI treatment, the concentration of 5-HT in the synaptic cleft may be increased twofold, but over the course of 2 weeks it may be increased sixfold.

THE DRUGS

The view that the antidepressant effects of SSRIs result from enhancement of 5-HT function is supported by the results of studies in which patients were depleted of brain 5-HT, by taking an amino acid drink low in L-tryptophan. This has the effect within 2 hours of causing a relapse of depressive symptoms in patients with depression who have recently remitted while taking an SSRI (but less so in those treated with desipramine).

A possible strategy to accelerate and to enhance antidepressant action with SSRIs would be to prevent the initial feedback inhibition by blocking the presynaptic autoreceptors with a 5-HT-1A antagonist. The beta-blocker pindolol has 5-HT-1A antagonist properties and has been tried in combination with SSRIs, particularly paroxetine. Controlled trials suggest that it does accelerate the antidepressant effect of SSRIs (see p. 379).

SSRIs – INDICATIONS FOR THEIR USE

The main diagnoses for which SSRIs are indicated are depressive illness, panic disorder, OCD and bulimia nervosa. They may also be effective in dysthymia, PTSD, premenstrual dysphoria, binge eating disorder and in some cases of body dysmorphic disorder. All SSRIs may not be equally effective in all conditions.

Acute depression

The treatment of moderately severe depressive illness is the prime indication for SSRIs. As a guide to severity, patients with a score of more than 20 on the 21-item Hamilton Depression Rating Scale (Hamilton, 1960) will generally show improvement compared with placebo, which is significant after 1–2 weeks. In milder depressive disorders, SSRIs have little advantage over placebo, although they might be considered if there is no response to supportive non-specific measures.

For those with more severe depression, and those who have melancholic or psychotic depressions (see chapter 11), an SSRI may be less effective than an antidepressant with a broader spectrum of pharmacological actions, such as amitriptyline or higher doses of the SNRI venlafaxine.

Between SSRIs there is no evidence for superior efficacy of a particular drug in depressive illness as a whole, except that some prescribers find fluvoxamine less useful, being less well tolerated than the other SSRIs in depression. Fluoxetine is sometimes found to have a slower onset of action than other antidepressants, but this is probably because its long half-life means that 1–2 weeks must pass before steady-state therapeutic plasma level is reached.

Dosage

For fluoxetine, dose-ranging studies have found no greater rates of improvement with doses exceeding 20 mg per day, but the incidence of side-effects increases sharply. For patients who have improved a little after 3 weeks, there may occasionally be improvement following an increase in dose, but there are better alternative strategies for refractory depression (see chapter 11).

Likewise, for sertraline a daily dose of 50 mg is sufficient for most patients, though higher doses are often used. The dose is less certainly defined for paroxetine, though 20 mg per day is usually as effective as higher doses. With citalopram the starting dose of 20 mg needs generally to be increased to 40 mg per day, although 20 mg is sufficient for most elderly patients. The dose range for fluvoxamine is more uncertain, with evidence that a dose as low as 25 mg may be sufficient in some patients, but higher doses often being used and being associated with more frequent side-effects than other SSRIs.

Continuation treatment of depression (relapse prevention)

For continuation treatment (for 6 months after remission), sertraline, paroxetine, citalopram and fluoxetine are effective, if continued in the same dose as for acute therapy. Reduced doses may be better tolerated but tend to be somewhat less effective. Hence the maxim is 'the dose that gets you well, keeps you well'. The drugs seem equally effective at preventing relapses.

Maintenance treatment (prophylaxis against recurrence)

The return of depressive illness more than 6 months after the episode has remitted is regarded as a recurrence rather than relapse (see chapter 11). Fluoxetine, paroxetine, citalopram and sertraline are effective in preventing recurrences. However, most studies of antidepressants in this context are flawed by the possibility of depressive recurrences being triggered in the placebo group by abrupt discontinuation of the previous treatment.

Tolerance to SSRIs

Cases have been reported of apparent loss of efficacy with fluoxetine and other SSRIs during long-term treatment. In some cases the improvement is restored by an increase in dose. In others, however, the problem may result from accumulation of high levels of the SSRI, and these should improve when the dose is reduced. It is speculated that excessive serotonin may suppress dopamine release, and thereby cause lethargy or loss of drive, in addition to anxiety.

Subtypes of depression

Melancholia and severe depression

In severe depression with scores of 30 or more using the 21-item Hamilton Depression Rating Scale, or in melancholia, fluoxetine, paroxetine and citalopram have been found less effective than broader-acting drugs such as the TCAs amitriptyline or clomipramine, or the SNRI venlafaxine.

Psychotic depression

TCAs in combination with antipsychotics are usually superior to TCAs alone; SSRIs can be of some limited use.

THE DRUGS

Depression with prominent anxiety

In general, depressed patients with high levels of agitation or anxiety do not show definite differences between SSRIs in their responses. In agitated depression fluoxetine may be less useful.

Depression with insomnia

Patients with depression often have reduced REM latency, increased REM sleep and poor sleep continuity, with increased waking and early morning waking. The SSRIs, like the TCAs and MAOIs, suppress REM sleep. They also affect sleep continuity, reducing total sleep time, with frequent brief awakenings during non-REM sleep. Daytime drowsiness may reflect less efficient sleep with these drugs. It is greatest with paroxetine.

Depressive illness in children

A study of fluoxetine in children and adolescents with depression is the first placebo-controlled trial to demonstrate the efficacy of any antidepressant drug in this age group (see Table 25.2). Perhaps surprisingly, TCAs have never been proven efficacious in a controlled trial in children (see chapter 18).

Depression in the elderly

All antidepressant classes appear of similar efficacy in older people. The improvement is less robust, perhaps because older patients require longer to respond to acute antidepressant treatment. The SSRIs generally do not impair cognition, lacking anticholinergic and anti-histamine actions. In the context of clinical trials, withdrawal rates are only slightly lower with SSRIs than with tricyclics. Higher NNTs have been reported for fluoxetine and for moclobemide. It is, however, more difficult in older subjects to extrapolate from clinical trials to clinical practice because many patients (the very old and the physically infirm) are excluded from trials. Case note review in primary care suggests that older patients are significantly less likely to have contraindications or serious side-effects to SSRIs than to TCAs.

Atypical depression

Like classical MAOIs, fluoxetine and sertraline are effective.

Bipolar depression

Both paroxetine and fluoxetine have been shown effective in at least a proportion of patients. The number switching into mania appears to be less with these drugs than with TCAs, on which about 10% of bipolar depressives switch. However, some individuals are very sensitive to switching when treated with SSRIs.

Depression in seasonal affective disorder; dysthymia

Fluoxetine and sertraline are both effective in winter depression in seasonal affective disorder (SAD), and during 3–6 months treatment

Table 25.2 Effects of selective serotonin reuptake inhibitors in depression and related conditions

Diagnosis	Drug	Duration	Criterion	Drug–placebo (%)	NNT	Reference
Depression (adult)	Fluoxetine	8 weeks	50% reduction in HRS	25	4	Stark & Hardison, 1985
Depression (child)	Fluoxetine	8 weeks	Much improved or very much improved (CGI)	23	4.3	Emslie et al, 1997
			Complete remission	8	12.5	Emslie et al, 1997
Seasonal affective disorder	Fluoxetine	5 weeks	50% reduction in HRS	25	4	Lam et al, 1995
Prevention of depression	Fluoxetine	1 year	No relapse or recurrence	31	3.2	Montgomery, 1989
	Sertraline	1 year	No relapse or recurrence	33	3	Doogan & Caillard, 1992
	Paroxetine	1 year	No relapse or recurrence	27	3.7	Montgomery & Dunbar, 1993
Dysthymia	Fluoxetine	3 months	50% reduction in HRS and CGI much or very much improved	22.5	4.5	Vanelle et al, 1997
PTSD (civilian)	Fluoxetine	12 weeks	Much improved or very much improved (CGI)	23	4.3	Davidson et al, 1997

NNT, numbers needed to treat; HRS, Hamilton Depression Rating Scale; CGI, clinical global impression; PTSD, post-traumatic stress disorder.

in dysthymia (see Table 25.2). TCAs may also be effective but are less well tolerated.

Brief recurrent depression

Fluoxetine and other SSRIs have not been proved to be effective.

Other conditions

PTSD

Short-term efficacy has been demonstrated for paroxetine and fluoxetine. However, the benefits appear somewhat less than from older TCAs (see chapter 20).

Premenstrual dysphoric disorder

Short-term efficacy has been demonstrated for fluoxetine 20 mg daily, and sertraline 50 mg daily. Improvement is felt within the first cycle and some benefit is observed even if dosing is limited to the 1-week luteal phase, before symptoms are expected.

Analgesic effects

SSRIs have generally proved less effective than TCAs, such as amitriptyline, as adjuncts to pain relief in conditions including neurogenic pain, fibromyalgia and diabetic neuropathy.

Panic disorder and social phobia

The second main indication for SSRIs is panic disorder, and this use is discussed in chapter 15.

OCD, Tourette's syndrome and body dysmorphic disorder

These uses of SSRIs are also discussed in chapter 15.

Bulimia nervosa, binge eating disorder and anorexia nervosa

The use of SSRIs in these conditions is discussed in chapter 23.

EFFECT SIZE AND RELIABILITY

The magnitude of the effect of treatment varies between indications (see Table 25.2 and chapters 15 and 23).

Complete remission as a result of treatment is unusual in all conditions, but in general the benefits of treatment are greater for depression and panic disorder than for bulimia; and although the benefit is reliable in OCD, it is relatively small. The effect in preventing recurrences of depression is one of the most robust, with a small NNT.

SIDE-EFFECTS OF SSRIs

The drug that has been the most widely studied is fluoxetine. Those side-effects that occur with a 5% greater incidence than on placebo,

Box 25.2 Side-effects of fluoxetine

Over 5% incidence above placebo	Less common
Nausea (10–30%)	Headache
Anorexia (7%)	Increased sweating
Insomnia (7%)	Akathisia
Nervousness (7%)	Dystonia
Fine tremor (10%)	Parkinsonism
Drowsiness (6%)	Rash/allergy/vasculitis
Diarrhoea (5%)	Inappropriate ADH secretion
Sexual dysfunction	Prolonged seizures in ECT
loss of libido	Bradycardia
erectile/lubrication	Yawning, spontaneous orgasm
orgasm/ejaculation	Psychiatric reactions – mania, psychosis

ADH, antidiuretic hormone; ECT, electroconvulsive therapy.

and those less common are listed in Box 25.2. The frequencies are only a rough guide.

Nausea, nervousness, insomnia and diarrhoea tend to subside with time, as does headache. Increased sweating may also occur.

Sexual side-effects include loss of libido, as well as erectile impotence and ejaculatory failure in men, and reduced lubrication and anorgasmia in women. A rare occurrence is the experience of repetitive yawning combined with spontaneous orgasmic feelings.

A fine tremor is a relatively common side-effect, but true EPS are less common.

The extent to which these side-effects are clinically significant can be gauged from the resulting drop-out rates in clinical trials. These are about 15% with fluoxetine, compared to 5% on placebo. Although the side-effect profile is less extensive than with TCAs (less sedation, hypotension, weight gain and anticholinergic effects), the drop-out rates with older TCAs in usual doses are only marginally higher at about 20%. Particular TCAs have lower drop-out rates, for instance lofepramine.

The possibility that fluoxetine may increase aggression or suicidality has been extensively scrutinised since the first reports. In general, placebo-controlled studies show aggressive feelings and impulses declining during treatment. However, in a small minority of patients, aggressive or suicidal thoughts linked to akathisia have occurred and reoccurred when the drug was reintroduced to the patient.

Fluoxetine may cause bradycardia, but no measurable effect on cardiac conduction in patients. Inappropriate antidiuretic hormone (ADH) secretion occurs more commonly in the elderly. Prolonged seizures during ECT are discussed in chapter 40.

Differences in side-effects between individual SSRIs

All the SSRIs have high rates of initial nausea, especially fluvoxamine.

Fluoxetine is associated with higher rates of nervousness, anorexia and headaches. Sertraline is associated with high rates of diarrhoea, dry mouth and ejaculatory abnormalities. Paroxetine is associated with

THE DRUGS

Box 25.3 Pattern of adverse effects of selective serotonin reuptake inhibitors (SSRIs)

Symptoms	Comments
Nausea	Common at first with all SSRIs, especially fluvoxamine, less so if taken with food
Anxiety/nervousness	More common and persistent with fluoxetine
Headaches	Common at first with fluoxetine (5%)
Dry mouth	More common with paroxetine, sertraline and citalopram
Somnolence	More common with paroxetine, fluvoxamine and citalopram
Diarrhoea	More common with sertraline
Reduced appetite	Mainly fluoxetine
Orgasmic/ejaculatory problems	More common with paroxetine and sertraline
Dystonia, Parkinsonism	More common with paroxetine; least common with sertraline

high rates of drowsiness, dizziness, constipation, urinary slowing, sweating, sexual side-effects and dystonia. Citalopram is relatively well-tolerated but produces nausea, somnolence and dry mouth.

Overall, the SSRIs show similar levels of acceptability, with the exception of fluvoxamine, which is more likely to be discontinued because of side-effects, mainly nausea, insomnia and drowsiness. The pattern is shown in Box 25.3.

Gastrointestinal side-effects

The anticholinergic property of paroxetine makes it more likely to cause constipation and less likely to cause diarrhoea than the other SSRIs.

Psychiatric side-effects

Anxiety, agitation and insomnia are more commonly reported with fluoxetine than with other SSRIs, but these are dose-dependent and occur more often with higher doses of the other drugs. Depersonalisation can also occur.

Weight changes

A recovery in body weight is traditionally viewed as an early sign of clinical improvement in depression. However, with TCAs some patients develop excessive weight, associated with carbohydrate craving. Weight gain is the most common reason for discontinuing long-term treatment with TCAs.

Both paroxetine and citalopram lead to weight gain, but only as depression improves. Citalopram may also cause carbohydrate craving. By contrast, fluoxetine tends to produce weight loss, although this anorexiant effect seems to wane after 6 months of treatment. Patients on sertraline gain less weight than those on paroxetine, but more than those on fluoxetine.

Sexual dysfunction

Sexual dysfunction is part of depressive illness, making the side-effects more difficult to recognise in depression than in panic disorder and OCD. Few trials have investigated this thoroughly.

Women with depression tend to report more frequent sexual dysfunction than men do, although this improves early during treatment with SSRIs. For patients with depression who continue on SSRIs there is an overall improvement of ratings of sexual function as their depression improves.

Reduction in libido may occur to a similar extent with all the SSRIs, but paroxetine is associated with higher rates of erectile and orgasmic problems. For instance, it had an overall placebo-adjusted rate of sexual side-effects of more than 20% in men, with figures of 8% for loss of libido, 7% for erectile impotence and 20% for ejaculatory problems, in patients with panic disorder or OCD. In women with panic disorder the rate of anorgasmia owing to paroxetine was about 8%. These effects were dose-related and lower figures occurred with a 20 mg dose.

Patients with pre-existing premature ejaculation tend to be content with the outcome, as do their partners, and SSRIs have been suggested for this indication.

Effects on cognitive function

The drowsiness reported by some patients on SSRIs does not appear to be associated with measurable evidence of psychomotor impairment in normal volunteers, such as might interfere with the ability to drive or operate machinery, except with high doses of paroxetine.

Cognitive impairment occurs in major depression and is particularly important in the elderly, who may already have cognitive deficits, as a result of ageing. Cognitive function tends to improve as patients respond to treatment, even using antidepressants with anticholinergic effects. However, in both elderly volunteers and older patients with depression, little cognitive impairment is seen with SSRIs, but significant impairment with TCAs.

EPS

Pattern and frequency

Akathisia appears as restlessness, irritability and dysphoria, which can be accompanied, in patients with depression, by increased suicidal ideation. It is underdiagnosed and may be mistaken for agitated depression. It may appear as jitteriness during the early stages of treatment in anxious patients, with reports of inner shakiness and insomnia.

SSRIs may cause acute dystonia or Parkinsonism. These are rare side-effects occurring in less than 1% of patients but are ones about which they should be warned.

The possible development of tardive dyskinesia has also been recorded during long-term treatment with SSRIs.

THE DRUGS

Pathogenesis

Serotonin interacts with dopamine pathways, tending to reduce dopamine release. In the nigro-striatal dopamine pathway, this may account for Parkinsonism and dystonia. In the meso-cortical pathway, it may account for akathisia, although increased noradrenalin acting on beta-receptors has also been suggested. There is also serotonin innervation of the motor neurons, in the brain stem and spinal cord, as well as the primary motor areas of the cortex, and the drugs may act there.

Predisposing factors

Recent or current treatment with a dopamine blocker such as an antipsychotic or metoclopramide increases the likelihood of developing EPS with SSRIs. A previous brain injury, for instance by stroke, also increases the risk and patients with incipient Parkinson's disease are also vulnerable. However, depression occurring as part of Parkinson's disease often responds well to SSRIs. Although antipsychotic drugs or lithium may increase the risk of EPS with SSRIs, these drugs can usually be combined effectively without such an interaction.

Differences between individual SSRIs

Dystonia has been most commonly reported with paroxetine. Akathisia seems to occur most frequently with fluoxetine; this drug differs from the others in being an agonist at 5-HT-2C receptors, stimulation of which can lead to anxiety and depersonalisation, as well as reduced appetite.

EPS with other antidepressants

Parkinsonism, dystonia and akathisia have been reported, less commonly, with the TCAs, MAOIs, bupropion, nefazodone, carbamazepine and lithium. They have also been reported during withdrawal from antidepressants, particularly SSRIs.

Management

These EPS can be reduced or avoided by using lower doses of SSRIs. Cessation and a change to a different drug should be the first action, but the addition of an anticholinergic drug can help symptomatically for dystonia; and for akathisia the beta-blocker propranolol or switching to a 5-HT-2 antagonist such as nefazodone or mirtazapine may be helpful. Benzodiazepines may relieve akathisia but are only suitable for short-term use.

Cardiovascular side-effects

Bradycardia may occur with other SSRIs as well as fluoxetine, but their general lack of anticholinergic or noradrenalin α-1 blocking properties is favourable, as is the lack of membrane-stabilising actions, in therapeutic doses.

Box 25.4 Four main groups of withdrawal symptoms of selective serotonin reuptake inhibitors

(1) Dizziness and vertigo
(2) Headaches, nausea, fatigue and 'flu-like symptoms
(3) Nervousness and insomnia
(4) Paraesthesiae and electric shock feelings

Withdrawl reactions with SSRIs

The SSRI withdrawal syndrome can develop after 5 weeks or more of treatment. Box 25.4 shows the four main groups of symptoms.

The syndrome is most common with the drugs with the shortest half-life, paroxetine and fluvoxamine, occurring in almost everyone, and 20% of patients experience more than one symptom. It is less common with fluoxetine, probably because of its slower metabolism.

The symptoms begin about 2 days after stopping paroxetine and last for 10 days. The most common symptoms are dizziness, paraesthesiae (electric feelings), nausea and fatigue – 'Seroxat flu' – which can develop, for instance, over a weekend if the drug is forgotten. Anxiety and mood changes are also frequently observed. Slow tapering of the dose, over more than 2 weeks, is necessary to avoid the problem. The symptoms are usually mild, but reintroduction of an SSRI will reverse them. A single dose of fluoxetine may be sufficient to relieve the problem, but symptoms may persist.

Toxicity and idiosyncratic reactions

Compared with other antidepressants, most of the SSRIs are extremely safe in overdose taken alone. Citalopram is the exception; convulsions and ECG abnormalities with widened QRS complexes occur in a third of overdoses of more than 600 mg and deaths have occurred. A metabolite, didemethylcitalopram, may be responsible.

With fluoxetine, an urticarial rash may appear after 2–3 weeks, associated with vasculitis and leading to arthralgia, lymphadenopathy and fever, a serum sickness-like condition. The drug must be stopped in such cases. Dyspnoea with fluoxetine may indicate the development of a rare pulmonary inflammation.

The control of diabetes may be altered by fluoxetine, lowering glucose levels.

The SSRIs should not be combined with MAOIs, because a dangerous serotonin syndrome is likely to result (see p. 87). An interval of 2 weeks should elapse between the use of fluvoxamine, paroxetine or sertraline and an MAOI; with fluoxetine there should be an interval of 5 weeks before an MAOI is commenced. Likewise the drugs should not be given until at least 2 weeks have elapsed after an MAOI has been stopped, except for moclobemide, which is usually eliminated within a day.

USE OF SSRIs IN PREGNANCY

The large database on fluoxetine shows that taken in the first trimester it is not associated with spontaneous abortion or major congenital abnormalities. Taken in the third trimester there is an increased risk of premature delivery, but the influence of depression, smoking and alcohol may account for this. No developmental complications at the pre-school stage were detected in children whose mothers had fluoxetine or TCAs during pregnancy. Babies breastfed by mothers on fluoxetine have drug levels of less than 10% of those of the mother, whereas during pregnancy the foetus receives the same dose as the mother – indicating the drug is safe in breastfeeding.

There is also a large database supporting the safety of fluvoxamine in pregnancy.

SSRI interactions

All SSRIs are metabolised in the liver and have the potential to affect the normal function of the hepatic cytochrome P450 enzymes (CYP) that are responsible for the metabolism of other drugs. In general, SSRIs are enzyme inhibitors; that is, they are able to decrease the functioning of certain cytochromes (see Box 25.5).

In doing this, they may slow the metabolism of other drugs and elevate their plasma levels. In many cases such alterations are clinically unimportant, but a few interactions are dangerous and a very few are potentially fatal.

Fluvoxamine is a potent inhibitor of CYP IA2, and a moderate inhibitor of CYP IIIA4. Inhibition of CYP IA2 can drastically increase plasma levels of clozapine, theophylline and some TCAs and so cause severe adverse effects. Inhibition of CYP IIIA4 by fluvoxamine may increase levels of co-administered alprazolam (drowsiness may result), as well as cisapride and terfenadine, drugs that may adversely affect cardiac rhythm. Norfluoxetine is similar in its effect on CYP IIIA4. Other drugs to be used cautiously with fluvoxamine are propranolol and phenytoin.

All SSRIs can inhibit CYP IID6, the enzyme most commonly involved in drug metabolism, usually as a hydroxylase. Fluoxetine and paroxetine

---

Box 25.5 Selective serotonin reuptake inhibitors (SSRIs) – cytochrome inhibition

Cytochrome	Substrate examples	Antidepressant inhibitors
CYP IA2	Theophylline, clozapine, R-warfarin	Fluvoxamine
CYP IID6	Quinidine, TCAs, opiates, antipsychotics (many others)	Fluoxetine, paroxetine, sertraline (weak)
CYP IIC9	S-warfarin	Fluvoxamine, fluoxetine, sertraline
CYP IIIA4	Carbamazepine, cisapride, terfenadine, alprazolam	Fluvoxamine, norfluoxetine

are the most potent inhibitors, sertraline is a moderate inhibitor and fluvoxamine and citalopram have virtually no effect at normal clinical doses. Potential interactions are numerous, but few are clinically important. Plasma levels of TCAs can be increased by more than 100% and this interaction is potentially fatal if high doses of TCAs are being given. Blood levels of phenothiazines can be increased but not markedly. Other drugs to be used with caution include carbamazepine, phenytoin, the anti-arrhythmics flecainide and encainide, and vinblastine.

SSRIs also interact with warfarin, although the mechanism is far from clear. Inhibition of CYP IIC9 may be involved, but pharmacodynamic mechanisms are also possible. The effect is unpredictable, but there are several reports of prolongation of clotting times.

Sertraline is 98% bound to plasma proteins and there may be interactions with other drugs that are highly protein bound, such as tolbutamide.

Pharmaco-economics

A few studies have addressed the economic outcome of prescribing SSRIs. However, pharmaco-economic trial methods are considerably less robust than those of clinical efficacy trials, and so results are variable and difficult to interpret. At present the only clear observation of note is that a consideration only of the purchase price of an antidepressant is inappropriate.

FURTHER READING

Reviews

DeVane, C. L. (1995) Comparative safety and tolerability of selective serotonin reuptake inhibitors. *Human Psychopharmacology*, **10**, S185–S193.

Edwards, J. G. & Anderson, I. (1999) Systematic review and guide to selection of selective serotonin reuptake inhibitors. *Drugs*, **57**, 507–533.

Nutt, D. J. (ed.) (1998) Selective serotonin reuptake inhibitors in depression: a decade of progress. *Journal of Psychopharmacology*, **12**(Suppl. B).

Pharmacodynamics

Sargent, P. A., Williamson, D. J. & Cowen, P. J. (1998) Brain 5-HT neurotransmission during paroxetine treatment. *British Journal of Psychiatry*, **172**, 49–52.

Smith, K. A., Fairburn, C. G. & Cowen, P. J. (1997) Relapse of depression after rapid depletion of tryptophan. *Lancet*, **349**, 915–919.

Normal subjects

Knutson. B, Wolkowitz, O. M., Cole, S. W., *et al* (1998) Selective alteration of personality and social behaviour by serotonergic intervention. *American Journal of Psychiatry*, **155**, 373–379.

Therapeutic uses

Mittman, N., Herrmann, T. R., Einason, V. O., *et al* (1997) The efficacy, safety and tolerability of antidepressants in late-life depression: a meta-analysis. *Journal of Affective Disorders*, **46**, 191–217.

Smith, A. J. (1998) The analgesic effects of selective serotonin reuptake inhibitors. *Journal of Psychopharmacology*, **12**, 407–413.

THE DRUGS

Verkes, R. J., Van der Mast, R. C., Hengeveld, M. W., *et al* (1998) Reduction by paroxetine
of suicidal behaviour in patients with repeated suicide attempts but not major
depression. *American Journal of Psychiatry*, **155**, 543–547.

Side-effects

Lane, R. M (1998) SSRI-induced extra pyramidal side effects and akathisia: implications
for treatment. *Journal of Psychopharmacology*, **12**, 192–214.

Studies quoted

Davidson, J. R; Malik, M. L. & Sutherland, S. N. (1997) Response characteristics to
antidepressants and placebo in post-traumatic stress disorder. *International Clinical
Psychopharmacology*, **12**, 291–296.
Doogan, D. P. & Caillard, V. (1992) Sertraline in the prevention of depression. *British
Journal of Psychiatry*, **160**, 217–222.
Emslie, G. J., Rush, A. J., Weinberg, W. A., *et al* (1997) A double-blind, randomized,
placebo-controlled trial of fluoxetine in children and adolescents with depression.
Archives of General Psychiatry, **54**, 1031–1037.
Lam, R. W., Gorman, C. P., Michalon, M., *et al* (1995)Multicenter, placebo-controlled
study of fluoxetine in seasonal affective disorder. *Americal Journal of Psychiatry*,
152, 1765–1770.
Leonard, B. & Richelson, E. (2000) Synaptic effects of antidepressants: relationship to
their therapeutic and adverse effects. In *Schizophrenia and Mood Disorders: The
New Drug Therapies in Clinical Practice*, pp. 67–84. Oxford: Butterworth Heinemann.
Montgomery, S. A. (1989) The efficacy of fluoxetine as an antidepressant in the short
and long term. *International Clinical Psychopharmacology*, **4** (Suppl 1), 113–119.
—— & Dunbar, G. (1993) Paroxetine is better than placebo in relapse prevention and
the prophylaxis of recurrent depression. *International Clinical Psychopharmacology*,
8, 189–195
Stark, P & Hardison, C. D. (1985) A review of multicenter controlled studies of of
fluoxetine *vs* imipramine and placebo in outpatients with major depressive disorder.
Journal of Clinical Psychiatry, **51**, 559–567.
Vanelle, J.-M., Attar-Levy, D., Poirier, M.-F., *et al* (1997) Controlled efficacy study of
fluoxetine in dysthymia. *British Journal of Psychiatry*, **170**, 345–350.

Rating scale quoted

Hamilton, M. (1960) A rating scale for depression. *Journal of Neurology, Neurosurgery
and Psychiatry*, **23**, 56–62.

NORADRENALIN REUPTAKE INHIBITORS

Of the older TCAs the most selective for inhibition of noradrenalin as opposed to 5-HT or dopamine reuptake was desipramine (with a ratio of about 240 for noradrenalin: 5-HT). The drugs now called noradrenalin reuptake inhibitors (NRIs) are devoid of the receptor-blocking actions of the TCAs, at H_1, acetylcholine-M, and noradrenalin-α-1 receptors. They should also lack membrane-stabilising activity. The first drug to be described as an NRI was reboxetine. However, the older tetracyclic drug maprotiline can be included in this category.

Mechanisms of action

Their primary pharmacological action of the NRIs is to inhibit noradrenalin reuptake and thereby increase the concentration of noradrenalin in the synaptic cleft, and increase the stimulation of noradrenalin α-1, noradrenalin α-2 and noradrenalin-β receptors. The action at pre-synaptic (α-2) autoreceptors tends to reduce noradrenalin cell firing (e.g. in the locus coeruleus), thereby reducing the release of noradrenalin. However, over several days, downregulation occurs in α- and β-receptors. The reduction in sensitivity of pre-synaptic auto-receptors tends to restore noradrenalin release, while the downregulation of postsynaptic β-receptors tends to reduce the post-synaptic response. Overall the level of transmission (which can be judged, for instance by nocturnal melatonin secretion from the pineal gland), is increased.

Noradrenalin is thought to be important in reward-driven behaviour (via the ventral noradrenergic bundle) and in arousal (via the locus coeruleus) (see chapter 7).

The view that enhanced noradrenalin function is important in the recovery of depressive illness using non-specific MARIs (such as the TCAs) is supported by findings with interventions designed to lower brain noradrenalin function acutely. The administration of α-methyl para-tyrosine, which inhibits tyrosine hydroxylase, lowers brain noradrenalin levels. This intervention leads to a relapse of depressive symptoms in patients who have improved on desipramine, though not in those who have improved on SSRIs.

Noradrenalin may be more involved in the symptoms of anergia, fatigue and loss of drive in depression, and 5-HT may be more involved in the alteration in subjective mood and anxiety, but there is as yet no consistent evidence that a particular clinical pattern of depressive illness is more likely to benefit from an NRI than from an SSRI.

A theoretical rationale does exist for using an NRI as augmentation in patients who have responded only partially to an SSRI, although this is not yet supported by clinical data. This strategy would appear preferable to, for instance, increasing the dose of an SNRI, which would lead to unnecessarily high levels of inhibition of serotonin reuptake, with a consequent increase in side-effects.

Maprotiline

This is a tetracyclic antidepressant, closely related in structure to the TCAs. Interestingly, it is not effective in panic disorder. Its use is also limited because it has a greater tendency than other antidepressants to lower the seizure threshold and to cause fits.

Reboxetine

Structure and mechanism of action

The molecule has chemical similarity to fluoxetine. However, it is relatively selective for inhibiting the reuptake of noradrenalin and is described as an NRI (see Table 26.1).

Clinical uses

In the acute treatment of major depression, reboxetine is of similar efficacy to fluoxetine. In one study, in out-patients with depression, reboxetine was more effective than fluoxetine in improving social functioning. This included greater improvement on items measuring work, spontaneous activity, family relationships and the ability to cope with finances. The use of reboxetine in the elderly has not been adequately explored, but the lack of postural hypotension may be an advantage.

Side-effects

These are mainly autonomic effects, probably representing sympathetic over-stimulation and central inhibition of the parasympathetic system (see Table 26.2). Insomnia and sweating are troublesome. Some tolerance to the side-effects may develop, as reboxetine has been well tolerated in long-term treatment.

Pharmacokinetics and dosage

Reboxetine is rapidly absorbed after oral doses. It is mainly metabolised in the liver and has an elimination half-life of about 13 hours. The starting dose is 4 mg, increasing to twice daily and a maximum dose of 12 mg a day. Reboxetine is not indicated for use in the elderly; if it is used, half these doses (2–4 mg a day) should be given.

Toxicity

No fatal overdoses have been reported.

Interactions

Reboxetine is highly protein-bound and may therefore interact temporarily with other protein-bound drugs, e.g. propranolol or dipyridamide.

Table 26.1 Affinities of antidepressants for reuptake sites and receptors of human brain

Drug	NRI	SRI	DRI	H₁	Acetylcholine-M	NA α-1	NA α-2	Serotonin-2A
Bupropion	0.002	0.01	0.2	0.2	0.002	0.02	0.001	0.0005
Maprotiline	9	0.02	0.1	50	0.2	1	.01	0.8
Mianserin	1	0.03	0.01	250	0.1	3	1.4	14
Milnacipran	1.2	11	0.001	0.008	0.002	0.007	NA	0.01
Mirtazepine	0.02	0.001	0.001	700	0.15	0.2	0.7	6
Nefazodone	0.3	0.5	0.3	5	0.01	4	0.02	30
Reboxetine	14	2	0.009	0.3	0.02	0.01	NA	0.02
Trazodone	0.01	0.6	0.01	0.3	0.0003	3	0.2	13
Venlafaxine	0.09	11	0.01	0	0	0	0	0

NRI, noradrenaline reuptake inhibition; SRI, serotonin reuptake inhibition; DRI, dopamine reuptake inhibition; H, histamine receptor; NA, noradrenalin; NA, not available. Affinity is expressed as $1/10^7 \times Kd$, where Kd is equilibrium dissociation constant in molarity. Thus, higher numbers indicate greater strength of that action. Ratios of different figures in the rows show how many times more potent the drug is in the two actions. Note that these figures are obtained in vitro and may be different from the effects of the drug and its metabolites in the body.

Adapted from Leonard and Richelson (2000).

Table 26.2 Common side-effects of reboxetine

Side-effect	Placebo-adjusted (%)
Dry mouth	11
Constipation	9
Insomnia	9
Sweating	7
Impotence	5
Tachycardia	3
Urinary hesitancy	3
Vertigo	2

In this and other tables the rate on placebo is subtracted from the rate on drug, so that a figure for numbers needed to harm (NNH) can be calculated (see chapter 5).

Discontinuation reactions

No discontinuation symptoms have been reported. Reboxetine is available as tablets of 4 mg.

SEROTONIN AND NORADRENALIN REUPTAKE INHIBITORS

These drugs block the reuptake of serotonin and noradrenalin (like TCAs such as amitriptyline) but differ from the TCAs by their lack of receptor-blocking activity at H_1, acetylcholine-M and noradrenalin α-1 and α-2 receptors. They should also lack membrane-stabilising activity. They should therefore not cause sedation or postural hypotension or fatality in overdose.

Venlafaxine

Structure and mechanism of action

Venlafaxine is a bicyclic compound. It is about five times more potent in blocking the reuptake of 5-HT than that of noradrenalin in the body (see Table 26.1). It has also a weak action blocking the reuptake of dopamine. At low doses (up to 75 mg daily) its actions resemble those of SSRIs, but at higher doses (up to 300 mg daily) it also blocks noradrenalin and to some extent dopamine reuptake.

Clinical uses

It has been studied mainly in depression. At low doses (75 mg daily) it is similar in efficacy to fluoxetine. However, at higher doses (150 to 300 mg daily) it is more effective than fluoxetine in severe depression including in-patients and those with melancholic depression. At these higher doses, it is similar in efficacy to the broader-spectrum TCAs such as imipramine and clomipramine. Venlafaxine is also effective in generalised anxiety disorder, where it is used at a dose of 75 mg daily

Table 26.3 Side-effects of venlafaxine

Side-effect	Placebo-adjusted (%)
Nausea	25
Somnolence	14
Dizziness	12
Dry mouth	11
Sweating	10
Sexual dysfunction	10
Insomnia	9
Constipation	9
Asthenia	7
Nervousness	7
Raised blood pressure	5 (at doses above 200 mg)
Seizures	0.3

Side-effects

Discontinuation rates for adverse events are similar to those for SSRIs at lower doses and almost as high as for TCAs at higher doses (see Table 26.3).

Pharmacokinetics and dosage

Venlafaxine is well-absorbed after oral administration. It is subject to first-pass metabolism, producing an active metabolite, desmethyl-venlafaxine, which is pharmacologically similar. Its elimination half-life of about 4 hours is short, and its active metabolite has a half-life of only about 8 hours. This means it is usually administered twice daily, and is liable to produce discontinuation problems. The starting dose is 37.5 mg twice daily. A sustained-release (XL) formulation (75 mg and 150 mg capsules) is also available for once daily use. The dose can be increased gradually to a maximum of 375 mg daily (225 mg for XL form).

Toxicity

Overdoses produce tachycardia and QT prolongation, and seizures (0.3%) have been reported. Fatality is rare.

Interactions

It is demethylated and also hydroxylated (by CYP IID6). It does not significantly inhibit cytochrome CYP enzymes. Toxic interactions (serotonin syndrome) with MAOIs are to be expected.

Discontinuation reactions

Severe discontinuation symptoms have been reported, resembling those of SSRIs (see chapter 25), even after missing only one or two doses. This may reflect both the short half-life and a stimulant action arising from dopamine reuptake inhibition. After 6 weeks or more of treatment or a higher dose for any period, gradual reduction over more than 2 weeks is advised.

Venlafaxine is available as tablets of 37.5 mg, 50 mg, 75 mg and XL 75 mg and 150 mg capsules.

Milnacipran

Structure and mechanism of action

This is not yet licensed in the UK. Milnacipran is an SNRI, which inhibits 5-HT and to a slightly lesser extent noradrenalin reuptake without affecting dopamine reuptake, and without blocking neurotransmitter receptors significantly (see Table 26.1).

Clinical uses

As an antidepressant, milnacipran is of comparable efficacy with imipramine and probably superior to SSRIs.

Side-effects

Dysuria is thought to result from increased noradrenalin function, but blood pressure is not raised (see Table 26.4).

Pharmacokinetics and dosage

It is rapidly absorbed and has a half-life of about 8 hours. It is mostly eliminated unchanged via the kidney. The usual dose is 50 mg twice daily.

Toxicity

No prolongation of the QT interval occurs. Overdoses produce nausea, vomiting, tachycardia, sweating and respiratory difficulties.

Interactions

It has no effects on the cytochrome CYP enzymes. Adverse interactions with MAOIs are expected.

Discontinuation reactions

None reported.

Table 26.4 Common side-effects of milnacipran

Side-effect	Placebo-adjusted (%)
Vertigo	5
Sweating	4
Anxiety	4
Hot flushes	3
Dysuria	2

Table 26.5 Common side-effects of mirtazapine

Side-effect	Placebo-adjusted (%)
Sedation, drowsiness	9–14
Dry mouth	9
Increased appetite, weight gain	9
Constipation, oedema, confusion, abnormal dreams, muscle pains, tremor, agranulocytosis	Uncommon

NORADRENERGIC AND SPECIFIC SEROTONERGIC ANTIDEPRESSANTS

This term was invented to describe a class of drugs with a complex pharmacology. The only member of the class available at present is mirtazapine, but mianserin has strong similarities.

Mirtazapine

Structure and mechanism of action

Mirtazapine has a tetracyclic structure similar to that of mianserin. It works by blocking noradrenalin α-2 autoreceptors, which results in enhanced release of noradrenalin from noradrenergic terminals, and by blocking α-2 heteroreceptors (receptors on 5-HT neurons), which increases 5-HT release from serotonergic terminals. The increased release of noradrenalin also increases the firing of serotonergic neurons through stimulation of α-1 receptors. Both noradrenalin and 5-HT function are increased. In addition, mirtazapine blocks postsynaptic 5-HT-2 and 5-HT-3 (but not 5-HT-1A) receptors; it is these actions that give rise to the description 'specific serotonergic'. The net result is to increase noradrenalin and 5-HT-1 transmission. Blockade of 5-HT-2 and 5-HT-3 receptors means that side-effects resulting from stimulation of these (insomnia, agitation, sexual dysfunction and nausea) should be minimised.

Mirtazapine also blocks histamine H_1 receptors very strongly, thus causing sedation, but has little effect on acetylcholine, dopamine or noradrenalin α-1 receptors.

Clinical uses

Mirtazapine is a sedative antidepressant and has comparable efficacy to amitriptyline and clomipramine in patients with depression, including severe depression. It may be more effective than trazodone or fluoxetine in severe cases.

In longer-term treatment it has efficacy comparable with amitriptyline in preventing relapses and recurrences, and similar rates of drop-outs.

Side-effects

The most common troublesome side-effects are sedation, and increased appetite with weight gain (see Table 26.5). Dry mouth is also common, but other anticholinergic features are not. The proportion of patients dropping out of treatment through side-effects (about 10%) is lower than on amitriptyline and slightly lower than on fluoxetine.

THE DRUGS

273

Pharmacokinetics and dosage

It is rapidly absorbed but after first-pass metabolism only about 50% reaches the systemic circulation. The elimination half-life is 20–40 hours (longer in the elderly), so that steady-state levels are reached after 4–9 days. Its metabolism in the liver is by four or more different cytochrome CYP enzymes, and the metabolites have little or no activity.

The starting dose is 15–30 mg. It is claimed that sedation is less with the higher dose. The optimal dose is 15–45 mg taken at night, for most patients.

Toxicity

Overdoses have resulted in sedation, but no reported cardiovascular or ECG changes. The rate of seizures reported is lower than for imipramine.

Interactions

Mirtazapine is only about 85% bound to plasma proteins, and only weakly inhibits cytochrome CYP enzymes. Its potential for pharmacokinetic interactions with other drugs is therefore low. It should not be prescribed with, or within 14 days of stopping, an MAOI.

It interferes pharmacodynamically with the actions of clonidine, which are exerted via α-2 receptors.

Discontinuation reaction

None has been reported and the long half-life should help avoid this problem. Mirtazapine is available as tablets of 30 mg.

Mianserin

Mianserin ('Bolvidon', 'Norval') was withdrawn from the UK market after the introduction of mirtazapine. It is sedative and produces weight gain. Bone marrow depression with agranulocytosis occurred in about one in 5000 patients and was more common in the elderly, tending to occur after 4–6 weeks of treatment and being usually reversible. Arthralgia, polyarthropathy and rashes also occurred.

SEROTONIN ANTAGONIST AND REUPTAKE INHIBITORS

Nefazodone has complex actions but its main ones have led to it being classed an SARI. Trazodone can be included in the same class. Both drugs block 5-HT-1A and 5-HT-2, as well as H_1 and noradrenalin α-1 and α-2 receptors.

Trazodone

Trazodone was developed in the 1970s from animal models based on aversive conditioning, and is not effective in other animal models of depression. It does not downregulate noradrenalin β-receptors as most other antidepressants do.

Structure and mechanism of action

It is a phenylpiperazine, with complex pharmacological actions (see Table 26.1). It blocks the reuptake of 5-HT, and blocks more potently 5-HT-2A and noradrenalin α-1 receptors, and less potently H_1 and noradrenalin α-2 receptors. It also blocks subtypes of 5-HT-1 receptors, but its metabolite meta-chlorophenylpiperazine (mCPP) is an agonist at 5-HT-1, -2A and -2C receptors and might otherwise increase anxiety. Trazodone lacks anticholinergic activity.

Clinical uses

It was used extensively in the US as an antidepressant before the introduction of SSRIs. Like the SSRIs, it tends to be less effective than broader-spectrum drugs such as venlafaxine and amitriptyline. It remains in use for its sedative properties, especially in depression, and it also improves anxiety. It has been shown to be effective in bulimia nervosa but not in OCD. The starting dose is 150 mg at night, increasing to at least 300 mg, with the maximum dose being 600 mg (for the elderly 100 mg increasing to 300 mg maximum).

Side-effects

The most common side-effects are sedation and postural hypotension. It reduces REM sleep. Sexual side-effects include persistent erections, and even dangerous priapism. This usually occurs early in treatment and men should be warned to discontinue trazodone if persistent erections occur spontaneously. In women, increased libido and spontaneous orgasm can occur.

Rarely reported side-effects include chronic active hepatitis and agranulocytosis.

Pharmacokinetics and dosage

It is more than 90% protein-bound in plasma and is metabolised in the liver partly by CYP IID6, with a half-life of 5–9 hours. The metabolites include m-CPP, which has a half-life of 4–14 hours.

Toxicity

Even with large overdoses fatalities are rare unless trazodone is taken in combination with another CNS depressant. Patients should have their blood pressure monitored.

Interactions

It potentiates other CNS depressants, and inhibits the actions of clonidine. It has potential to contribute to serotonin syndrome, but this has been rare.

Discontinuation reactions

Withdrawal should be tapered over one month, as reactions occur with malaise, myalgia, nausea and restless legs. Trazodone is available

THE DRUGS

as tablets of 150 mg; CR tablets of 150 mg; capsules of 50 mg and 100 mg; and liquid at 50 mg/5 ml.

Nefazodone

Structure and mechanism of action

This is also a phenylpiperazine, related to trazodone. It potentiates 5-HT (and to a lesser extent noradrenalin) transmission by inhibiting reuptake, and it blocks 5-HT-2A receptors. The overall effect is to increase 5-HT-1 (and 5-HT-3) function. Blocking H_1 receptors, it is sedative but less so than trazodone. It also blocks noradrenalin α-1 and α-2 receptors. It has active metabolites, with similar properties, and also mCPP.

Clinical uses

It is an antidepressant with sedative properties. It also improves anxiety, including panic disorder. It improves sleep with an increase in REM sleep.

Side-effects

The main ones are somnolence, postural hypotension, those associated with SSRIs, weight gain, weakness and palinopsia (visual streaking). Blocking 5-HT-2A receptors. It is distinguished by its lack of sexual side-effects and can help to counteract sexual side-effects experienced on other drugs (see Table 26.6).

Pharmacokinetics and dosage

It is rapidly absorbed but extensively metabolised, and mCPP is a metabolite; this is an agonist at 5-HT-1, -2A and -2C receptors and can cause anxiety. More is formed if the CYP IID6 enzyme is reduced either genetically or by other drugs such as SSRIs.

The half-life of nefazodone is 2–4 hours, but longer for the metabolites. The initial dose is 100 mg twice daily (50 mg in the elderly), increasing by 50–100 mg twice daily each week to a dose of 300–600 mg daily (less in the elderly). It can also be given as a single dose at night.

Toxicity

It appears to be safe in overdose and for use in epilepsy. There is little information on its use in pregnancy.

Table 26.6 Common side-effects of nefazodone

Side-effect	Placebo-adjusted (%)
Dry mouth	8
Somnolence	6
Dizziness	6
Nausea	6
Constipation	3
Blurred vision	3
Postural hypotension	3

Interactions

It is a weak inhibitor of CYP IID6 and IA2. It is a potent inhibitor of CYP IIIA4, and should not be given with terfenadine, cisapride or cyclosporin, and used cautiously with alprazolam and perhaps other benzodiazepines. It should not be combined with MAOIs.

Discontinuation reactions

It should be withdrawn slowly, because of its short half-life and serotonergic properties. Nefazodone is available as tablets of 100 mg and 200 mg and a starter pack with 50 mg.

DOPAMINE AND NORADRENALIN REUPTAKE INHIBITORS

The first DNRI was nomifensine, but it was withdrawn. Bupropion is another DNRI, used in the US as an antidepressant, and also used as an aid to stop smoking.

Bupropion

Structure and mechanism of action

It is a unicyclic aminoketone. Bupropion does not have a tricyclic structure. As a result it has little blocking effect on receptors. Bupropion itself inhibits the reuptake of dopamine and noradrenalin but weakly. It is metabolised to hydroxybupropion, which is a more potent inhibitor.

Clinical uses

It is preferred for use in bipolar depression and retarded or atypical depression, because it has activating properties. It may carry less risk of inducing mania. It is used (as amfebutamone) to assist in the discontinuation of cigarette smoking, its only licensed indication in the UK. It may improve ADHD in children and adults.

Side-effects

These are mostly due to dopamine over-stimulation. They include nausea, insomnia, agitation, dry mouth, dizziness, weight loss and psychosis. It produces fewer sexual side-effects than any SSRI. It does not reduce REM sleep.

Pharmacokinetics and dosage

It is metabolised mainly by CYP IID6 and the terminal half-life is about 14 hours. The maximum dose is 400 mg daily.

Toxicity

It lowers the seizure threshold in a dose-dependent manner, and fits occur in up to 0.5% of people over 2 years. Overdoses lead to fits, hallucinations, tachycardia and loss of consciousness; deaths have occurred. Those severe adverse reactions seem to occur more frequently during use in smokers.

Interactions

It should be used cautiously with other drugs that may lower the seizure threshold, including other antidepressants. It should not be used in combination with dopamine agonists or MAOIs. It increases valproate levels. Its own level is decreased by carbamazepine.

Discontinuation reactions

It should be withdrawn slowly. It is available as tablets ('Zyban': modified release) 150 mg.

FURTHER READING

Berman, R. M., Narasimhan, M., Anand, A., *et al* (1999) Transient depressive relapse induced by catecholamine depletion. *Archives of General Psychiatry*, **56**, 395–403.

Leonard, B. & Richelson, E. (2000) Synaptic effects of antidepressants: relationship to their therapeutic and adverse effects. In *Schizophrenia and Mood Disorders: The New Drug Therapies in Clinical Practice*, pp. 67–84. Oxford: Butterworth Heinemann.

Sachs, G. S., Lafer, B., Stoll, A. L., *et al* (1994) A double-blind trial of bupropion versus desipramine for bipolar depression. *Journal of Clinical Psychiatry*, **55**, 391–393.

Wilens, T. E., Spencer, T. J., Biederman, J., *et al* (2001) A controlled clinical trial of bupropion for attention deficit hyperactivity disorder in adults. *American Journal Psychiatry*, **158**, 282–288.

The discovery of the psychotropic effects of MAOIs dates from 1952 when iproniazid given to patients for tuberculosis was found to lift their mood. Isoniazid, still widely used for TB, has no activity as an MAOI; although it produces psychotic reactions in some tuberculosis patients, it is thought to do so by a different mechanism. Iproniazid was introduced as an antidepressant in 1957.

The uses of MAOIs in psychiatry do not fall into neat categories. They have been described as sedatives, psychic energisers, euphoriants, antidepressants and anti-phobics. Some patients are undoubtedly helped by MAOIs, some specifically by only one drug of the group. The indications are depressive illness, especially atypical depression; anxiety states, including panic disorder; social phobia and OCD; and where MARI antidepressants have failed. Selegiline is also used in Parkinson's disease.

Most MAOIs are hydrazine derivatives and contain the chemical grouping -NH-NH- in the side-chain. Hydrazines such as phenelzine ('Nardil') are inactivated by acetylation in the liver, by which -NH-NH- is converted to -NH-NH-CO-CH$_3$. The speed of acetylation is genetically determined, some individuals being fast and others slow acetylators.

The non-hydrazine derivatives include amphetamine (only weak as an MAOI) and more particularly its relative tranylcypromine ('Parnate').

Most MAOI drugs combine irreversibly with monoamine oxidase (MAO) and therefore inactivate the enzymes that oxidise serotonin, noradrenalin, dopamine, tyramine and other amines. These amines may be neurotransmitters, substances in foods or ingredients of medicines. The MAO enzymes are found in many parts of the body, for instance the intestinal wall, liver, platelets, the heart, kidney and lung, and the brain. There are two main enzymes, MAO-A and -B. MAO-A oxidises serotonin and noradrenalin. MAO-B oxidises dopamine. Both enzymes oxidise tyramine. MAO-A is inhibited reversibly by moclobemide ('Manerix'), MAO-B by selegiline ('Eldepryl') and both are inhibited by the older MAOIs, phenelzine, isocarboxazid and tranylcypromine.

Within the brain MAO is present in mitochondria pre-synaptically in the nerves that release noradrenalin, 5-HT or dopamine. It is thought that MAOIs increase the storage and release of these transmitters. Enzymes are proteins that are continually being broken down and resynthesized during life. When an enzyme is irreversibly inhibited and hence functionally destroyed, fresh enzyme is gradually resynthesised in the course of 2–3 weeks and eventually replaces all that has been destroyed, unless fresh inhibitor is continually added. During treatment, free MAOI disappears by metabolism and excretion, leaving inactivated enzymes that take time to be replaced. This time for recovery is why it is advisable to wait 2 weeks after stopping an MAOI before starting another drug (e.g. a TCA), and also why measurement of an MAOI drug blood level may tell little about the degree of enzyme inhibition. The activity of the enzyme in platelets can, however, be usefully measured.

Apart from amine oxidases, the drugs inactivate other enzymes, particularly liver hydroxylases. The drugs may also inactivate pyridoxal, a coenzyme derived from vitamin B6 (pyridoxine), which plays a part in many processes, in the metabolism of organic acids and of the neurotransmitter GABA. These inactivations are rapid, whereas the clinical effects are slow – so it is difficult to know how the drugs act.

Interactions and side-effects

Because of the numerous effects of MAOIs, caution and watchfulness are required: caution in deciding to use them and to mix them with other drugs, and watchfulness for the physical signs of side-effects and of toxicity. They are frequently hypotensive, especially in causing postural hypotension, but paradoxically facilitate hypertensive episodes, sometimes with severe headache, particularly when amine-rich foods are eaten. This occurs because amines such as tyramine in food are normally metabolised by MAO in the gut wall and liver, and do not reach the general circulation. If they do, they enter sympathetic nerve endings and cause the release of noradrenalin, leading to vasoconstriction, cardiac stimulation and hypertension. The last can be so severe as to produce cerebral or subarachnoid haemorrhages. Patients should be advised not to eat any cheese – especially highly fermented ones such as Gorgonzola – hung game, caviar, sauerkraut, pickled herrings or chicken liver, and to avoid meat or yeast extracts – Bovril, Oxo, Marmite. Alcohol is best avoided, especially heavy red wines, but even non-alcoholic beers may cause problems. Bananas and broad beans, except the pods, are safe.

The pharmacy will provide patients prescribed an MAOI with clear warning cards. Patients should carry this card explaining they are taking an MAOI, so that other practitioners, including anaesthetists and dentists, may know and prescribe their drugs with appropriate caution to avoid unpleasant or dangerous interactions.

The MAOIs may cause ankle oedema and puffy hands because of fluid retention. They may be hypoglycaemic because they inhibit the breakdown of insulin. They may cause jaundice. They prevent the metabolism and so enhance the effect of morphine, pethidine, nefopam and dextromethorphan, and likewise of anti-Parkinsonian drugs, TCAs, barbiturates and phenytoin. If an MAOI is added to the prescription of a patient already stabilised on one or more of these other drugs, the stability may be upset and a toxic overdose develop. But the fact remains that, in spite of many potential risks, troubles are uncommon in practice when care is taken.

MAOIs are unsafe combined with amphetamines or methyldopa, or with other drugs that increase 5-HT function. With the latter a serotonin syndrome is liable to develop (see p. 87). Such drugs include SSRIs, clomipramine, serotonin agonists such as buspirone and carbamazepine.

The selective MAO-A or -B inhibitors produce much less interaction with foodstuffs and other drugs because tyramine can be metabolised by either enzyme.

Phenelzine

Phenelzine ('Nardil') may be used for depressive states, especially those with atypical features (see p. 109); depressions unresponsive to TCAs, including combined treatment; and anxiety states – panic disorder, social phobia, OCD.

Phenelzine is started with 15 mg three times daily (twice daily in older people) and after 1 week increased to 60 mg daily if side-effects are not marked. Raise to 75 mg daily after a second week (except for the elderly, in whom 60 mg is the maximum dose usually given). For younger patients up to 90 mg daily may be required.

Combination with MARIs

Depressive illness which has not responded to a TCA or MAOI alone, may do so with combined treatment, but only certain TCAs are safe to combine. Either amitriptyline or imipramine may be used. Start the TCA first in a low dose, for example 100 mg at night, or not more than 150 mg daily (clomipramine or SSRI must not be used). Then introduce phenelzine 15 mg twice and then thrice daily. Enquire carefully for side-effects and measure blood pressure (which may fall) after 2 or 3 days, at 1, 2 and 3 weeks, and whenever the patient is seen thereafter. If the patient is already taking phenelzine, it is possible to start a TCA with it by small doses at night, very slowly increasing. There is no evidence from controlled trials attesting to the efficacy of this combination for refractory depression.

Combination with lithium

Drug-resistant depression may respond to phenelzine 15 mg thrice daily, plus lithium carbonate to give a plasma concentration of lithium of 0.5–0.8 mmol/l.

Side-effects and interactions

The drug has some sedative action and may quickly counteract insomnia in some states of tension. It should not be given during infective hepatitis, obstructive jaundice, liver cirrhosis or congestive cardiac failure. It should not be used in cerebrovascular disease and should be used cautiously in the elderly. Patients must be told to avoid all self-medication, for instance for colds, because of the risk of interactions with ephedrine and other sympathomimetics.

Common side-effects are sweating, dry mouth, weakness and faintness, especially from postural hypotension. Less frequent are tingling paraesthesia in upper or lower limbs (for which pyridoxine, 50 mg daily, is sometimes given), ankle oedema and tremor.

Toxic reactions include hyperpyrexia, convulsions, agitation and confusional states in which hallucinations may be prominent. Patients with depression may swing into hypomania while on the drug. In cases of hypertensive crisis phentolamine (5–10 mg intravenously) is given.

Because of drug interactions avoid sympathomimetic amines (amphetamine, fenfluramine, ephedrine), including those sometimes present in proprietary cold cures and cough medicines, anti-hypertensive drugs (such as methyldopa, guanethidine) and antihistamines. Note that preparations of local anaesthetic sometimes contain sympathomimetic amines.

Sensitivity to insulin may be increased, perhaps by blocking insulin destruction, and hence increased sensitivity to oral anti-diabetic drugs resulting in unexpected hypoglycaemia. Morphine, pethidine and dextromethorphan (in 'Actifed' cough linctus) are contraindicated, but not other analgesics. Metabolism of many drugs by the liver, for instance barbiturates, and phenytoin, may be interfered with. Phenelzine is available as tablets of 15 mg.

TRANYLCYPROMINE

Although tranylcypromine ('Parnate') has less marked MAOI activity than phenelzine, it is strongly sympathomimetic and has side-effects and interactions similar to phenelzine. The same drugs and foods must be avoided. Liver damage is less likely.

In a dose of 10 mg twice or three times daily it is used for depressions where phenelzine might be prescribed. However, like amphetamine, to which it is chemically related, tranylcypromine has some immediate euphoriant effect and may cause insomnia, so is best taken in the morning. The immediate effect encourages the patient, but can lead to dependence. It is available as tablets of 10 mg.

MOCLOBEMIDE

Moclobemide ('Manerix') is a benzamide derivative and a RIMA. Tyramine taken with it can still be metabolised by MAO-B. Also, because of its reversibility, large quantities of tyramine or other substrates will displace moclobemide from the enzyme. It is thus relatively free of interactions with foodstuffs, but patients should avoid very large quantities of tyramine-rich foods and certain drugs.

Moclobemide is an effective and well-tolerated antidepressant in doses of 300 mg or more daily. It is of less use than older MAOIs for social phobia and has not proved effective in panic disorder.

Side-effects are less common than with the older MARIs but include insomnia, headache, dizziness and nausea. It may rarely cause reversible confusional states. It is not sedative, lacks anticholinergic effects and is safe in overdose.

Start on 300 mg daily with food, adjusting the dose to 150–600 mg daily according to response.

Interactions

Because of its reversibility and short half-life, a switch to other drugs can be made after only 24 hours. However, it should not be started after an MARI, which blocks serotonin reuptake, until the other drug has had time to leave the body (4–5 half-lives). Serotonin syndrome may result if it is co-administered with an SSRI, SNRI or other MARIs such as clomipramine, which have strong effects on 5-HT reuptake.

Patients should avoid cough remedies containing drugs like ephedrine or dextromethorphan. Pethidine or codeine should not be administered with it. It is metabolised by hepatic mono-oxygenase, and blood levels are increased by drugs such as cimetidine, so that a lower dose is needed. It is available as tablets of 150 mg.

SELEGILINE

Selegiline ('Eldepryl') is a selective MAO-B inhibitor that potentiates dopamine function in the brain. It is used in Parkinson's disease. It does not produce a tyramine reaction and no dietary restrictions are required. It has not been found useful as an antidepressant except at high doses (30 mg per day), at which it is not selective for MAO-B and tyramine intake must be restricted.

Side-effects include hypertension and nausea, and it can cause confusional states and psychotic reactions, as might be expected from its potentiation of dopamine transmission.

Particular interest surrounds selegiline because of the occurrence of a Parkinson-like condition caused by the synthetic heroin contaminant methylphenyltetrahydropyridine (MPTP). MPTP is converted by MAO-B to another compound, MPP, that enters nigrostriatal dopamine neurons selectively, and destroys them. Selegiline gives full protection against this toxic action of MPTP in animals. It was also be found to delay the development of disability in Parkinson's disease, but recent reports of increased overall mortality have led to a decline in its use. It is available as tablets of 5 mg and 10 mg.

FURTHER READING

Sunderland, T., Cohen, R. M., Molchan, S., *et al* (1994) High dose selegiline for refractory depression in old age. *Archives of General Psychiatry*, **51**, 607–615.

Quitkin, F. M., Harrison, W., Steward, J. W., *et al* (1991) Response to phenelzine and imipramine in placebo non-responders with atypical depression. *Archives of General Psychiatry*, **48**, 319–323.

THE DRUGS

These are drugs used primarily in the treatment of schizophrenia, and for mania. Some may be used as hypnotics, or in small doses to treat anxiety and tension. Chemically they form several distinct groups. The phenothiazines and the thioxanthenes resemble the tricyclics in having a three-ring structure, but the central ring has only six atoms instead of seven and one of them is sulphur: typical drugs are chlorpromazine and flupentixol . Then there are the butyrophenones (e.g. haloperidol) related to the analgesic pethidine, and the phenylbutylpiperidines (e.g. pimozide).

THE DEVELOPMENT OF ANTIPSYCHOTICS

The first effective antipsychotic, chlorpromazine, was synthesised in 1950 by Charpentier of Rhône-Poulenc laboratories in France, investigating a series of antihistamines for use in anaesthesia. The surgeon Laborit noticed its unusual properties of tranquillisation in 1951 and indicated these to psychiatric colleagues; its use in psychosis was first reported by Delay and Deniker in 1952 (see chapter 1). This drug, called 'Largactil' because of its large number of pharmacological actions, was the first of a number of phenothiazines introduced into psychiatry. A few years later Janssen and colleagues, investigating derivatives of pethidine in animals, discovered haloperidol; noting its ability to antagonise the effects of amphetamine, they studied it in schizophrenia and found it to be useful. It was introduced clinically in 1957. The mechanism of action of the antipsychotic drugs began to be clarified in 1963 when Swedish workers Carlsson and Linqvist noted increased levels of the dopamine metabolite HVA in the CSF; they postulated that haloperidol and chlorpromazine blocked dopamine receptors. The receptors themselves were first identified by their binding to radioactively labelled haloperidol. It was shown that all known antipsychotics had in common the ability to bind these dopamine receptors and that their potency in doing so correlated highly with their potency in schizophrenia. It became widely believed that all antipsychotic effects were due to blockade of dopamine receptors. Drugs were then developed to be more specific in blocking dopamine and not other transmitters – for instance pimozide and sulpiride.

More recently two important developments have occurred. First, dopamine receptors have been recognised as having subtypes (see p. 70). Blockade of D_2 receptors is thought to be important for antipsychotic effects, and the benzamide drugs, sulpiride and amisulpride, are specific D_2 antagonists. However, D_2 receptors themselves can be further subdivided (to include D_3 and D_4), and the antipsychotics differ in the extent to which they block these different subtypes. Clozapine, for instance, is able to block D_4 receptors that are not blocked by haloperidol or the benzamides; benzamides tend to block D_3 receptors preferentially (see chapter 30). The fact that the different subtypes are located in different proportions in the basal ganglia (more D_2 receptors) and the limbic areas (more D_3 receptors) indicates the importance of the selectivity of drugs for the different subtypes in determining their clinical effects.

Secondly, the blockade of other transmitters may be important. For instance, blockade of noradrenalin α-1 and H_1 receptors contributes to the early sedative effects and behavioural control by antipsychotics. Blockade of 5-HT-2 receptors may modify the effects of D_2 blockade, and produce a greater improvement in some of the symptoms of schizophrenia with fewer EPS, as claimed for risperidone and olanzapine (see chapter 30).

PET scans and receptor occupancy

The technique of PET allows the visualisation of the number and distribution of receptors in the living brain. A drug, which is selective for a particular class of receptors, is labelled with a positron emitting atom and injected intravenously. PET then shows the distribution of the labelled drug, as it attaches to receptors in the brain. This method can be used when the patient is receiving treatment with other drugs, to determine by how much the uptake of the labelled drug is reduced; from this can be calculated the occupancy of the receptors by the other drug. In this way it has been shown that classical antipsychotics must block 70–85% of D_2 receptors (as measured in the basal ganglia) in order to treat acute schizophrenia effectively. By contrast, clozapine, in clinically effective doses, occupies only about 50% of D_2 receptors, but also occupies a similar proportion of D_1 receptors, and presumably of other subtypes of dopamine receptors (D_3 and D_4). Similarly, Parkinsonian side-effects in young patients occur only when D_2 receptor occupancy in the basal ganglia reaches 75% or more.

Side-effects

Dopamine receptors are members of the large class of receptors linked to G-proteins, and other members of the receptor class share much of the same peptide structure. It is not surprising that some drugs that block dopamine receptors bind also to receptors for other members of the class, in particular H_1 receptors, acetylcholine-M, 5-HT-2, and noradrenalin α-1 and α-2 receptors (see chapter 7). The side-effects of the antipsychotics can be largely understood in relation to their pharmacological actions (Box 28.1). Thus, blockade of dopamine receptors causes EPS (see chapter 17) and NMS, reduced drive and hyperprolactinaemia. It probably also contributes to weight gain. Blockade of acetylcholine-M receptors causes atropinic side-effects, dry mouth, constipation, blurred vision, urinary retention and impaired concentration; it may, however, protect against Parkinsonism, dystonia and akathisia. Blockade of α-1 receptors contributes to sedation and postural hypotension, especially in the first few days of treatment, and ejaculatory impotence or retrograde ejaculation. H_1 blockade produces sedation and possibly weight gain. 5-HT-2C blockade may contribute

---

Box 28.1 Pharmacological and clinical effects of antipsychotics

D_1-like blockade	Synergistic or antagonistic to D_2 blockade
	Blunts cocaine euphoria
D_2-like blockade	Antipsychotic, antimanic
	Parkinsonism, dystonia, akathisia
	Mental dulling, reduced drive
	Hyperprolactinaemia
	Neuroleptic malignant syndrome
	Weight gain
Acetylcholine-M blockade	Dry mouth, constipation, blurred vision
	Urinary retention, impaired concentration
	Protects against Parkinsonism, dystonia
Acetylcholine-M4 agonism	Hypersalivation, etc.
H_1 blockade	Sedation
Noradrenalin α-1 blockade	Postural hypotension
	Transient initial sedation
	Ejaculatory problems
Noradrenalin α-2 blockade	Antidepressant
5-HT-1 blockade	Hypothermic
5-HT-2A blockade	Reduces Parkinsonism and dystonia
	Increases slow-wave sleep
	Improves mood
	Delayed ejaculation, blurred vision
5-HT-2C blockade	Weight gain
5-HT-3 blockade	Anti-emetic
Blocking cardiac potassium channels	Delayed cardiac repolarisation
	Prolonged QT interval
	Dysrhythmia

to weight gain, while 5-HT-2A blockade may reduce Parkinsonism and dystonia, and also confer beneficial effects on mood and sleep.

Hyperprolactinaemia due to antipsychotics results in blood levels of prolactin up to 10 times normal but seldom above 3000 mU/l. By contrast, even higher levels are seen in people with prolactinomas. Associated clinical features are galactorrhoea, amenorrhoea and reduced libido. Chronic hyperprolactinaemia can lead to hypogonadism, with oestrogen deficiency and osteoporosis, but this does not appear to occur with antipychotics. Galactorrhoea may be mild and tolerated, but, if it is problematic, a switch to olanzapine or quetiapine is indicated (see chapter 30). The use of dopamine agonists such as bromocriptine to counteract it, carries a theoretical risk of exacerbating the psychosis, although this happens rarely.

Toxic and allergic reactions

Rashes may occur but are seldom a major problem. They indicate a need for blood count and liver funtion tests.

Abnormal liver function tests and cholestatic jaundice occur with phenothiazines in about 1% of patients and occasionally with haloperidol and zuclopenthixol. It is prudent to assess liver function tests before and during the first 2 weeks of treatment. If the tests become abnormal, a switch to a different class of antipsychotic is preferable. The reaction is allergic and usually begins about 10 days after starting the drug, with malaise or 'flu-like symptoms, and with an increase in eosinophils, followed a week later by a marked rise in alkaline phosphatase and then by transaminase and bilirubin. Most cases recover fully in 8 weeks after withdrawal. On chlorpromazine a few develop chronic cholestasis, with jaundice or abnormal liver function tests, taking up to 3 years to recover. If there is uncertainty about which drug is involved, blood tests should be monitored daily, and the least suspect drug should be reintroduced.

Agranulocytosis occurs rarely with phenothiazines, usually after 10–90 days of treatment. Because of its rarity and suddenness, occasional blood tests are of little value in detecting this, but signs of infection early in therapy should lead to an immediate full blood count. The neuroleptic malignant syndrome is described in chapter 8.

Cardiac toxicity and sudden death

Reports of sudden death in patients on antipsychotics and sedative medication have caused considerable recent concern. The older literature indicated that high doses of phenothiazines, particularly thioridazine, were associated with sudden cardiovascular collapse. Pimozide in high doses affects cellular calcium and potassium channels and produces ventricular tachycardia (seen in the ECG as Torsade de Pointes with varying QRS complexes) that can progress to ventricular fibrillation. More recently cases of sudden death have been reported involving the high-potency antipsychotics haloperidol and droperidol, often used in disturbed young males by injection, sometimes in high doses and in combination with a benzodiazepine. A number of mechanisms may be involved. The accumulation and subsequent sudden release of drugs given intramuscularly is possible. Some patients on long-term treatment have tardive dyskinetic symptoms affecting the oesophagus, which interfere with swallowing and lead to aspiration of food and asphyxia. Other cases are unexplained. Respiratory death through laryngeal spasm and dystonia or respiratory depression may be involved in a small number. Unsuspected NMS causing respiratory distress is another possibility. However, the majority are probably owing to cardiac dysrhythmias. Phenothiazines, especially thioridazine, and high-potency drugs such as droperidol and some atypical antipsychotics in high doses can increase the QT interval or produce T-wave flattening indicative of abnormal repolarisation. This is because of an action blocking the potassium channels known as the delayed rectifier in cardiac cells, and it predisposes to ventricular dysrhythmia and fibrillation. Other factors predisposing to dysrhythmia are hypokalaemia and high levels of catecholamines, as in a patient who is struggling under restraint.

Care should be exercised in prescribing antipsychotics to patients with a history of cardiac disease, and in administering parenteral medication to control behavioural disturbance (see chapter 14).

THE DRUGS

The Royal College of Psychiatrists has published a Consensus Statement on the use of high doses of antipsychotics in schizophrenia (Thompson, 1994). It is recommended that, in general, psychiatrists should use doses of antipsychotic medication for schizophrenia within the limits of dose advised by the *BNF* or the Association of the British Pharmaceutical Industry data sheet. Higher doses should only be prescribed on the advice of a consultant, and a second opinion should be obtained; the ECG should be checked, with attention to the QT interval, and blood taken for measurement of electrolytes and glucose.

Pharmacokinetic interactions of classical antipsychotics

The development of these drugs predates detailed understanding of metabolism by cytochrome P450 (CYP) enzymes. However, the phenothiazines induce enzymes that increase their own metabolism, requiring higher doses to be given after a few weeks. Orphenadrine can also induce these enzymes. Conversely the phenothiazines and tricyclic MARIs compete for hydroxylase enzymes (CYP IID6) in the liver, so increasing the blood levels of the tricyclics. Propranolol interferes with the metabolism of phenothiazines, leading to increased blood levels. Carbamazepine induces liver enzymes and has been shown to lower blood levels of haloperidol by half within 3 weeks. Phenothiazines can induce phenytoin toxicity by inhibiting its metabolism.

Discontinuation effects

Abrupt withdrawal of antipsychotics may lead to nausea, agitation and insomnia and possibly to a rebound exacerbation of the underlying psychosis. A condition resembling NMS with pyrexia has also been reported. Those with anticholinergic properties may be more liable to produce discontinuation problems.

PHENOTHIAZINES

This bewilderingly large group of drugs, of which chlorpromazine was the first to be used in psychiatry, all have molecular structures on the same ground plan and broadly similar therapeutic effects, differing mainly in their side-effects.

The modifications to the molecule that vary the clinical effects are in the atoms attached at the $\star$ and the side-chain R (Figure 28.1). The liability to induce sleep for instance, or Parkinsonism, is altered by changing R. Attachments of fluorine atoms at the $\star$ increases the potency of a drug. Figure 28.1 will help an understanding of the inter-relations of some commonly used phenothiazines.

The drugs with the first type of (aliphatic) side-chain are low potency, and have a broad spectrum of pharmacological actions, causing sedation and hypotension but less Parkinsonism. Drugs with the second and third types of side-chain – the piperazines – are high potency, and produce less sedation and hypotension but more acute EPS. Thioridazine has a piperidine side-chain and no halogen, is low potency, has a broad spectrum of pharmacological actions and is less liable to produce Parkinsonism.

Figure 28.1 The basic structures of PHENOTHIAZINES, and roughly equivalent doses

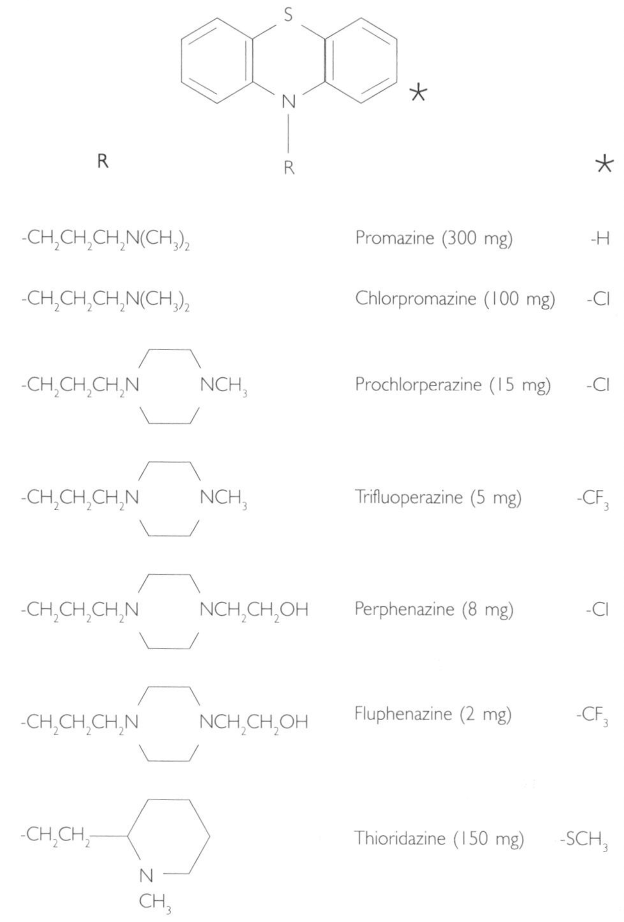

R		*
-CH$_2$CH$_2$CH$_2$N(CH$_3$)$_2$	Promazine (300 mg)	-H
-CH$_2$CH$_2$CH$_2$N(CH$_3$)$_2$	Chlorpromazine (100 mg)	-Cl
-CH$_2$CH$_2$CH$_2$N◯NCH$_3$	Prochlorperazine (15 mg)	-Cl
-CH$_2$CH$_2$CH$_2$N◯NCH$_3$	Trifluoperazine (5 mg)	-CF$_3$
-CH$_2$CH$_2$CH$_2$N◯NCH$_2$CH$_2$OH	Perphenazine (8 mg)	-Cl
-CH$_2$CH$_2$CH$_2$N◯NCH$_2$CH$_2$OH	Fluphenazine (2 mg)	-CF$_3$
-CH$_2$CH$_2$— (piperidine ring, N-CH$_3$)	Thioridazine (150 mg)	-SCH$_3$

A long-acting (depot) phenothiazine, fluphenazine decanoate ('Modecate'), is made by esterifying the R side-chain terminal, -OH-, with a long-chain fatty acid, decanoic acid, which increases its lipid solubility, and dissolving it in a vegetable oil. A single intramuscular dose may be effective for 2–5 weeks (or longer in the elderly).

Clinical use

The elderly are much more sensitive to phenothiazines; therefore use smaller doses to avoid sedation and hypotension, and use less potent drugs to avoid Parkinsonism. Healthy adults become drowsy on small doses that would not affect a patient with schizophrenia or mania. Patients with brain damage may be unusually sensitive to phenothiazines. The tendency to have fits may be slightly increased in epilepsy, but the drugs are valuable for controlling the special irritability and aggression that sometimes occur in epilepsy. Chlorpromazine is acutely ictogenic in a dose-related fashion.

For control of florid psychotic illnesses it is best not to be timid or tentative but to start with quite big doses, chlorpromazine 100 mg or trifluoperazine 5 mg, each three times daily, and soon adjust the dose up or down as required. The occasional patient finds the acute dose too big, and feels very drowsy. Others may rather quickly develop a dystonic reaction (which may be misjudged as hysterical), twisting of a limb, arching of the back, torticollis and spasm of the tongue. This must be treated with an anti-Parkinsonian drug and may need an adjustment of the dose. Many clinicians give an anti-Parkinsonian drug prophylactically, especially when prescribing haloperidol or trifluoperazine.

When one phenothiazine in full dosage as syrup or by injection has not been successful, another is unlikely to do much better. It is preferable to change to a butyrophenone or another class of antipsychotic. All of them take time, even several weeks of continuous administration to abolish schizophrenic symptoms, but are often quick to control mania. They differ in their sedative effects, which are evident from the start, but show little difference in true antipsychotic effect.

CHLORPROMAZINE

Chlorpromazine ('Largactil') may be used for:

- control and maintenance therapy of schizophrenia and other psychoses
- treatment of mania
- control of the violent patient
- impulsivity, for example in borderline personalities
- insomnia
- tension, anxiety and agitation
- nausea and vomiting
- appetite stimulation in anorexia nervosa.

For acutely disturbed states, chlorpromazine is the classic drug of choice (equal with haloperidol), having a prolonged quietening effect without impairment of consciousness. Chlorpromazine is therefore used to control manic states, acute disturbance in schizophrenia, delirium and confusional states and to prevent aggressive outbursts in epilepsy. Large doses are tolerated and indeed required, as it is important to gain control quickly. Chlorpromazine syrup 100 mg repeated 4–6 hourly for 3–6 doses usually achieves control; initially in the most severe, a deep intramuscular injection of 50–100 mg repeated as necessary used to be recommended, converting (by overlapping) to an oral dose as soon as cooperation is achieved. Intramuscular chlorpromazine is less widely used now as it is painful and produces postural hypotension, and alternative means of acute tranquillisation are preferred (see chapter14). This route avoids first-pass metabolism, which can be extensive (see below). Tranquillising effects should be evident within 6–24 hours and doses of 300–800 mg a day are continued. Once the abnormal behaviour is controlled, start reducing the dose.

Acute disturbance apart, chlorpromazine can still be used for the treatment of schizophrenia, especially paranoid and catatonic types. The antipsychotic effect begins after 3–6 days but is more marked from 2 weeks, and delusions lessen, auditory hallucinations diminish or cease and thought disorder is less marked. Start with oral chlorpromazine 150 mg daily, which may need to be raised in 150 mg daily steps, at intervals. The *BNF* maximum is 1000 mg daily. Increasing the dose too quickly in the initial stages may induce hypotension; a high dose at 2–3 weeks may induce Parkinsonism and akathisia.

A dose of 25–100 mg at night produces an early hypnotic effect. Small doses, 25–50 mg three times daily, reduce nausea and vomiting and similar doses or higher are used in anorexia nervosa to stimulate appetite and weight gain. Ten to 25 mg three times daily suppresses tension and anxiety; higher doses can lessen OCD symptoms.

Side-effects

Common early side-effects are sedation, hypotension (dizziness), dry mouth, indigestion and blurred vision – all usually improving over 2 weeks.

Uncommon early side-effects include dystonia. Sudden appearance of torticollis, arching of back, tongue protrusion and oculogyric crisis are all easily mistaken for hysterical reactions or for the onset of acute neurological damage. Treat by giving parenteral anticholinergic drugs. Relief begins in a few minutes. Continue with oral anticholinergics.

In the Medium term, common side-effects are:

- mild rash at 10–14 days, usually trivial and quickly fades
- tiredness, weakness, internal restlessness (akathisia or 'jitters'), insomnia at night but drowsy by day and Parkinsonism developing – stiffness of arms and legs, tremor, loss of facial mobility and expression, sometimes salivation. These do not spontaneously resolve. Treat with anti-Parkinsonian drugs or by reduction of phenothiazine dose
- weight gain, by degrees, of 6 kg or more to a plateau by 18 months. This reverses slowly when phenothiazine dose is reduced or stopped; attention to diet is advisable
- galactorrhoea, which can be distressing, and sometimes amenorrhoea. In these cases it may be possible to reduce the dose if the psychosis has improved; otherwise a switch to olanzapine or quetiapine will avoid the problem
- reduced libido, which may result from raised prolactin levels
- ejaculatory problems and erectile impotence
- photosensitivity: some patients on chlorpromazine are liable to sunburn easily. Avoid direct exposure (shady hats and gloves) or use an ultraviolet-blocking skin cream with a high strength. Consider changing to another drug that does not cause photosensitivity

THE DRUGS

- pigmentation of exposed skin, with a metallic grey-mauve colour occurs occasionally, especially in females after 4 years of treatment. Deposits in the cornea and lens may occur with higher doses but rarely impair vision
- frostbite – fingers are more liable to freezing and frostbite in very cold weather, and patients should wear warm gloves when outside
- epileptic fits, which require a change of drug or the addition of an anticonvulsant
- jaundice – if liver function tests deteriorate, or cholestatic jaundice develops, chlorpromazine should be stopped. Treatment should be resumed later with a different drug, not a phenothiazine
- when continued in large doses in patients with constipation, perforation of the bowel may occur as a result of ischaemic necrosis
- agranulocytosis occurs rarely.

A late side-effect is tardive dyskinesia; after a year or more of continuous drug treatment, especially in the elderly or where there is brain damage (neurological disease, head injury, dementia or alcoholism), spontaneous writhing movements appear, especially around the mouth and tongue (see chapter 17).

Metabolism of phenothiazines

All the drugs are rapidly metabolised in the gut wall and liver by oxidation of the sulphur atom in the central ring, by hydroxylation of the side rings and by changes in the side-chains. Most of the metabolites are clinically inactive. Sulphoxides and hydroxy-derivatives are excreted to some extent in urine and predominantly through the liver into the gut and then out in the faeces. The microbial flora of the gut is capable of reducing inactive sulphoxide back to active drug, which can then be reabsorbed and circulate again. Drug metabolites continue to be excreted for some months after drug-taking has stopped.

There is much variation from patient to patient in the speed of metabolism of the same drug, especially between the drug-naive patient and one who has already received large doses for a long time. Metabolism begins in the gut wall even before absorption into portal hepatic blood, and continues on arrival in the liver. Metabolism is speeded up after 2–3 weeks of continued use. For these reasons injected drug may be several times more effective than oral. The increased rate of metabolism declines in about 2 weeks on stopping phenothiazines.

Contraindications and interactions

Chlorpromazine is broadly compatible with other drugs and with ECT.

It blocks the liver metabolism of some drugs, such as morphine, pethidine, TCAs, and increases blood levels. It is contraindicated where the patient is already semi-comatose from alcohol, or is known to have a liver disease such as cirrhosis, or immediately following an attack of hepatitis. Large doses may diminish symptoms of acute abdomen and of fevers, making physical diagnosis harder.

It is available as tablets (10 mg, 25 mg, 50 mg and 100 mg), syrup (25 mg per 5 ml), forte suspension (100 mg per 5 ml), injection (intramuscular 25 mg per ml in 1 ml and 2 ml ampoules) and suppositories (100 mg).

THIORIDAZINE

Thioridazine ('Melleril') was subject to a change in its licence in the US and UK in 2000 as a result of evidence that it prolongs the QT interval and because there has been an excess of deaths of people on this drug, mainly elderly people. It was particularly useful in calming agitation and restlessness, but otherwise was used for the same purposes as chlorpromazine, although there was no injectable form. For control of psychosis a dose one-and-a-half times that of chlorpromazine was used. It was used in the elderly because, of all the phenothiazines, it is the least likely to produce extrapyramidal signs, having pronounced anticholinergic properties. Dizziness resulting from hypotension, especially postural hypotension, and muzziness might occur, particularly at the start of treatment. Doses above 600 mg a day, particularly for longer than 4 weeks, carry the risk of pigmentary retinopathy and blindness.

Thioridazine was widely, indeed too widely, used to control behavioural disturbance in people with dementia. Its major effect is non-specific sedation; it can cause marked EPS and falls, as well as increasing confusion. Non-drug approaches and atypical antipsychotics are usually preferable.

It is now indicated for second-line treatment of schizophrenia in adults under specialist supervision. The ECG should be recorded before starting and for any dose increase, and electrolytes should be checked. It should not be given to people with cardiac disease, an abnormal ECG or those on other medication that may cause ECG changes, or may inhibit its metabolism via CYP IID6.

PROMAZINE

Promazine is much less potent as an antipsychotic than chlorpromazine; it is now occasionally used as a hypnotic or sedative for the elderly, where drug-induced confusional states are a risk. Beware of producing oversedation, urinary and faecal incontinence, disorientation and lowered temperature.

Orally give 25–100 mg once, or up to four times daily; intramuscularly give 50 mg, repeatable after 6 hours. It is available as tablets of 25 mg and 50 mg, suspension (50 mg per 5 ml) and injection (50 mg per ml in 1 ml ampoules).

TRIFLUOPERAZINE

Trifluoperazine ('Stelazine') is much more potent (i.e. it can be used in lower doses) than chlorpromazine; it produces little sedation or hypotension but is more liable to produce dystonia, akathisia and

Parkinsonism. It is more suitable for the patient with less behavioural disturbance, for instance out-patients.

For paranoid psychosis and schizophrenia give 15 mg (range 10–30 mg) daily by mouth, in divided doses, or as a spansule at night. For symptomatic anxiety, give 1–5 mg once or more daily. Anti-Parkinsonian drugs are likely to be needed; they may either be given from the start – especially if there is a risk of alienating the patient through an EPS – or the patient should be warned of the possible need and be ready to take them if the side-effect develops. Review the question of need after 2, 4 and 8 weeks' continuous treatment, since the need may disappear as the psychosis settles, or if the dose is reduced for maintenance treatment.

It is available as tablets of 1 mg and 5 mg, spansules of 2 mg, 10 mg and 15 mg, syrup (1 mg per 5 ml), liquid concentrate (10 mg per ml for dilution) and injection (1 mg per ml, in 1 ml ampoules).

PERPHENAZINE

The use and side-effects of perphenazine ('Fentazin') are as for chlorpromazine, but it is less sedative and more prone to induce Parkinsonism. Give 4–8 mg three times daily as tablets. For anxiety, give 2 mg twice or three times daily, and upwards. Has been successfully used for intractable hiccough.

PERICYAZINE

Pericyazine ('Neulactil') is used for treating psychoses and behavioural disturbance, in doses of 15–30 mg by mouth for psychoses, but up to 300 mg daily for severe behavioural disturbance due to psychosis or mental handicap. Side-effects are as for chlorpromazine but pericyazine is more sedative.

RELATED PHENOTHIAZINE

Methotrimeprazine ('Noxinan') is used for pain in terminal care and prochlorperazine ('Stemetil') is used as an anti-emetic, and for nausea and vertigo. Both have antipsychotic activity.

FLUPHENAZINE AND ITS DECANOATE

Fluphenazine hydrochloride ('Moditen', 'Prolixen') is the most potent of the phenothiazines. Fluphenazine decanoate ('Modecate') is fluphenazine esterified in the side-chain with decanoic acid, a long-chain fatty acid, and dissolved in sesame oil with benzyl alcohol, for injection. A single dose will continue to give therapeutic benefit for 1–6 weeks (and the drug lasts longer in long-term treatment, being detectable for several months). The drug is injected into a muscle, where it remains as a fatty depot; from this depot the drug is gradually removed via the lymphatic system, including the action of phagocytes, and the active drug is released. The injection is eminently suitable for long-term treatment of chronic schizophrenia, particularly in out-patients who may not be able, or willing, particularly if they feel well, to take tablets regularly for very long periods, or for patients suspicious of tablets. It is also useful in preventing frequently recurrent attacks of mania or hypomania in bipolar disorder (see chapter 12).

Fluphenazine hydrochloride need only be taken orally once a day, in a dose of 1–10 mg. At least 5 mg a day is usually required to treat psychosis. There is considerable individual variation in absorption of the drug.

Fluphenazine decanoate is given by deep intramuscular injection, usually into the gluteal muscle. When starting depot treatment a test dose of 12.5 mg (6.25 mg in the elderly) is given, to detect any allergic response to the vehicle and to familiarise the patient with the drug. Three to 7 days later the patient starts on a regular dose of 25 mg weekly (maximum 50 mg weekly), which continues for 4–6 weeks during which time previous oral medication is gradually withdrawn. The frequency is then reduced. The onset of EPS suggests that a sufficient blood level has already been reached; blood levels will continue to rise until steady-state is reached unless the dose is reduced. The maintenance dose of fluphenazine decanoate varies for individuals between 6.25 mg and 100 mg given every 2–6 weeks. Lower doses are required in females, people over the age of 50 and with longer periods since the last relapse. The most common dose is 25 mg a fortnight or the equivalent. Dystonic reactions, tremor and restlessness may occur, especially in the 2 days after the injection, as a portion of free fluphenazine is released from the depot. During this time the patient may need anticholinergic medication. Some patients continue to experience such side-effects throughout the course of the injections and need to continue on anticholinergic drugs. Side-effects can sometimes be avoided by halving the dose and giving the injection twice as often. Minor degrees of side-effects, especially drowsiness or flatness, and restlessness, are not uncommon and it may, unfortunately, take some months for the patient to adjust to.

Sometimes in otherwise well-controlled patients symptoms seem to worsen or to begin to reappear towards the end of the third or fourth week after the injection; if true, this suggests the need to shorten the interval between injections or to increase the dose a little. The aim is to find the optimal interval and the smallest dose that will achieve control.

After a relapse has been brought under control it is possible to reduce the dose over the following 6 months. After that, if the patient is stable, the dose may be reduced to one that has previously been found to maintain stability. If it is known that a patient has previously relapsed when the dose is reduced below a certain level, then he/she should be advised to continue on that dose or a higher one. When planning a reduction of dose with the patient remember that for pharmacokinetic reasons the full effect of the reduction will not occur until 4–6 months after the prescription is changed, and there is an increased risk of relapse for up to 2 years. Most will do well on 25 mg fortnightly; some need more, some manage on even less. Patients feel better on lower doses and have fewer Parkinsonian and other side-effects. The patient should therefore be supervised regularly and not too infrequently. This can be done if the injection is administered by a CPN who arranges for the patient to be reviewed by the doctor. Even the most stable patient should be reviewed at least once a year and the review should preferably include a doctor who knows the patient. Team reviews or community ward rounds enable information to be shared and experience to be gained.

Fluphenazine is available as fluphenazine hydrochloride ('Moditen') tablets of 1 mg, 2.5 mg and 5 mg; fluphenazine decanoate ('Modecate'), injection (25 mg/ml) in 0.5 ml, 1.0 ml and 2.0 ml ampoules, and ready-filled disposable 1.0 ml and 2.0 ml syringes; and fluphenazine decanoate ('Modecate Concentrate') injection (100 mg/ml) of 0.5 ml and 1.0 ml ampoules.

PIPOTHIAZINE PALMITATE

Pipothiazine is a phenothiazine available for use only as a depot formulation of the palmitic acid ester in sesame oil ('Piportil'). The same practical considerations apply to its clinical use as those just described for fluphenazine decanoate (also see chapter 13). It is structurally similar to thioridazine, but no clinical advantages over fluphenazine decanoate have been shown.

BUTYROPHENONES

These drugs, related chemically to the analgesic pethidine, are mostly used in psychiatry for the control of schizophrenia, mania and acute brain syndrome, especially when aggression and excitement are present. Haloperidol blocks dopamine D_2 receptors, and to a lesser extent noradrenalin α-1 receptors. Although chemically quite distinct from phenothiazines, their therapeutic effects are similar, but some individual patients may do better with one type of drug than with the other.

HALOPERIDOL

Haloperidol ('Serenace', 'Haldol', Figure 28.2) may be used for:

- severe excitement, overactivity or aggression, especially associated with mania or schizophrenia
- continuous treatment of mania, schizophrenia and paranoid psychosis
- restlessness and agitation in the elderly
- acute confusional states (see chapter 16)
- Gilles de la Tourette's syndrome.

For the acutely excited and overactive patient begin with 5–10 mg intramuscularly repeated 2-hourly up to 60 mg total over 12 hours if necessary. This dosage controls most states, and when it does the dose can be reduced to 5–10 mg thrice daily orally and then further reduced in a few days depending on the response. Because of the side-effects, oral procyclidine 10 mg up to thrice daily may need to be given. If

Figure 28.2 The structure of haloperidol

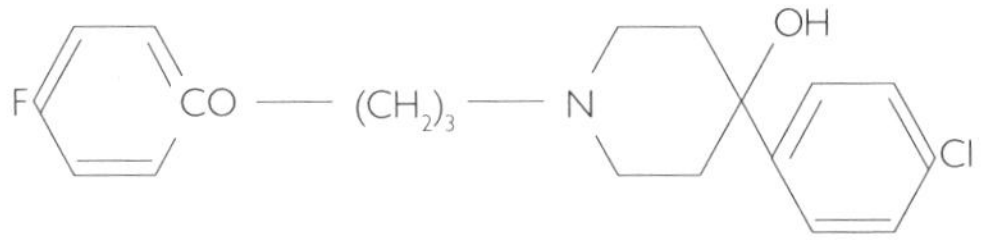

intravenous haloperidol is given, then intravenous procyclidine 10 mg may be given at the same time but in a separate syringe. These high doses of haloperidol are required in severe manic, drug-induced and schizophrenic excitements, but lower doses may be quite adequate for acute brain syndromes.

In continued treatment for mania and schizophrenia 2–5 mg thrice daily is usually adequate, but a frequent check for psychotic symptoms and side-effects should guide. Bigger doses may be needed and may be well tolerated. Claims are made that doses of up to 80 mg a day are effective in resistant cases, but this is not supported by research evidence, which in general shows that higher doses are less effective (see also p. 142). The drug is also used in depot form (haloperidol decanoate) for maintenance therapy.

For agitation in the elderly the appropriate starting dose is 0.5 mg twice daily. Children with Gilles de la Tourette's syndrome should be maintained on the lowest effective dose, which is likely to be around 0.1 mg/kg a day. Pimozide (see below) is an alternative (0.05–0.20 mg/kg).

Side-effects

EPS are common, more so than with chlorpromazine, and can come on at any stage of treatment. Stiffness, rigidity or extreme restlessness are the most frequent. The elderly and those with basal ganglia disease are especially prone to these.

Side-effects can occur with remarkable suddenness even after a single small dose, although these are more likely with larger doses. They may appear as excitement lessens. Side-effects may persist for 3 months or longer after stopping haloperidol, and commonly do so for 10 days. Intravenous procyclidine 10 mg relieves acute symptoms, and an anticholinergic should be continued orally. Test at intervals, by gradual withdrawal, whether it continues to be needed during long-term treatment.

Haloperidol is available as tablets of 1.5 mg, 5 mg, 10 mg and 20 mg; capsules (0.5 mg); liquid (2 mg per ml, 10 mg per ml); and injection (5 mg in 1 ml, 10 mg in 1 ml, 20 mg in 2 ml).

Haloperidol decanoate is used similarly to fluphenazine decanoate with intervals of up to 4–6 weeks, but with about twice the dose. Local pain at the site of injection is more often a problem than with other depot injections. Start with a test dose of 50 mg deeply intramuscular, followed by 100–200 mg every 1–4 weeks, depending on the urgency. Maintenance doses of 100 mg four weekly are common, more than 300 mg unusual.

Haloperidol is available as haloperidol decanoate in sesame oil in ampoules of 50 mg in 1 ml and 100 ml in 1 ml.

Droperidol

Droperidol ('Droleptan') was withdrawn voluntarily by the manufacturer in 2001, following evidence that it prolongs the QT interval and concerns about sudden death. It is a more sedative drug than haloperidol, by virtue of its greater potency in blocking noradrenalin α-1 and histamine H_1 receptors. It was used for acute tranquillisation and mania, but was not licensed for the treatment of psychosis. Tolerance develops to its sedative effects. It is metabolised with a half-life of 4 hours, and consequently had to be administered at more frequent intervals than haloperidol.

Related drugs

Benperidol ('Anquil') is licensed for the control of deviant and antisocial sexual behaviour, although it is probably not more specific than other antipsychotics for this (see chapter 22).

Thioxanthenes

Thioxanthenes resemble phenothiazines closely, but have a carbon atom in place of the nitrogen atom of the middle ring to which the side-chain is attached. The side-chain is usually linked to this carbon atom by a double bond, which makes the molecule look a little like a TCA with a sulphur atom (but with a six – not a seven – atom central ring). The thioxanthene analogue of fluphenazine is flupentixol. Chlorprothixene is the analogue of chlorpromazine but is not licensed in the UK. Zuclopenthixol has a chlorine atom, but a side-chain like flupentixol . Both flupentixol and clopenthixol are available as decanoates for depot injection. The thioxanthenes are pharmacologically different from phenothiazines in that they block both D_1 and D_2 receptor types. (Figure 28.3).

Flupentixol

By deep intramuscular injection, flupentixol decanoate ('Depixol') is effective against schizophrenic symptoms (20–100 mg every 2–4 weeks), comparable with fluphenazine decanoate but less sedative. It tends to be preferred in the more lethargic patient or one with a history of depression. Begin with a test dose of 20 mg intramuscularly. Rarely, doses can go up to 400 mg weekly. The depot injection may also be tried to control bipolar disorder when other treatments have failed (40–80 mg weekly). The higher dose tablet ('Depixol') is used for psychosis (3–9 mg twice daily). Like other antipsychotics, oral flupentixol ('Fluanxol') can be given in smaller doses (0.5–1.5 mg morning and midday) for anxiety and is also licensed for depression. Older reports suggest that flupentixol may give rise to overactivity, albeit rarely.

It should be noted that flupentixol has stereoisomers; whereas the depot injection contains only the zu-flupentixol isomer, the tablets contain the racemic mixture. It has been shown that only the zu- form (which blocks dopamine receptors) has antispychotic activity. It is available as tablets ('Fluanxol') of 0.5 mg and 1 mg; 'Depixol' 3 mg. Cis(Z-)flupentixol decanoate in thin vegetable oil is 'Depixol' – 2% ampoules (clear) 20 mg in 1 ml, 40 mg in 2 ml; 10% ampoules (amber) 100 mg in 1 ml; 20% ampoules (amber) 200 mg in 1 ml.

Zuclopenthixol

Zuclopenthixol ('Clopixol') is more sedative than flupentixol and is more suitable for the patient who is behaviourally disturbed. Oral doses begin with 20–50 mg daily to a maximum of 150 mg daily. Acutely disturbed patients who consistently refuse oral medication and would require repeated doses of simple intramuscular injections may be given zuclopenthixol acetate ('Acuphase') by deep intramuscular injection with a duration of action of 3 days. Start with 50–150 mg, repeated after 1–3 days to a maximum of 400 mg in total. The onset of full action takes about 2–8 hours. Zuclopenthixol decanoate can be used to follow this, or for longer-term treatment. Start with 100 mg intramuscular gluteal injection, and increase to 200–500 mg every 1–4 weeks. The maximum dose is 600 mg a week. Zuclopenthixol Di HCl (oral) ia available as tablets of 2 mg, 10 mg and 25 mg; zuclopenthixol acetate ('Acuphase') injection (50 mg/ml) in 1 ml and 2 ml ampoules; zuclopenthixol decanoate ('Clopixol')injection (200 mg/ml) in 1.0 ml ampoule and 10 ml vial; and concentrate injection (500 mg/ml) in 1.0 ml ampoule with needle.

BUTYLPIPERIDINES

Pimozide

Pimozide ('Orap') is more selective for dopamine receptors than haloperidol, and less sedative. It may be used for schizophrenia and paranoid psychosis; mania; Gilles de la Tourette's syndrome; and monosymptomatic delusional hypochondriasis. In the last condition, pimozide may be uniquely effective when other drugs have failed. It

Figure 28.3 A thioxathene and a phenothiazine compared

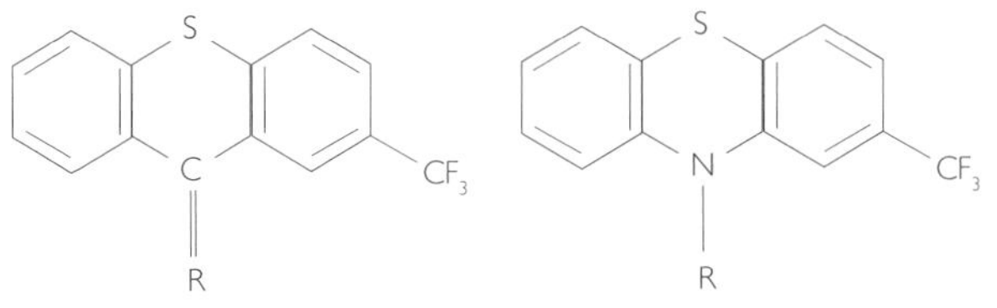

(a) flupentixol

(b) fluphenazine

has a long duration of action with a half-life averaging 53 hours and does accumulate during regular doses.

Pimozide is more potent than other antipsychotics as a calcium antagonist, and fatal dysrhythmias (Torsade de Pointes) can occur with high doses. An ECG should be done before starting treatment and annually, and with particular care in those on more than 16 mg daily. Pimozide is contraindicated if there is a prolonged QT interval or any history of cardiac arrhythmia. Other drugs that prolong the QT interval should be avoided in combination, particularly cisapride and the anti-histamines astemizole and terfenadine, but also TCAs and other antipsychotics. Diuretics that alter electrolytes should also be avoided.

For acute psychosis it is given once daily in a starting dose of 6 mg, which can be increased by weekly steps of 2 or 4 mg to a maximum of 20 mg. For other indications start with 2 mg and increase gradually by 2 mg steps to a maximum of 16 mg. Its advantages are that it is fairly free of sedative and hypotensive side-effects. Parkinsonism, dystonia and akathisia occur frequently. Its long half-life means that its plasma concentration changes rather slowly, and even missing a day's dose will not alter the level much. Some patients can be well treated by weekly supervised dosing.

In monosymptomatic delusional hypochondriasis, for instance delusional parasitosis, the dose should start at 2 mg daily, increasing to 16 mg. It is available as tablets of 2 mg, 4 mg and 10 mg.

Pregnancy

Chlorpromazine, trifluoperazine, haloperidol and both fluphenazine decanoate and flupentixol decanoate have been used in large numbers of women, including throughout pregnancy. In general the risks of continuing these drugs during pregnancy will outweigh the risks (to the mother and future child) of untreated psychotic illness. Antipsychotic drugs for which less clinical experience has been obtained should not be prescribed when pregnancy is planned. However, many pregnancies are unplanned, and the newer antipsychotics tend to increase the fertility of people with schizophrenia.

Equivalent doses of antipsychotic medication

It is impossible to generalise accurately about the equivalent doses of different antipsychotics because of the variation in metabolism of the same drug between individuals, and because different drugs have different half-lives and therefore accumulate to different extents. However, some very rough guides are available.

Depot antipsychotics

The principles of depot medication for schizophrenia are discussed in chapter 13. The depot formulations are less affected by individual metabolic differences than oral drugs, because they avoid first-pass

Table 28.1 Approximately equivalent doses of depot antipsychotics

Depot drug	Equivalent doses (mg)	BNF maximum (mg/week)
Fluphenazine decanoate	25	50
Haloperidol decanoate	50	75
Pipothiazine palmitate	25	50
Flupentixol decanoate	40	400
Zuclopenthixol decanoate	200	600

metabolism in the gut and liver. See Table 28.1 for approximately equivalent doses.

The first three can be given every 2–6 weeks, and have an apparent plasma half-life of about 3 weeks. The last two have a shorter duration and may need to be given more often, every 2–3 weeks, and in the case of zuclopenthixol sometimes weekly. In the elderly different doses apply for each drug; fluphenazine decanoate in particular is needed in progressively lower doses after the age of 50.

Box 28.2 Disadvantages of classical antipsychotics

Limited efficacy
delayed effects
resistant positive symptoms
residual negative symptoms
secondary negative symptoms
cognitive symptoms
secondary depression

Acute pharmacological side-effects
extrapyramidal side-effects
Parkinsonism
acute dystonia
akathisia
postural hypotension
anticholinergic effects
impotence
cardiotoxicity

Long-term pharmacological side-effects
hyperprolactinaemia:
    galactorrhoea
    amenorrhoea
    low libido
weight gain
tardive dyskinesia
tardive dystonia

Idiosyncratic reactions
Neuroleptic malignant syndrome
rash
hepatitis
agranulocytosis

THE DRUGS

Conclusion

Box 28.2 summarises the shortcomings of classical antipsychotic drugs. These represent challenges for new drug development and we shall return to them in chapter 30.

Further reading

Clinical studies

Johnstone, E. C., Crow, T., Frith, C. D., *et al* (1978) Mechanism of the antipsychotic effect in the treatment of acute schizophrenia. *Lancet*, **i**, 848–851.

Johnstone, E. C., Crow, T. J., Ferrier, I. N., *et al* (1983) Adverse effects of anticholinergic medication on positive schizophrenic symptoms. *Psychological Medicine*, **13**, 513–527.

Spivak, B., Gonen, N., Mester, R., *et al* (1996) Neuroleptic malignant syndrome associated with abrupt withdrawal of anticholinergic agents. *International Clinical Psychopharmacology*, **11**, 207–209.

Taylor, D. (1999) Depot antipsychotics revisited. *Psychiatric Bulletin*, **23**, 551–553.

Tranter, R. & Healy, D. (1998) Neuroleptic discontinuation syndromes. *Journal of Psychopharmacology*, **12**, 401–406.

PET scan evidence on blockage of D_2 receptors

Farde, L., Nordstom, A. L., Wiesel, F. A., *et al* (1992) Positron emission tomographic analysis of central D_1 and D_2 dopamine receptor occupancy in patients treated with classical neuroleptics and clozapine. *Archives of General Psychiatry*, **49**, 538–544.

Sudden deaths and ECG effects

Appleby, L., Shaw, J., Amos, T., *et al* (2000) Sudden unexplained deaths in psychiatric in-patients. *British Journal of Psychiatry*, **176**, 405–406.

Reilly, J. G., Ayis, S. A., Ferrier, I. N. *et al* (2001) Sudden death and thioridazine. Proceedings of the British Pharmacological Society, Clinical Pharmacology Section, University of Birmingham, 18–21 December 2000. *British Journal of Clinical Pharmacology*, **51**, 363.

—, —, — *et al* (2000) QTc interval abnormalities and psychotropic drug therapy in psychiatric Patients. *Lancet*, **355**, 1048–1052.

Royal College of Psychiatrists (1997) *The Association Between Antipsychotic Drugs and Sudden Death*. Report of the Working Group of the Royal College of Psychiatrists' Psychopharmacology Sub-Group. Council Report CR57. London: Royal College of Psychiatrists.

Consensus statement

Thompson, C. (1994) The use of high dose antipsychotic medication. *British Journal of Psychiatry*, **164**, 448–458.

EPS encountered in psychiatric practice are nearly all drug-induced (see chapter 17). Only a small number result from primary basal ganglia disease, although the ageing or damaged brain is predisposed to both Parkinsonian side-effects and tardive dyskinesia. Phenothiazines with a piperazine side-chain (R in Figure 28.1, p. 289), such as trifluoperazine, and the butyrophenones are the two groups of antipsychotic drugs that most commonly cause Parkinsonism and other EPS. On occasion TCAs in high dose or SSRIs may also be responsible. Lithium will also provoke such reactions, mainly when added to an antipsychotic or an antidepressant, but sometimes alone in toxic doses.

Parkinson's disease itself was first successfully treated with the atropine group of drugs that block cholinergic activity. Subsequently atropine-like synthetic drugs, also antihistaminic in action, were developed, and then drugs that improve dopaminergic transmission in the basal ganglia, such as L-dopa, bromocriptine and amantidine. None of these latter drugs are useful in drug-induced Parkinsonism, but they are relevant to psychiatric practice because of their side-effects or their occasional use for primary Parkinsonism in psychiatric patients. Fifteen per cent of patients taking L-dopa develop significant psychiatric symptoms and may present with a toxic confusional state (acute brain syndrome), depression, hypomania or paranoid state or with vivid visual or auditory hallucinations. L-dopa may then have to be reduced or stopped. Dopamine agonists such as bromocriptine, lysuride and pergolide can produce psychotic reactions. Amantidine is less of a problem, but in a few patients, especially those who have had a previous psychiatric illness, psychotic states with confusion and hallucinations occur. The MAO-B inhibitor selegiline may also give rise to psychosis and agitation.

The synthetic anticholinergic drugs procyclidine, orphenadrine and benzhexol and more sedative ones like benztropine and biperiden can control or modify drug-induced EPS so that antipsychotic medication may be maintained. Anti-Parkinsonian drugs should not be prescribed routinely to patients on antipsychotic drugs (with the exception of haloperidol and trifluoperazine), but only when side-effects appear. The therapeutic action of antipsychotics may be modified by anti-Parkinsonian drugs. If EPS do appear, consider reducing the level of antipsychotic drug before prescribing an anti-Parkinsonian drug long-term.

With most atypical antipsychotics, anti-Parkinsonian drugs are not required, unless high doses are used. Exceptions include sometimes modest doses of risperidone and amisulpride. In addition, the co-administration of a typical antipsychotic (an undesirable practice) often provokes the need for anticholinergic medication.

ANTICHOLINERGIC DRUGS

These block acetylcholine-M receptors. In the caudate and putamen, dopamine normally acts to inhibit acetylcholine neurons. Most antipsychotic drugs block this action of dopamine, and thereby increase release of acetylcholine. In addition to their anti-muscarinic or atropinic actions, the drugs are also to varied extents antihistaminic, and block dopamine reuptake. The latter action, along with the central anticholinergic action, causes stimulant effects and a risk of abuse and dependence. High doses cause confusional states or psychotic reactions.

The synthetic anticholinergic drugs used in large doses, especially in the elderly, can produce an acute brain syndrome. Their anticholinergic activity can interfere with the treatment of narrow-angle glaucoma, and provoke acute retention of urine in men with prostatic hypertrophy. Side-effects may appear before the optimal dose for controlling Parkinsonian symptoms is achieved.

Abrupt discontinuation of anticholinergic drugs can cause a rebound syndrome with nausea, insomnia and anxiety.

Procyclidine is discussed in some detail as typical of the group. Others are described briefly. Despite similar action, one of these drugs may suit a patient better than others, so that if side-effects develop, an alternative should be tried.

Procyclidine

Procyclidine ('Arpicolin', 'Kemadrin') is widely used to relieve drug-induced EPS and (intravenously) to relieve acute dystonia. The drug is well absorbed from the gut and is metabolised rapidly. Intravenous or intramuscular procyclidine, usually 10 mg, relieves acute dystonia within 5–10 minutes (longer if intramuscular) and gives relief for 30 minutes to 4 hours. The half-life is 12 hours and often oral doses twice daily are enough.

When beginning typical antipsychotic medication, try to do without anti-muscarinic drugs until side-effects show; then start with procyclidine 5 mg twice daily, gradually increasing every 2–3 days up to 5–10 mg three times daily. Once the side-effects are controlled, try slowly to reduce the drug every 3–4 months and, if possible, withdraw. Alternatively, the antipsychotic may be able to be reduced to a level with fewer side-effects. Many clinicians now advocate switching to an atypical antipsychotic if EPS occur, or even the first-line use of atypical drugs, especially in patients with a history of severe Parkinsonism or dystonic reaction, but also in newly diagnosed patients.

A patient with acute disturbance may need high doses of typical antipsychotics quickly and then giving concurrent procyclidine avoids potential additional stress from unpleasant side-effects. It also can help with later compliance.

Side-effects, typical of all anti-muscarinic drugs, include drowsiness (insomnia with procyclidine and bezhexol), dry mouth, blurred vision, dilated pupils, nausea and constipation. Higher doses, especially in the elderly, can cause confusion and hallucinations. Anti-muscarinics can also worsen the cognitive symptoms of schizophrenia. Avoid their use in narrow-angle glaucoma or where prostatic hypertrophy is likely, as an acute obstruction can occur. Sound rules are to keep to the lowest dose possible to relieve EPS and if changing dose, to do it gradually. Sudden stoppage can produce acute side-effects (akinesia, rigidity, salivation and urinary retention) and may precipitate a cholinergic rebound (nausea, diarrhoea, abdominal pain, restlessness and insomnia). In the latter syndrome, post-synaptic cholinergic receptors have become sensitised by long-term muscarinic blockade (i.e. they are upregulated and more sensitive to acetylcholine). When the blockade is abruptly removed, cholinergic transmission is vastly increased and parasympathetic overdrive occurs.

Patients may experience a pleasurable 'buzz' with procyclidine and more so with benzhexol. Some hoard, or trade tablets with others, to get a large supply. In many inner-city areas, anticholinergics have a street value. Higher doses produce euphoria and, rarely, hallucinations. A useful sign is fixed dilated pupils. It is available as a tablet of 5 mg, syrup in 2.5 mg/5 ml and 5 mg/5 ml strength and an injection of 5 mg/ml.

Benzhexol

Benzhexol ('Artane', 'Broflex') is used similarly to procyclidine. Start with a low dose, 1 mg daily, and increase slowly, allowing 2–3 days to elapse between each increase. An effective dose is usually between 4 and 15 mg daily. It has more pronounced stimulant effects than procyclidine and is perhaps more prone to abuse. (Preference for different drugs appears to depend on geography as well as pharmacology.) Higher doses may well precipitate an excited and abnormal mental state; another drug should then be tried. It is available as tablets of 2 mg and 5 mg and syrup at a strength of 5 mg/5 ml.

Benztropine

Benztropine ('Cogentin') is longer acting than other drugs and, probably because of this, is frequently prescribed in the US. Start with a low dose (0.5–2 mg) once daily for the first few days and increase gradually to 6 mg daily, if necessary. Some patients do better on divided doses, some on a single daily dose. Acute dystonic reactions are relieved by 2 mg given intramuscularly or intravenously. It is available as a tablet of 2 mg and an injection of 1 mg/ml.

Orphenadrine

Orphenadrine ('Biorphen', 'Disipal') is usually well tolerated by patients and is less prone to abuse than benzhexol or procyclidine. Start with 50 mg three times daily and increase, if necessary, up to 200 mg daily. Orphenadrine is a potentially toxic drug, with strong membrane-stabilising activity, and large overdoses can be fatal. Recent naturalistic research indicating high toxicity makes orphenadrine a poor choice for patients at risk of overdose or suicide. It is available as a tablet of 50 mg and an oral solution ('Elixir'), 25 mg/5ml.

Biperiden

Biperiden ('Akineton') is similar to, but more sedative than, orphenadrine. Start with 1 mg twice daily and increase up to 6–12 mg daily. The parenteral preparation may cause hypotension; if intravenous, give slowly in a dose of 2.5–5 mg. It is available as a tablet of 2 mg and an injection of 5 mg/ml.

Tetrabenazine

Tetrabenazine ('Nitoman') is used for the control of abnormal movement disorders such as Huntington's chorea and tardive dyskinesia. It works by depleting neuronal stores of biogenic amines, including dopamine; this is similar to the action of reserpine but less pronounced. The use of tetrabenazine has declined markedly over the past two decades. The dose starts with 25 mg daily and gradually increases to 25 mg three times daily, up to a maximum of 200 mg daily. If there is no improvement after 7 days of high-dose treatment, do not persist with the drug. Drowsiness, indigestion, hypotension and Parkinsonism occur as side-effects, at high doses. If depression occurs, an MARI may be given; MAOIs must be avoided because of the risk of a confusional state. It is available as a tablet of 25mg.

OTHER ANTICHOLINERGICS

Hyoscine

Hyoscine hydrobromide has profound peripheral effects that can be useful in clozapine-induced hypersalivation. The dose is 300 μg up to three times daily. The tablets (trade name 'Kwells', used for motion sickness) can be sucked or chewed, which may provide a topical effect.

Pirenzepine

Pirenzepine is also used for clozapine-induced hypersalivation. At a dose of 25 mg three times daily, it is usually effective and well tolerated. Pirenzepine blocks muscarinic receptors, particularly the M_4 receptors that occur in glandular tissue and are stimulated by clozapine but also M_1 receptors. It is no longer marketed in the UK, but is available through pharmaceutical importers.

FURTHER READING

Buckley, N. & McManus, P. (1998) Fatal toxicity of drugs used in the treatment of psychotic illness. *British Journal of Psychiatry*, **172**, 461–464.

Caulfield, M. P. (1993) Muscarinic receptors – characterisation, coupling and function. *Pharmacology and Therapeutics*, **58**, 319–379.

Horn, A. S., Coyle, J. T. & Snyder, S. H. (1971) Catecholamine uptake by synaptosomes from rat brain: structure activity relationships of drugs with differential effects on dopamine and norepinephrine neurones. *Molecular Pharmacology*, **7**, 66–88.

Jellinek, T., Gardos, G. & Cole, J. J. (1981) Adverse effects of antiparkinson drug withdrawal. *Archives of General Psychiatry*, **35**, 483–489.

Mintzer, J. & Burns, A. (2000) Anticholinergic side-effects of drugs in elderly people. *Journal of the Royal Society of Medicine*, **93**, 457–462.

Szabadi, E. (1997) Clozapine-induced hypersalivation (letter). *British Journal of Psychiatry*, **171**, 89.

Box 28.2 (p. 301) summarised the shortcomings of the classical antipsychotic drugs. New drugs have been developed with the aim of overcoming these problems.

Animal models exist for acute EPS, and most new drugs have been selected as having a reduced propensity to cause them. The term atypical is used in various ways but is best reserved to describe antipsychotic drugs that are relatively lacking in EPS. Among the classical antipsychotics, those with intrinsic anticholinergic activity, such as thioridazine, are less likely to cause acute EPS. However, there are at least three other ways in which drugs can act as antipsychotics without producing acute EPS. These mechanisms are used to classify the atypical drugs (see Box 2.1, p. 17).

Firstly, drugs may block subtypes of D_2-like receptors, including those in the corpus striatum, in such a way that fewer EPS occur. The benzamide drugs (sulpiride and amisulpride) are examples. According to one hypothesis, these and other atypicals dissociate rapidly from the D_2 receptor, allowing endogenously released brief pulses of dopamine to compete with these drugs for occupancy of the receptor, despite the drugs appearing to have high occupancy in PET scans.

Secondly, drugs that potently block 5-HT-2A as well as D_2 receptors (SDRAs) seem to enhance dopamine release and thereby to avoid producing EPS, except at higher doses (sometimes above the licensed range) when their D_2 blocking effects predominate. Examples are risperidone, sertindole and ziprasidone; but others such as clozapine, olanzapine, zotepine and quetiapine share the property of blocking 5-HT-2A receptors.

Thirdly, drugs with a broad range of receptor blocking actions – PRAs but whose dopamine receptor-blocking actions appear to be exerted particularly on dopamine receptors in the limbic brain areas (nucleus accumbens, amygdala, cortex) as opposed to the extrapyramidal areas (basal ganglia, corpus striatum, etc.). Examples are clozapine, olanzapine, quetiapine and zotepine.

This chapter describes the newer drugs and examines to what extent they overcome the shortcomings of the classical antipsychotics. As will be seen, these new drugs tend to produce fewer EPS and some produce very much less (or placebo-level). For some there is also evidence of less tardive dyskinesia. All can cause NMS. They vary in the extent to which they block acetylcholine-M, histamine H_1 and noradrenalin α-1 receptors.

There is growing interest in their ability to cause less mental dulling than older drugs, and to improve cognitive function in schizophrenia, and also in their beneficial effects upon mood.

Unfortunately, concerns remain about their interactions with ion channels and their effects upon the cardiac electrical impulse. Blocking the delayed rectifier potassium channels in the heart prolongs the QT interval (see p. 287). Information about this is scanty, but a study conducted for the FDA in patients given standard doses of six drugs found the greatest prolongation with thioridazine; slight lengthening also occurred with ziprasidone and quetiapine, but little with olanzapine, risperidone or haloperidol.

None of the other atypicals is associated with the high risk of bone marrow suppression seen with clozapine. Information about other idiosyncratic reactions may yet arise.

THE CLINICAL TRIALS

For regulatory approval, the new drugs must be shown to be effective by comparison with placebo. Some trials include a classical antipsychotic as an active comparator. In order to demonstrate subtle advantages over the classical drug, large numbers of patients must be included. A common trial design includes patients who have generally responded only partially to previous treatments, and treats them with either one of several fixed doses of the new drug or haloperidol or placebo. During the study there is usually only modest improvement even on the active treatments (see Table 30.1). For example, half those on active treatment show a 20% reduction in score on the Positive and Negative Syndrome Scale (PANSS; Kay *et al*, 1987), and only 10% of those on placebo do so. There tend, however, to be more early drop-outs through side-effects in the patients on haloperidol, and through lack of improvement in those on placebo. This biases the analysis, using the intent-to-treat method with last observation carried forward (see p. 36). The bias is in favour of the treatment with fewer early drop-outs. A further problem is that the new drug is tested in a range of doses but most trials use only one fixed dose of the comparator, usually haloperidol, and this may not be the optimal dose. In particular, doses of haloperidol of 20 mg/day and more are associated with a less good outcome in groups of patients than doses of 10 mg/day.

BENZAMIDES

The discovery that clinical efficacy in schizophrenia is highly correlated with potency in binding D_2 receptors (see p. 284) drove a strategy for drug development based on selective antagonism of dopamine, and at D_2 (as opposed to D_1) receptors. The benzamides represent the outcome of that drive. In general they produce fewer EPS than classical antipsychotics. There are differences among the benzamides in the extent to which they block the different subtypes of D_2-like receptors. At therapeutic doses these drugs do occupy a high proportion of D_2-like receptors in the basal ganglia, as do classical antipsychotics, but cause less EPS. It is probable that at the same time they produce substantial blockade of limbic D_2-like receptors (including the D_3 subtype).

Sulpiride

Pharmacology

Sulpiride ('Dolmatil', 'Sulpitil') is a benzamide and selective for D_2 receptors, including the D_3 subtype (see Figure 30.1). At low doses it

Figure 30.1 The structure of sulpiride, a benzamide

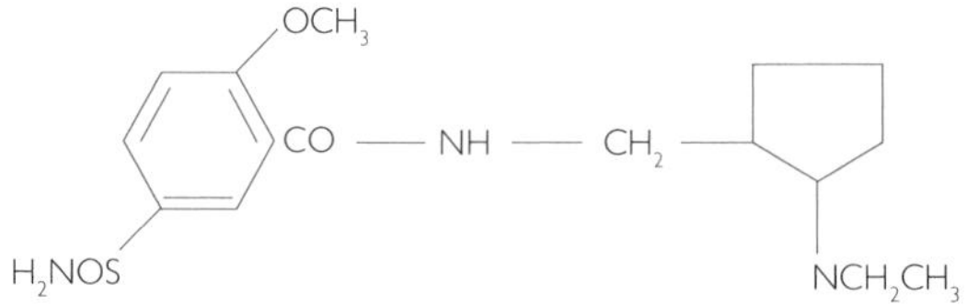

has activating effects thought to be due to blockade of presynaptic D_2-like autoreceptors. It is particularly potent in blocking dopamine receptors in the pituitary and increasing prolactin levels. Sulpiride is not metabolised to any extent but is excreted unchanged in the urine.

Clinical effects

At the higher doses needed to suppress positive symptoms, the activating effect is lost. It is particularly suitable for those with schizophrenia who will adhere to oral medication, and who do not need sedation, and for those troubled by acute EPS with other drugs. Higher doses have also been found effective in mania.

Its activating effect in low doses is not specific for schizophrenia; it has also been used in low doses as an antidepressant and for dysthymia. It can also be effective as an adjunct to clozapine in treatment-resistant schizophrenia. It is used as an adjunct to SSRIs in OCD.

Adverse effects include tiredness, restlessness and weight gain. Parkinsonism, if it occurs, is mild. The incidence of tardive dyskinesia is still uncertain. Anticholinergic side-effects are minimal. Poisoning by overdose can produce restlessness and clouding of consciousness, leading on to coma and low blood pressure, but there have been no deaths reported and recovery is quick. In women side-effects arise from hyperprolactinaemia: amenorrhoea and galactorrhoea. These limit the drugs' widespread use.

Dose

For positive schizophrenic symptoms, start with 400 mg twice daily, rising to a maximum of 1200 mg twice daily. For negative symptoms try reducing the dose of 400 mg towards 200 mg twice daily. In general, do not change dose more often than once per week. It is available as tablets of 200 mg and 400 mg.

Amisulpride

Pharmacology

Amisulpride ('Solian') is a substituted benzamide. It differs from sulpiride in being slightly more potent, and having greater selectivity for pre- rather than post-synaptic dopamine receptors in animals. Like sulpiride it blocks D_2 and D_3, but not D_1, D_4 or D_5 receptors, or receptors for acetylcholine, 5-HT, H_1 or noradrenalin.

Table 30.1 Schizophrenia: efficacy of atypical antipsychotics v. chlorpromazine or haloperidol

Diagnosis	Treatments and daily dose (n patients)	Duration	Criterion of improvement	Drop-outs for inefficacy (%)	Drop-outs for AEs (%)	Response (%)	ARR (%)	NNT (95% CI)
Treatment-resistant schizophrenia Mean BPRS=43 Kane et al, 1988	Clozapine up to 900 mg (126)	6 weeks	20% less BPRS and CGI 3 (mild) or less	1	12	30	26	4 (3–6)
	Chlorpromazine up to 1000 mg plus benztropine (139)					4		
Schizophrenia Mean BPRS=45 Arvanitis et al, 1997	Quetiapine 300–750 mg (155)	6 weeks	20% less BPRS	36	15	46	30	4 (3–6)
	Haloperidol 12 mg (50)			33	33	38	8	NSD
	Placebo (51)			59	10	16	22	5 (3–6)
Acute on chronic schizophrenia Mean BPRS=36 Marder & Meibach, 1994	Risperidone 6 mg (63)	8 weeks	20% less PANSS	17	28	57	35	3 (2–6)
	Haloperidol 20 mg (64)			38	20	30	27	4 (3–10)
	Placebo (64)			62	6	22	8	NSD

Acute on chronic schizophrenia/intolerant Mean BPRS=33 Tollefson et al, 1997	**Olanzapine** 5–20 mg (1336)	6 weeks	40% less BPRS	21	12	52		
	Haloperidol 5–20 mg (660)	6 weeks		32	21	34	18	5 (5–8)
Acute relapse: responders Mean BPRS=43 Moller et al, 1997	**Amisulpride** 800 mg (95)	6 weeks	CGI much improved or very much improved	12	15	62		
	Haloperidol 20 mg (96)			12	29	44	18	5 (4–25)

AEs, adverse events; ARR, absolute risk reduction; NNT, numbers needed to treat; CI, confidence interval; NSD, not statistically significant; CGI, clinical global impression; PANSS, Positive and Negative Syndrome Scale; BPRS, brief psychiatric rating scale.

It should be noted that the patients selected for each study had different characteristics. The level of severity of illness can be judged by the mean BPRS scores at entry. One study used patients who were proven to be treatment-resistant. One study excluded such patients. One study included patients on the basis that they were intolerant of previous typical antipsychotics.

The NNT in comparisons with placebo represents the pharmacological advantage of prescribing the drug at all. By contrast the NNT in comparisons of an atypical with a classical drug represents the advantage of prescribing the atypical instead of the classical drug.

The plasma half-life is about 12 hours; the drug is mainly excreted unchanged in the urine and bile, so lower doses are needed in the elderly or those with renal impairment.

Clinical effects

In acute schizophrenia it is as effective as haloperidol in reducing positive symptoms, but it produces Parkinsonian side-effects in fewer patients, for example 50% as against 70%, a small advantage. It reduces depression and anxiety more than classical antipsychotics, as do other atypicals.

In patients with predominantly negative symptoms (hebephrenic, disorganised or residual schizophrenia) amisulpride in low doses (50 or 100 mg) reduces negative symptoms, without exacerbating positive symptoms, but it has not been shown to be superior to low doses of classical antipsychotics.

Adverse effects include insomnia, anxiety and agitation. It produces a similar degree of weight gain to haloperidol, and a greater elevation of prolactin levels, leading to galactorrhoea, and amenorrhoea in a quarter of premenopausal women. Although ECG changes have not been seen at therapeutic doses, overdoses have led to fatal ventricular fibrillation.

Dose

For acute schizophrenia the dose is 600–1000 mg/day. For patients with predominantly negative symptoms use 50–300 mg/day. It is available as tablets of 50 mg and 200 mg.

Clozapine

Clozapine ('Clozaril') is a dibenzodiazepine first produced in 1959. It has a tricyclic structure with seven atoms in the central ring (see Figure 30.2); as such it resembles the tricyclic antidepressants.

It carries a risk of agranulocytosis in up to 3% of those who take it, but this is greatly reduced to about 0.6% if weekly blood counts are performed to detect the onset of neutropenia. However, it is useful in schizophrenia that has shown resistance to other antipsychotics. It also produces few or no acute EPS and can lead to improvement in severe tardive dyskinesia.

It can only be used orally and the patient must agree to weekly blood counts for 18 weeks, then every 2 weeks until 1 year, then monthly as long as treatment continues. Treatment is monitored in the UK by the Clozaril Patient Monitoring Service(CPMS) with which the doctor and pharmacist must register the patient before the pharmacy can dispense.

Pharmacology

It has a very broad spectrum of pharmacological activity at class II neurotransmitter receptors (see p. 67), blocking all types of dopamine receptor (D_{1-5}, including D_4, which is blocked very little by other antipsychotics), H_1, acetylcholine-M and noradrenalin α-1 and α-2, and

Figure 30.2 Chemical structures of antipsychotics

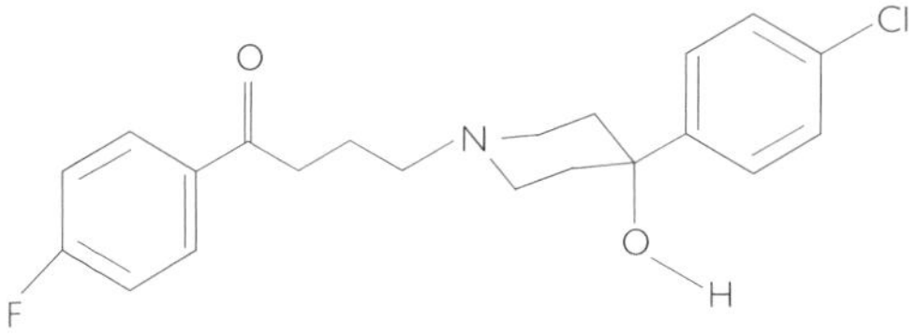

Haloperidol

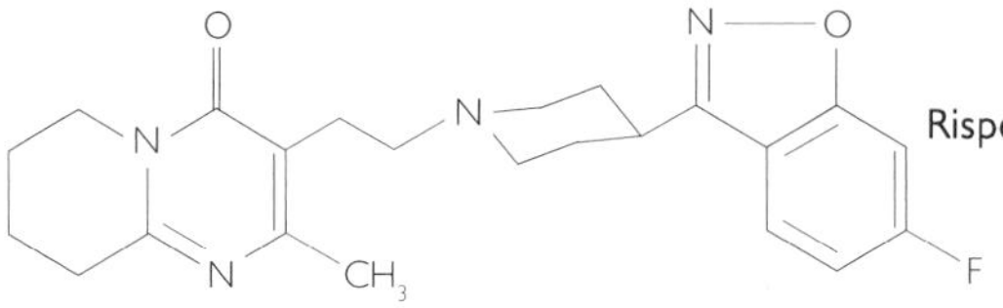

Risperidone

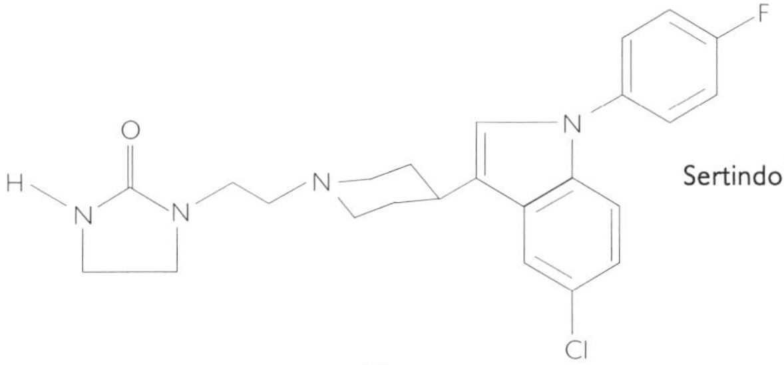

Sertindole

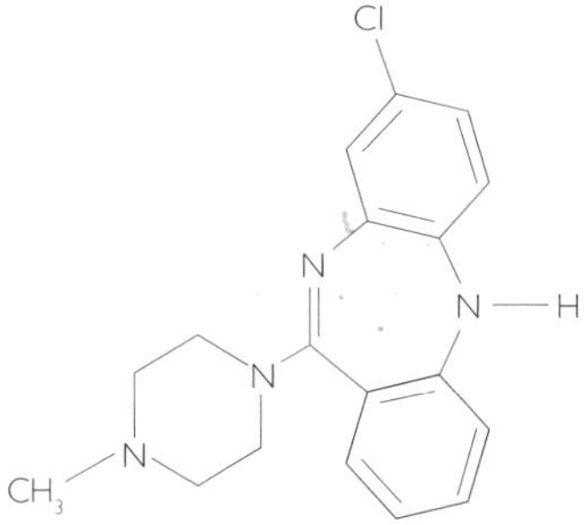

Clozapine

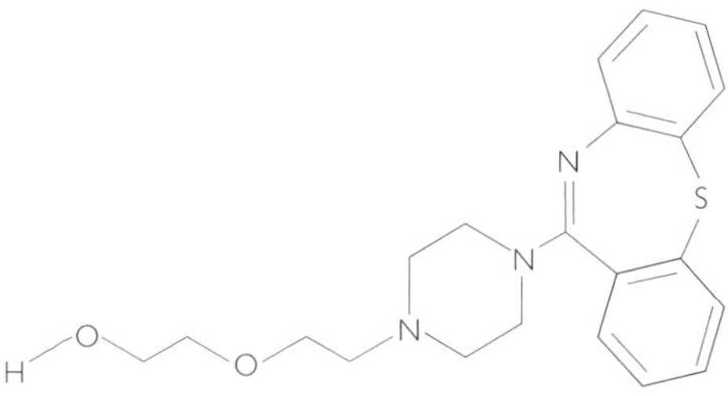

Quetiapine

Figure 30.2 continued

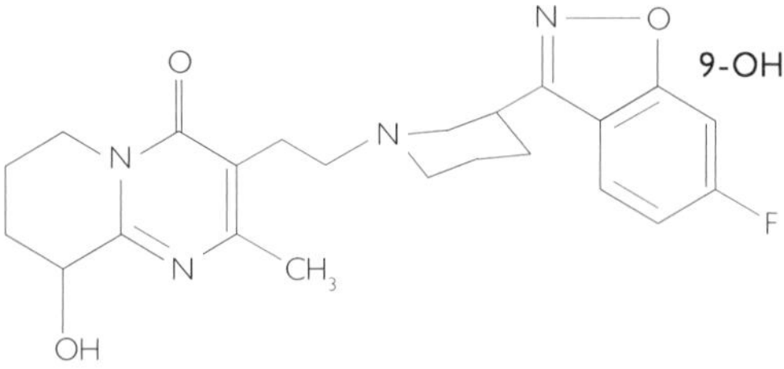

9-OH risperidone

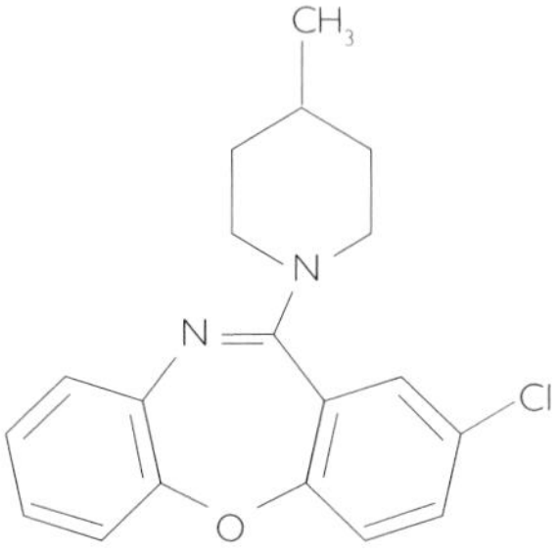

Loxapine

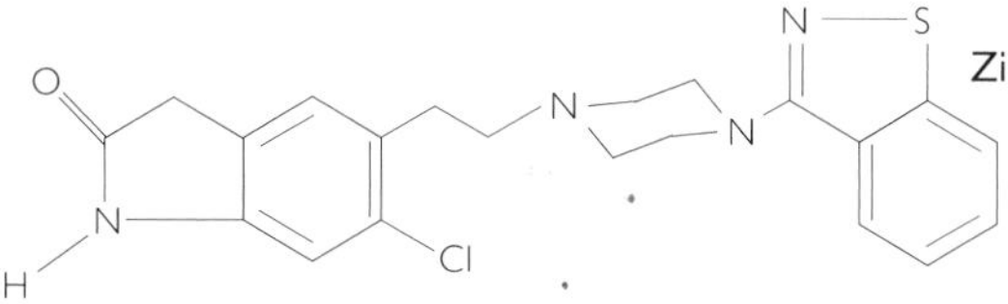

Ziprasidone

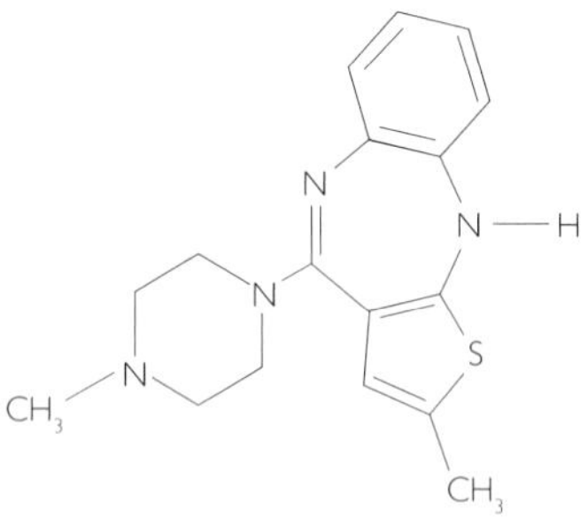

Olanzapine

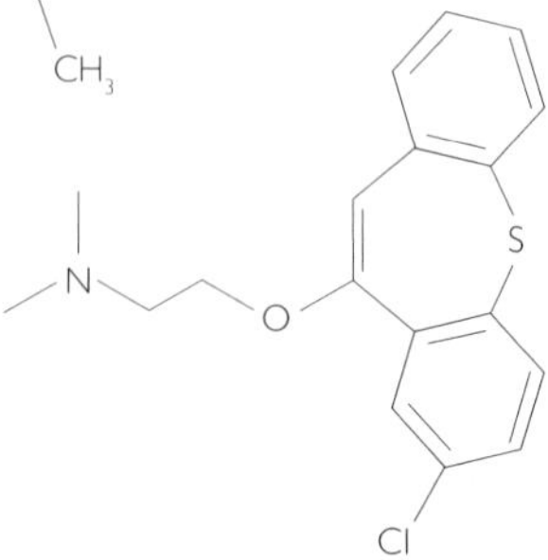

Zotepine

has a potent action at 5-HT-2A and 5-HT–2C receptors. It is unusual in having agonist activity at a subtype of acetylcholine-M receptor, the M_4 receptor of glandular tissues, including salivary glands. Of great interest is the finding in PET studies that clozapine exerts its therapeutic effects while blocking a much lower proportion (40–60%) of D_2 receptors in the striatum that is the case with classical antipsychotics, which occupy over 75%.

Metabolism

Its metabolism is complex (see Table 30.2 and below).

Clinical effects

Patients selected for treatment should have had an unsatisfactory improvement despite the use of adequate doses of other antipsychotics (see p. 144–145); also those who have had severe neurological side-effects limiting the use of other antipsychotic drugs.

Improvement continues to develop for up to 1 year, but most improvement occurs in the first 12 weeks, and patients should not normally continue treatment beyond 4–6 months if there is no response. About 60% of such patients benefit. Patients with paranoid symptoms seem to benefit most, as do those with an onset after the age of 20. Both positive and negative symptoms and depression improve, along with social functioning, but the primary negative or core deficit symptoms persist, as do a lot of cognitive impairments. Beneficial effects on violence in treatment-resistant patients have also been seen. It is less clear that the overall functioning of the patient improves markedly, so as to result in earlier discharge from hospital.

The improvement in severe tardive dyskinesia begins within the first few months and continues for 3 years.

During long-term treatment clozapine is associated with a reduced suicide rate in schizophrenia. It is also used for treatment-resistant mania and rapid-cycling bipolar disorder.

Despite the advantages of clozapine (see Box 30.1), adverse effects are numerous and marked. They include sedation, hypotension (occasionally hypertension), nausea, vomiting and fits. Although atropinic side-effects occur, clozapine commonly produces troublesome

THE DRUGS

Box 30.1 Summary of advantages of clozapine over classical antipsychotics

Greater efficacy on positive symptoms in treatment-resistant patients
Fewer secondary negative symptoms
Improvement in some cognitive symptoms in treatment-resistant patients
Greater improvement in depression and anxiety
Improvement in violence
Fewer or no acute extrapyramidal side-effects
Less tardive dyskinesia
Reduced suicide risk
Asymptomatic rise in serum prolactin

Table 30.2 Metabolic interactions of atypical antipsychotics

Drug	Primary metabolic enzyme	Secondary metabolic enzymes	Major metabolites (inactive unless stated)	Drugs reducing plasma levels	Drugs increasing plasma levels	Comments
Clozapine	CYP1A2	CYP2D6 CYP3A4?	Norclozapine (?active) Clozapine-N-oxide	Smoking, carbamazepine, phenytoin	Fluvoxamine, other SSRIs, caffeine, ketoconazole	Complex metabolic pathways Inhibition interactions potentially dangerous
Risperidone	CYP2D6	CYP3A4	9-OH risperidone (active)	Carbamazepine	SSRIs, nefazodone	Parent and major metabolite have equal activity Difficult to determine clinical effects
Olanzapine	CYP1A2	CYP2D6 CYP2C19 FMO3	Norolanzapine Glucuronide	Smoking, carbamazepine	Fluvoxamine ? other 1A2 inhibitors	Dose changes not usually required
Quetiapine	CYP3A4	CYP2D6	Hydroxy compounds (?active)	Thioridazine, phenytoin, carbamazepine	?Nefazodone and other 3A4 inhibitors	Dubious clinical significance
Amisulpride	Renally excreted	Renally excreted	None	None	None	
Zotepine	CYP3A4	CYP2D6 CYP2C19 CYP1A2	Zotepine-N-oxide, zotepine-S-oxide norzotepine (active)	? smoking	Inhibitors of CYP3A4 – benzodiazepines	
Ziprasidone	CYP3A4	Not known	Ziprasidone sulphoxide, ziprasidone sulphone	None reported ? carbamazepine	None reported ?Ketoconazole	Potential for interaction with CYP3A4 inducers and inhibitors

hypersalivation; this may need the addition of an anticholinergic drug for M_4 receptors; pirenzepine is available to pharmacies although not now marketed. Alternatively, high doses of hyoscine can be helpful. The mechanism of the hypersalivation may include reduced swallowing of saliva, as it is not always the case that salivary production is increased.

To counteract nausea, metoclopramide may be used. Clozapine also causes reflux oesophagitis, and omeprazole may be needed.

Fits occur in up to 4% of patients at doses above 600 mg per day. The anticonvulsant to use in combination with clozapine is valproate. The occurrence of fits may, however, signify the development of a generalised encephalopathy, which has a characteristic EEG pattern, and is accompanied by intellectual deterioration. Any patient on clozapine whose condition appears to deteriorate after an increase of dose, should be suspected of having this complication; an EEG should be performed to confirm the picture, although minor changes in the EEG are common. The encephalopathy is reversible on dose reduction. Sometimes myoclonic jerks occur as manifestations of epilepsy or encephalopathy with clozapine.

Parkinsonian symptoms are rare and then mild, and the risk of tardive dyskinesia is much lower than with other drugs. The rise in prolactin levels is also very small, transient and asymptomatic.

Weight gain occurs and can be substantial, and diabetes may develop in 30% in 5 years. NMS has been recorded, but is less common with clozapine.

Clozapine tends to worsen or to cause obsessional symptoms, and if this happens an SSRI may be needed; fluvoxamine should be avoided.

Concurrent use of other drugs should be kept to a minimum, especially avoiding those affecting the bone marrow, such as carbamazepine. If possible, depot antipsychotics should be avoided because of their long duration. If necessary an oral antipsychotic such as haloperidol may be continued, though only sulpiride has been proven to augment the response to clozapine.

So far about 3% of patients treated have developed neutropenia and had their treatment stopped; 0.6% of patients developed agranulocytosis. These cases occurred mostly at between 4 and 20 weeks of starting treatment. Asians and older people are at greater risk. Patients should be reminded to report if they develop an infection, fever or sore throat, so that a full blood count may be done immediately.

Withdrawal problems

Abrupt discontinuation of clozapine can lead to a florid relapse that is difficult to control with other antipsychotics. This may be partly a cholinergic rebound (see p. 304), and partly rebound exacerbation of the psychosis.

Dose

Before treatment, which invariably starts as an in-patient to allow monitoring of adverse effects, the patient should have a full blood count. The starting dose is 12.5 mg daily, increasing by 25–50 mg daily to 300 mg daily within 2 weeks or longer. This gradual increase helps to reduce the incidence of intolerable side-effects. The dose is then adjusted to between 200 and 450 mg per day in most cases, with a maximum of 900 mg per day. If treatment is stopped it should be done gradually because of the risk of rebound exacerbation of psychosis, which is difficult to control with other antipsychotics. Plasma levels can be helpful. Trough (pre-dose) levels of 350 μ/l are associated with clinical response. It is available as tablets of 25 mg and 100 mg.

THE 5-HT AND DOPAMINE RECEPTOR ANTAGONISTS

5-HT-2/D$_2$ Antagonists (SDRAs)

The confirmation in 1988 that clozapine is effective in treatment-resistant schizophrenia, with very little EPS, marked a turning point in strategies for antipsychotic drug development. Far from being a selective dopamine blocker, clozapine has a very broad spectrum of pharmacological actions. It is more effective than other antipsychotics in blocking the D$_4$ subtype of D$_2$ receptors, but its most potent blocking actions are on 5-HT-2A receptors and histamine receptors. Evidence has accrued suggesting that the combination of strong blockade of 5-HT-2A with moderate blockade of D$_2$-like receptors confers advantages, including less severe EPS, and less cognitive impairment than classical drugs. A series of novel atypical antipsychotics has since been developed that share this combination of receptor-blocking actions. The first to be marketed was risperidone. Another, sertindole, was withdrawn because of concerns about its effects upon the heart. Ziprasidone is licensed in the US and parts of Europe for patients under 65. All three are structurally similar to haloperidol with its central ringed (piperidine) nitrogen (see Figure 30.2).

Risperidone

Pharmacology

Risperidone ('Risperdal') is a benzizoxazole. It resembles clozapine in that it is a potent 5-HT-2A and D$_2$ antagonist, but differs in that it has less affinity for D$_3$ and D$_4$ receptors. It also blocks H$_1$, noradrenalin α-1 and α-2 but not acetylcholine receptors. It is effective in schizophrenia, with a much lower incidence of EPS than haloperidol.

The drug is metabolised partly by liver hydroxylase (CYP2D6) and has an active metabolite hydroxyrisperidone with similar properties that is excreted by the kidneys. The combined half-life is about 24 hours.

Clinical effects

In chronic schizophrenia with persistent symptoms it provides a slightly greater overall improvement than older antipsychotics. However, these advantages are greatest in a narrow range of doses, 4–8 mg daily. It may therefore be most suitable for patients who are maintained on modest doses of other antipsychotics but have persistent symptoms or Parkinsonism.

The advantage over haloperidol on negative symptoms is due in part to the lesser incidence of EPS, and greater improvement in depression. Comparisons with haloperidol have also shown that risperidone produces greater cognitive improvement, so that attention and working memory improve. It is also associated with less severe depressive symptoms during short-term follow up. It should be effective in long-term treatment, but the results of trials are awaited.

Risperidone does not have the same marked benefit in treatment-resistant patients as clozapine. There is preliminary evidence that it produces less tardive dyskinesia than classical antipsychotics, in the elderly.

Risperidone can worsen or occasionally induce obsessional symptoms in patients with schizophrenia. However, it can be helpful as an adjunct to an SSRI in the treatment of OCD (see chapter 15).

In bipolar disorder risperidone is of comparable efficacy to haloperidol in mania. However, it can occasionally lead to mania in patients with schizoaffective disorder. It is not yet licensed for use in bipolar disorder.

Risperidone is superior to haloperidol in controlling behavioural disturbance (particularly aggression) in patients with severe dementia. The optimal dose for this is 1 mg; doses of 2 mg or higher are associated with high rates of EPS.

Adverse effects of postural hypotension and mild sedation can be avoided by increasing the dose gradually. At doses above 6 mg/day there is an increasing incidence of EPS. Weight gain occurs to a greater extent than with haloperidol, and occasionally impairment of ejaculation or orgasm, and blurred vision. It blocks D_2 receptors in the pituitary and increases prolactin levels to a slightly greater extent than haloperidol. There is a correlation between raised prolactin levels and reduced libido.

Dose

Treatment starts gradually, to avoid postural hypotension, with 1 mg twice daily, increasing to 2 mg twice daily and 3 mg twice daily on the next 2 days. The optimal dose is 2–4 mg twice daily. Doses above 10 mg daily confer no added benefit but increase the occurrence of EPS, and doses of more than 16 mg a day should not be used. It is available as tablets of 1 mg, 2 mg, 3 mg and 4 mg.

Risperidone long acting injection

Risperidone has been formulated for long-acting intramuscular injection. It is encapsulated in microspheres of a biodegradable polymer, glycolic acid-lactate that is also used for sutures. Gradual hydrolysis of the polymer at the site of injection gives a slow release of risperidone, beginning three weeks after the first injection, achieving peak blood levels between 4 and 6 weeks. A dose of up to 50 mg is given as an aqueous suspension, every 2 weeks.

Ziprasidone

Pharmacology

Ziprasidone ('Zeldox') is a benzothiazolylpiperazine. It binds most strongly to 5-HT-2A, D_2 and D_3 receptors and slightly less strongly to D_4, noradrenalin α-1 and 5-HT-C receptors. It has weak affinity for acetylcholine-M and histamine H_1 receptors. In addition it is an agonist

THE DRUGS

319

at 5-HT-1A receptors and has a slight action as a serotonin and noradrenalin reuptake inhibitor, all of which might confer beneficial effects on mood.

PET scans in normal volunteeers show that at therapeutic doses it produces more blockade of 5-HT-2 (85%) than of D_2 (65%) receptors.

Its absorption is increased by food. It is metabolised by CYP3A4 and other paths, and has a half-life of 5–10 hours. No clinically relevant interactions are known.

Clinical effects

It improves the positive, negative and depressive symptoms of acute schizophrenia. It is sedative only at higher doses (160 mg/day) and it lacks anticholinergic side-effects. An intramuscular injection is effective in acute tranquillisation at a dose of 10–20mg.

The main adverse effects of drowsiness, nausea, dyspepsia and dizziness are infrequent. It is generally well tolerated. It produces only slightly more EPS than placebo. Abnormal ejaculation has not been found. Of particular interest, it produces less short-term weight gain than haloperidol, and longer-term effects on body weight are also favourable in comparison to other atypical antipsychotics. At the higher dose it produces only a slight transient rise in plasma prolactin.

Dose

The absence of postural hypotension means that the drug can be introduced easily. It should be taken twice daily, in a dose of up to 160 mg/day. It is available as tablets of 20 mg, 40 mg, 60 mg and 80 mg and an intramuscular formulation (mesylate trihydrate) of 20 mg/ml.

Sertindole

Although withdrawn because of cardiac side-effects, this drug was well investigated and remains of interest.

Pharmacology

It is a phenyl indol and has a narrow range of receptor blocking activity, being potent at 5-HT-2A, D_2, D_3, 5-HT-2C, and noradrenalin α-1 receptors. It produced significant lengthening of the QT interval in about 5% of people, probably by blocking potassium channels (the delayed rectifier).

Clinical effects

It is as effective as haloperidol in acute schizophrenia, but produces no significant EPS in the doses studied, up to the maximum of 24 mg/day. It appears to be more effective than haloperidol against the negative symptoms, perhaps because it produces less severe secondary negative symptoms.

Its most common adverse effects are nasal congestion (reported in up to 40%), a decrease in ejaculatory volume (but not retrograde ejaculation) in up to 20% of men (both probably related to noradrenalin α-1 blockade) and weight gain (attributed in part to blockade of 5-HT-

2C receptors). Less common side-effects are dizziness, dry mouth, nausea (probably related to 5-HT blockade), oedema, paraesthesia and QT prolongation. Drowsiness was not reported, and other aspects of sexual function (libido, erection and orgasm) were not affected. Prolactin levels are elevated by only a small amount, of little clinical significance.

PLURIPOTENT D_2-SPARING RECEPTOR
ANTAGONISTS — THE TRICYCLIC ATYPICAL ANTIPSYCHOTICS

The limited resemblance between the clinical effects of clozapine and those of risperidone or ziprasidone suggests that mechanisms other than 5-HT-2 blockade may be important, and drugs have been developed with greater structural similarity to clozapine. The tricyclic molecular form is shared by olanzapine, quetiapine, zotepine and loxapine, but only olanzapine shares the central diazepine ring. Like clozapine, these drugs have affinity for a wide range of neurotransmitter receptors (pluripotent). All are potent blockers of 5-HT-2 receptors. They share with clozapine the ability to exert antipsychotic effects while occupying a relatively low proportion of D_2 receptors in the basal ganglia (D_2-sparing). This may occur through their ability to block D_2-like receptors, which predominate in limbic areas of the brain; for example D_3 and D_5 receptors. SPET scans using the ligand epidepride (which binds to D_2-like receptors, including D_3) measure the blocking activity of these drugs in limbic areas.

Olanzapine
Pharmacology

Olanzapine is a thienobenzodiazepine. It has potent affinity for dopamine (D_{1-4}) receptors, as well as serotonin (5-HT 2-A, 2-C, 3 and 6), acetylcholine (M_{1-5}), noradrenalin (α-1) and histamine (H_1) receptors. It is metabolised by CYP1A2 and other enzymes.

Clinical effects

It is one of the most extensively investigated of all the atypical drugs, in clinical trials. It is effective in acute episodes of schizophrenia, in long-term treatment and in reducing relapses. It is also effective in acute mania.

Compared with haloperidol, it produces a greater degree of overall improvement and much less EPS. There is also a greater improvement in depressive symptoms. Secondary negative symptoms are therefore much less, and there is also greater improvement in cognitive functions, particularly attention. It is not as effective as clozapine in treatment-resistant schizophrenia.

Adverse effects are mainly increased appetite, weight gain, drowsiness and occasionally dry mouth. At higher doses (20 mg/day or more) other anticholinergic side-effects such as constipation and dizziness can occur. Acute EPS, with Parkinsonism, dystonia or akathisia, are not usually seen until the dose exceeds 20 mg/day. Parkinsonism is then usually mild, but akathisia may be problematic. In long-term

THE DRUGS

treatment, tardive dyskinesia develops in far fewer patients than on haloperidol. Obsessional symptoms sometimes emerge during treatment, but are not necessarily worsened by olanzapine. Plasma prolactin rises very little even with higher doses, and symptoms from this are rare. Early transient increases in liver transaminase enzymes occur in about 8% of patients. Peripheral oedema occurs in 3% of patients. Weight gain is pronounced over the course of 18 months. The mechanism includes increased appetite, which can amount to bulimic eating. There is also a change in glucose tolerance, with hyperglycaemia, hyperlipidaemia and diabetes, sometimes even in the absence of obesity.

Dose

The dose starts with 5 mg daily taken at night, because of the sedative effect. First episode patients may need no more than this, but for others the dose is increased gradually, according to response. The licensed maximum dose is 20 mg daily. Most patients require between 10 and 20 mg. Smokers, and others with induced liver metabolism, need the higher doses. Women may need lower doses.

Quetiapine

Pharmacology

Quetiapine is a benzothiazepine. It binds most strongly to noradrenalin α-1, 5-HT-2A, acetylcholine-M_1, histamine H_1 and dopamine D_2 and D_3 receptors, and to a lesser extent to 5-HT-2C and D_4 receptors.

SPET scans suggest a low occupancy (22–68%) of striatal D_2 receptors at therapeutic doses, but greater occupancy of limbic D_2/D_3 receptors.

It has a half-life of about 6–8 hours, and twice daily dosing is advised. It is metabolised by CYP3A4.

Clinical effects

It is a moderately sedative antipsychotic with very low incidence of acute EPS and is generally well tolerated. In comparison with haloperidol, quetiapine is as effective in improving the positive and negative symptoms, but with far fewer drop-outs. It does not produce EPS more than placebo at doses of up to 750 mg /day.

The main adverse effects are drowsiness and dyspepsia at high doses, postural hypotension, headache, dry mouth and constipation; nasal congestion is occasionally a problem. It does not raise prolactin levels. It does increase body weight more than haloperidol in the short-term, but over months it is less liable to cause weight gain than olazapine or clozapine. It can produce a transient increase in liver transaminase enzymes.

Dose

The dose is increased gradually from 50 mg on the first day to 300 mg by the fourth day, and then adjusted to between 300 and 450 mg/day, with a maximum of 750 mg/day. In the elderly these doses should be halved. It is available as tablets of 25 mg, 100 mg, 150 mg and 200 mg.

Zotepine

Pharmacology

Zotepine is a dibenzothiepine tricyclic drug, with an active metabolite, norzotepine. It binds strongly to histamine H_1, 5-HT-2A, noradrenalin α-1 and D_2, D_3 and D_4 receptors, but weakly to acetylcholine-M receptors. In addition it binds to D_1 and D_5 receptors and to 5-HT-2C, 5-HT-6 and 5-HT-7 receptors. It also blocks noradrenalin reuptake, and hence may have antidepressant effects, and produces side-effects such as dry mouth. In animals, it blocks phencyclidine (PCP) effects and has proconvulsant effects (see p. 77).

It has a half-life of about 14 hours in young adults, 20 hours in the elderly. It is metabolised by CYP1A2 for demethylation to the active norzotepine and CYP3A4. It occupies about 60% of striatal D_2-like receptors on SPET in therapeutic doses.

Clinical effects

Although the drug has been used very widely in other parts of the world, and is licensed for use in schizophrenia in the UK, there are few large well-controlled trials.

It is sedative. It produces much less EPS than haloperidol, and only slightly more than placebo. It is slightly more effective than haloperidol, with limited evidence of a greater improvement in secondary negative symptoms and cognitive symptoms. During long-term treatment it helps in preventing relapses.

Its effects in treatment-resistant schizophrenia remain to be clarified.

It has antimanic effects. The main adverse effects are dry mouth, constipation, weight gain, drowsiness and dizziness. Transient increases in liver enzymes occur. Uric acid excretion is promoted. There is a dose-related incidence of seizures, the risk being especially high above 300 mg/day. It produces a sustained rise in plasma prolactin levels. QT prolongation also may occur.

Dose

Starting at 50–75 mg/day, the dose is increased to a maximum of 300 mg/day (150 mg in the elderly). It is available as tablets of 25 mg, 50 mg and 100 mg.

Loxapine

Loxapine ('Loxapac') has a similar dibenzoxapine structure, but carries risks of dystonia, Parkinsonism, epileptic fits, hypotension and drowsiness. It does not have the advantages of clozapine. This demonstrates that minor structural differences in the molecule can confer huge clinical differences.

EVIDENCE FROM PET AND SPET SCANS

Using labelled raclopride and PET to visualise D_2 receptors in the striatum (see p. 285), it has been found that classical antipsychotics need to block 60–90 % of the D_2 receptors in order to have therapeutic effects.

THE DRUGS

However, doses blocking more than 80% of the receptors produce acute EPS, even in young physically healthy people. Clozapine, on the other hand, produces its therapeutic effects while blocking only 30–65% of these receptors. This may signify that clozapine exerts its therapeutic effects through other receptors that are not labelled by raclopride, which is a benzamide drug; clozapine causes less EPS because it blocks such as small proportion of dopamine receptors in the basal ganglia. (An alternative view regards these findings in scans as misleading, because drugs that dissociate more slowly from the receptors will produce greater blockade of short pulses of endogenous dopamine).

Using labelled setoperone to visualise 5-HT-2 receptors, it is known that clozapine, risperidone and olanzapine produce substantial blockade of 5-HT-2 receptors in the brain, approaching saturation at even the lowest therapeutic doses such as 5 mg of olanzapine. With risperidone, doses of 2–6 mg/day occupy 65–80 % of the D_2 receptors visualised by raclopride; higher doses occupy more than 80% of the receptors and are liable to produce EPS. With olanzapine, the D_2 occupancy, measured with raclopride, rises from about 40–65% at 5 mg/day, to 75–80% with 20 mg/day, and 80–90% with doses of 30–40 mg/day.

Using iodobenzamide to visualise D_2 receptors in the striatum with SPET, it seems that olanzapine and quetiapine produce less occupancy of D_2 receptors than classical antipsychotics, but more occupancy than clozapine. These findings help to explain why clozapine and the PRAs produce less EPS than typical antipsychotics, but they do not explain how they exert their therapeutic effects.

Using epidepride as the label for SPET, limbic dopamine receptors in the temporal lobe can be visualised. This compound binds to the D_3 and D_4 subtypes that predominate in these areas. Clozapine has five times greater affinity for D_4 than for D_2 receptors on assays in test tubes. In therapy, clozapine occupies 90% of the temporal lobe dopamine receptors visualised with epidepride, but only 60% of those in the striatum. Likewise, quetiapine and olanzapine produce greater occupancy in temporal areas than in the striatum. This evidence supports the role of D_3 and D_4 blockade in the antipsychotic effects of atypical drugs.

PHARMACOKINETIC INTERACTIONS

Atypical antipsychotics are involved in some important interactions (Table 30.2). Plasma levels of clozapine can be dangerously increased by fluvoxamine (which inhibits 1A2) and other SSRIs (that inhibit 2D6, but not citalopram, see p. 264), and decreased by carbamazepine and by smoking (both induce 3A4). With olanzapine, smoking and carbamazepine can reduce plasma levels. Zotepine levels are increased by diazepam and by fluoxetine.

SWITCHING FROM TYPICAL TO ATYPICAL ANTIPSYCHOTIC

Patients may be suitable for a switch from a classical to an atypical drug for the following reasons:

- persistent akathisia or Parkinsonism
- persistent negative symptoms

Table 30.3 Summary of actions of atypical antipsychotics

Action	Clozapine	Sulpiride	Amisulpride	Risperidone	Olanzapine	Quetiapine	Zotepine	Ziprasidone
Greater efficacy than classical drug								
Positive symptoms	+++	0	0	+	+	+/0	0	+
Negative symptoms	++	+	+	++	++		+	++
Cognitive symptoms	+	+	++	++	++		+	++
Depression	++	+	++	++	++			++
Treatment-resistant schizophrenia	+++	0	0	+	+		0	
Acute pharmacological side-effects								
EPS Parkinsonism	+/0	++	++	+	+	0	+	+
Acute dystonia	0	++	++	+	+	0	+	+
Akathisia	+/0	++	++	++	+	0	+	+
Hyperprolactinaemia	0	+++	+++	+++	+/0	+/0	++	+/0
Long-term pharmacological side-effects								
Weight gain	+++	+	+	++	+++	+	+++	0
Tardive dyskinesia	0			+	+			
Sedation	+++	+	0	+	++	+++	+++	+
Anticholinergic	+++	0	0	0	++	++	0	0
α-1 block	+++	0	0	++	+	++	++	+
Impaired glucose tolerance	++	0	0	+	++	+	0/+	0

+, evidence of mild effect, or advantage only in relation to high doses of comparator; ++, definite effect or advantage; +++, evidence of marked effect or advantage; 0, no side-effect, or no benefit; blank, no Information; EPS, extrapyramidal side-effects.

- subjective cognitive impairment
- persistent affective symptoms (depression, anxiety)
- persistent positive symptoms
- hyperprolactinaemia causing symptoms (amenorrhoea, galactorrhoea).

It is unwise to switch in patients for whom a relapse poses unacceptable risks to themselves or to others, or those who have recently recovered from an acute psychotic episode and are stable on the same medication, or who are stable on depot medication but have a recent history of poor compliance with oral treatment. Table 30.3 summarises the comparison of the atypical antipsychotics.

Switching to clozapine is indicated when the patient has persistent and disabling positve symptoms with or without negative symptoms, despite adequate doses of at least three other antipsychotics including at least one atypical drug, given for sufficient time, and in patients with tardive dystonia or severe tardive dyskinesia. Suitable patients will usually have been severely ill for over a year. They must be willing to have the necessary blood tests, and there must be consent or MHA authorisation (see p. 97). The problems that may be encountered are:

- difficulty in finding the optimal dose
- transient exacerbation of psychosis
- symptoms from discontinuation of anticholinergic drugs
- Parkinsonism, akathisia or dystonia from persistence of classical drug and cessation of anticholinergic
- initial worsening of tardive dyskinesia
- poor compliance with oral medication.

It may be difficult to know whether new symptoms are side-effects or the result of discontinuation, or relapse owing to insufficient dose of the new drug, or represent anxiety about changing. Tapering the reduction of the previous antipsychotic while introducing the new one helps to minimise these. In the case of depot medication, the new drug can be started soon after the last injection is given.

Discussion of the implications of switching (possible benefits, new side-effects and discontinuation problems) should include the carers because they may perceive changes in a different way to the patient or doctor.

Changing medication in a patient recently joining a different doctor poses a special problem. It may be perceived by the patient as a criticism of the previous doctor or as ending part of their relationship.

Discontinuing clozapine is particularly difficult because there may be a rebound exacerbation of the psychosis, that cannot be readily controlled with an alternative antipsychotic. This may result in part from cholinergic rebound, but the fact that clozapine blocks a wider range of receptors than other drugs may mean that upregulation of these is also important. It should be discontinued gradually if possible, but may have to be stopped abruptly if neutropenia develops.

FURTHER READING

Pharmacological evidence

Leysen, J. E., Janssen, P. M. F., Heylen, L., *et al* (1998) Receptor interactions of new antipsychotics: relation to pharmacodynamic and clinical effects. *International Journal of Psychiatry in Clinical Practice*, **2**, S3–S17.

Kapur, S. & Seeman, P. (2001) Does fast dissociation from the dopamine D_2 receptor explain the action of atypical antipsychotics? A new hypothesis. *American Journal of Psychiatry*, **158**, 360–369.

Evidence from scans

Farde, L., Nordstom, A. L., Wiesel, F. A., *et al* (1992) Positron emission tomographic analysis of central D_1 and D_2 dopamine receptor occupancy in patients treated with classical neuroleptics and clozapine *Archives of General Psychiatry*, **49**, 538–544.

Kapur, S., Zipursky, R. B., Remington, G., *et al* (1998) 5-HT-2 and D_2 receptor occupancy of olanzapine in schizophrenia: A PET investigation. *American Journal of Psychiatry*, **155**, 921–928.

Bigliani, V., Mulligan, R. S., Acton, P. D., *et al* (1999) In vivo occupancy of striatal and temporal cortical D_2/D_3 dopamine receptors by typical antipsychotic drugs. [123I]-epidepride single photon emission tomography (SPET) study. *British Journal of Psychiatry*, **175**, 231–238.

Stephenson, C. M. E., Bigliani, V., Jones, H. M., *et al* (2000) Striatal and extra-striatal D_2/D_3 dopamine receptor occupancy by quetiapine *in vivo*: [^{123}I]-epidepride single photon emission tomography (SPET) study. *British Journal of Psychiatry*, **177**, 408–415.

Amisulpride

Loo, H., Poirier-Littre, M. F., Theron, M., *et al* (1997) Amisulpride versus placebo in the medium-term treatment of the negative symptoms of schizophrenia. *British Journal of Psychiatry*, **170**, 18–22.

Danion, J.-M., Rein, W., Fleurot, O., *et al* (1999) Improvement of schizophrenic patients with primary negative symptoms treated with amisulpride. *American Journal of Psychiatry*, **156**, 610–616.

Moller, H. J., Boyer, P., Fleurot, O., *et al* (1997). Improvement of acute exacerbations of schizophrenia with amisulpride: a comparison with haloperidol. *Psychopharmacology*, **132**, 396–401.

Clozapine

Breier, A., Buchanan, R. W., Kirkpatrick, B., *et al* (1994) Effects of clozapine on positive and negative symptoms in outpatients with schizophrenia. *American Journal of Psychiatry*, **151**, 20–26.

Kane, J., Honigfeld, G., Singer, J., *et al* (1988) Clozapine for the treatment-resistant schizophrenic: a double-blind comparison with chlorpromazine. *Archives of General Psychiatry*, **45**, 789–796.

Lieberman, J. A., Saltz, B. L., Johns, C. A., *et al* (1991) The effects of clozapine on tardive dyskinesia *British Journal of Psychiatry*, **158**, 503–510.

Goldberg, T. E., Greenberg, R. D., Griffin, S. J., *et al* (1993) The effect of clozapine on cognition and psychiatric symptoms in patients with schizophrenia. *British Journal of Psychiatry*, **162**, 43–48.

Meltzer, H. Y. & Okayli, G. (1995) Reduction of suicidality during clozapine treatment of neuroleptic-resistant schizophrenia: impact on risk-benefit assessment. *American Journal of Psychiatry*, **152**, 183–190.

Munro, J., O'Sullivan, D., Andrews, C., *et al* (1999) Active monitoring of 12,760 clozapine recipients in the UK and Ireland. Beyond pharmacovigilance. *British Journal of Psychiatry*, **175**, 576–580.

THE DRUGS

Olanzapine

Beasley, C. M., Dellva, M. A., Tamura, R. N., *et al* (1999) Randomised double-blind comparison of the incidence of tardive dyskinesia in patients with schizophrenia during long-term treatment with olanzapine and haloperidol. *British Journal of Psychiatry*, **174**, 23–30.

Tollefson, G. D. & Sanger, T. M. (1997) Negative symptoms: A path analytic approach to a double-blind, placebo- and haloperidol-controlled trial with olanzapine. *American Journal of Psychiatry*, **154**, 466–474.

——, Beasley, C. M., Tran, P. V., *et al* (1997) Olanzapine versus haloperidol in the treatment of schizophrenia and schizophreniform disorders: Results of an international collaborative trial. *American Journal of Psychiatry*, **154**, 457–465.

——, Sanger, T. M. & Thieme, M. E. (1998) Depressive signs and symptoms in schizophrenia: A prospective blinded trial of olanzapine and haloperidol. *Archives of General Psychiatry*, **55**, 250–258.

Risperidone

Kleinberg, D. C., Davis, J. M., De Coster, R., *et al* (1999) Prolactin levels and adverse events in patients treated with risperidone. *Journal of Clinical Psychopharmacology*, **19**, 57–61.

Marder, S. R. & Meibach, R. C. (1994) Risperidone in the treatment of schizophrenia. *American Journal of Psychiatry*, **151**, 825–835.

Peuskens, J. (1995) Risperidone in the treatment of patients with chronic schizophrenia: a multi-national, multi-centre, double-blind, parallel-group study versus haloperidol. The Risperidone Study Group. *British Journal of Psychiatry*, **166**, 712–726.

Quetiapine

Arvanitis, L. A., Miller, B. G. & the Seroquel Trial 13 Study Group (1997) Multiple fixed doses of "Seroquel" (quetiapine) in patients with acute exacerbations of schizophrenia: a comparison with haloperidol and placebo. *Biological Psychiatry*, **42**, 233–246.

Sertindole

Zimbroff, D. L., Kane, J. M., Tamminga, C. A., *et al* (1997) Controlled, dose–respose study of sertindole and haloperidol in the treatment of schizophrenia. *American Journal of Psychiatry*, **154**, 782–791.

Zotepine

Prakash, A. & Lamb, H. M. (1998) Zotepine: a review. *CNS Drugs*, **9**, 153–117.

Ziprasidone

Daniel, D. G., Zimbroff, D. L., Potkin, S. G., *et al* (1999) Ziprasidone 40 mg bid and 80 mg bid in the acute exacerbation of schizophrenia and schizoaffective disorder: results of a 6-week placebo-controlled trial. *Neuropsychopharmacology*, **20**, 491–505.

Meta-analysis

Geddes, J., Freemantle, N., Harrison, P., *et al* (2000) Atypical antipsychotics in the treatment of schizophrenia: systematic overview and meta-regession analysis. *BMJ*, **321**, 1371–1376.

Mir, S. & Taylor, D. (2001) Atypical antipsychotics and hyperglycaemia. *International Clinical Psychopharmacology*, **16**, 63–74.

Scale quoted

Kay, S. R., Fiszbein, A. & Opler, L. A. (1987) Positive and Negative Syndrome Scale (PANSS) for Schizophrenia. *Schizophrenia Bulletin*, **13**, 261–276.

Principally used to treat affective disorders and especially to prevent their recurrence, lithium salts also sometimes suppress schizoaffective symptoms and some states of aggression, including those in people with learning disabilities.

Lithium, the smallest metal ion, is an element closely related to sodium and potassium (in group 1 of the Periodic Table of elements) and to calcium and magnesium (group 2). It is widely distributed as salts in nature, in rocks, spa waters and in the fluids of plants and animals. Traces are found normally in the human body, at about one-thousandth of the therapeutic level. The lithium ion penetrates cell membranes and is distributed throughout the body water. The intracellular concentration is slightly less than extracellular, because lithium is less efficiently pumped out of cells than sodium. By contrast, sodium is predominantly extracellular and potassium intracellular.

Lithium has numerous effects on bodily systems, especially at high concentrations. At the dilution present in normal untreated people, or resulting from drinking spa water, lithium can have no clinical effect. The narrow gap or overlap between therapeutic and toxic blood levels necessitates careful monitoring of blood lithium levels, usually based on samples taken 12 hours after the last dose. Understanding how lithium levels vary is important.

The lithium ion is readily absorbed from the stomach and intestine into the blood and enters most tissues; it soon begins to appear in the urine. It also appears in sweat, but not in the faeces unless there is diarrhoea or failure of the lithium tablet to disintegrate. The amount circulating in the blood at any time depends mainly on the balance between the rate of intake by mouth and of excretion in the urine. There is usually a rapid rate of absorption and a rapid excretion, provided renal function is normal. Lithium is excreted by glomerular filtration, with some reabsorbtion from the proximal tubule, as for sodium but much less efficiently. Renal blood flow, as decided by blood pressure, degree of vasoconstriction, hydration and sodium intake, is therefore important. A diet low in sodium, heavy sweating or pyrexia, dehydration, salt depletion and hypotension from any cause decrease urinary lithium and raise it in the blood, during constant oral dosing.

When a tablet of lithium carbonate is swallowed, providing it disintegrates and dissolves, the lithium concentration in the blood plasma rises rapidly to a sharp peak in 1–4 hours, followed by distribution in body fluids and slow penetration of the intracellular spaces of brain and bone. Disintegration is the rate-limiting step and slow-release tablets simply disintegrate slowly. Elimination is largely by the kidney and follows an exponential time course. The plasma half-life depends on renal excretion and varies from 7 to 20 hours in physically healthy individuals, but is longer in the elderly or physically unwell. On a regular dose, steady-state levels would be reached after

5 half-lives (between 2 and 9 days). After starting or changing the dose of lithium the blood level should be measured 3 days later to allow time for accumulation to occur. If lithium is taken once or twice daily, the blood concentration swings between a high level for a short time, and much lower levels for a considerable time, and is always changing. This has two important practical consequences. First, unpleasant side-effects such as vomiting and diarrhoea, or polydipsia with polyuria, are produced more by higher levels.

Secondly, it is essential to note the time when a blood sample for lithium measurement is taken, and the time when the last dose was taken also. Otherwise, the lithium value obtained by the laboratory cannot be correctly interpreted. To guide treatment the lithium is measured only when it is rather slowly changing near the latter part of its fall. So the blood should be taken at least 8 hours, preferably 12 hours, after the last dose, or just before taking the first dose of the day, if this is more convenient. If the dose is taken at 10.00 p.m. the blood test can be done the following morning, and any morning dose should be omitted until blood is taken. This gives a trough concentration of plasma lithium and treatment is guided by these troughs, and not by the peaks. On the other hand, side-effects and toxic signs (see below) depend more on the heights. Where more than one dose is given in the 24 hours the doses should be equally spaced, for example two, 12 hours apart; or three, 8 hours apart. This will prevent a big peak at one part of the day, while providing a satisfactory basal lithium level. Another way of avoiding peaks is to prescribe sustained-release tablets, which let out their lithium more slowly than ordinary tablets and so spread out and soften the peak time. Slow release leads to lower peaks and fewer side-effects. But it may still be necessary to give them 12-hourly, or more often, to split a big daily dose.

As dose follows dose the concentration of lithium in the 40 litres or so of body water tends to increase until the urinary excretion rate equals the lithium intake. The concentration then reaches a steady state that persists for very long periods provided the daily dose remains the same and the individual remains healthy. An intercurrent illness, anaesthesia or surgery will change the steady state and, therefore, require new blood tests and possibly a dose change. It does not necessarily mean that lithium must be stopped, but that closer control is needed. But once a steady state is achieved there is not the same need for frequent testing that there is when beginning treatment. Provided there is no change in health, once in 3 or 6 months will be enough. There are no absolute contraindications to lithium, but caution is required in renal failure, heart failure, recent myocardial infarction, electrolyte imbalance, the elderly and in patients who are unreliable taking medication or prone to dehydration.

Poor renal function, as in the elderly or those with kidney disease (including some who may be on regular renal dialysis) means more care in choosing the daily dose to be taken and more frequent monitoring of the lithium by blood tests. People with congestive cardiac failure with fluctuating renal function and excess variable body water, perhaps with signs of oedema, are unlikely to be suitable for lithium because of the difficulty in establishing and keeping control.

MECHANISMS OF ACTION

Ionic mechanisms

As the smallest alkaline cation, lithium can substitute for sodium, potassium, calcium and magnesium in several ways. It penetrates cells through sodium channels and other channels but is extruded less efficiently by active transport, so that the plasma : intracellular concentration ratio is about two in red cells. Within the cell lithium interacts with systems that normally involve other cations, including transmitter-release and second-messenger systems.

Second-messenger systems

Many transmitters and hormones (including thyroid stimulatory hormone (TSH), antidiuretic hormone (ADH) at vasopressin receptors, dopamine at D_1 receptors, and noradrenalin at β receptors) interact with receptors that use cyclic-AMP (c-AMP) as the second (intracellular) messenger (see p. 68). Lithium inhibits cAMP production in these systems. This action on ADH receptors contributes to the polyuria and polydipsia (nephrogenic diabetes insipidus), and at TSH receptors to goitre and hypothyroidism, which are side-effects.

Another second-messenger system is the phosphoinositide cycle, which controls intracellular calcium levels. This system is linked to acetylcholine-M_1 and M_3 receptors, noradrenalin α-1, 5-HT-2 and TRH receptors and some of these are inhibited by therapeutic levels of lithium. This system appears particularly sensitive to blockade by lithium when in its most activated state. Lithium also lowers levels of the intracellular messenger PKC.

Effects on 5-HT and receptor regulation

Lithium is thought to potentiate 5-HT responses in man by increasing the release of 5-HT and by increasing the sensitivity of 5-HT receptors. This may contribute to its antidepressant effect. Tryptophan depletion (see p. 254) does not impair mood in euthymic bipolar patients maintained on lithium, suggesting that a different mechanism underlies the mood-stabilising effect of lithium.

Lithium also reduces the development of receptor super-sensitivity, which occurs as a compensatory phenomenon, for instance during exposure to receptor blocking agents. This may be relevant to its augmenting effects with other agents.

LITHIUM SIDE-EFFECTS

The majority of patients on lithium will experience at least one side-effect, depending on the dose used and all should be informed about side-effects and signs of toxicity. Side-effects contribute to non-compliance and some require an intervention. Some side-effects occur quickly; diarrhoea and occasionally vomiting may result from direct local action in the gut. But most effects, therapeutic or otherwise, take some days to begin to appear because lithium build-up in the

THE DRUGS

brain is slower than in other tissues and some of its actions involve delayed responses.

Gastrointestinal

About a third of patients experience mild abdominal discomfort, sometimes with loose motions, during the first few weeks of treatment, especially with higher doses. By using divided doses these may be avoided. A slow-release preparation may be better tolerated but occasionally these themselves irritate the lower bowel. Severe or persistent diarrhoea suggests toxicity, as does vomiting.

Thyroid

Lithium tends to reduce thyroid function. The most sensitive laboratory index increased TSH occurs in a quarter of patients, thyroid enlargement (goitre) in about 5% and clinical hypothyroidism in 5–10% of patients. Those with pre-existing thyroid antibodies or a family history of thyroid disease are more likely to develop hypothyroidism. The development of hypothyroidism is often signalled by weight gain and lethargy and should be distinguished from depression. Treatment with thyroxine is usually straightforward and lithium can be continued. If lithium is withdrawn, thyroid function usually returns in about 2 months. Thyrotoxicosis may develop during lithium treatment, and there may be a rebound exacerbation when lithium is discontinued.

Kidney

Polydipsia is noted by about a third of patients on lithium and excessive thirst with polydipsia; they are usually reversible but after long-term treatment are not always so. Giving lithium once daily as opposed to divided doses usually makes no difference to total daily urine volumes but may occasionally be helpful. For patients in whom a reduction in dose is not appropriate, amiloride or the loop diuretic frusemide with or without potassium supplement may be helpful. In 1977 histological changes were reported in patients on lithium, including glomerular damage, interstitial fibrosis and tubular atrophy (chronic interstitial nephritis). Similar findings were later made in bipolar patients who had received no lithium treatment. Much further work has shown that during long-term treatment with lithium, monitored at therapeutic doses, no deterioration occurs in glomerular filtration rate in the vast majority of patients. However, occasional cases of chronic renal failure (and chronic interstitial nephritis) have been reported and attributed by nephrologists to lithium, even in patients whose lithium levels have been monitored carefully; this is thought to be a rare idiosyncratic reaction occurring over several years. Episodes of acute lithium toxicity can produce renal damage with reduced glomerular filtration rates.

Central nervous system

A fine tremor of the hands occurs in up to a quarter of patients and is similar to that in anxiety. It can be worsened by antidepressants. Beta-blockers such as propranolol (starting at 10 mg twice daily) reduce this and are best taken intermittently. Lithium can increase EPS (Parkinsonism) in patients on antipsychotic drugs, and can itself produce cogwheel rigidity in a few patients. In contrast to antipsychotic-induced Parkinsonism, this does not improve with anticholinergic drugs.

Mental and cognitive effects

Memory problems are frequently affirmed by patients interviewed about possible side-effects, but objective tests usually show little change. Some successful artists and professionals do not want to continue lithium because they sense a reduction in creativity, but the majority, although missing some hypomanic swings, consider their long-term productivity and creativity are higher under lithium treatment.

In therapeutic doses lithium does not impair psychomotor coordination and is not a bar to driving private motor vehicles. However, a diagnosis of manic depressive illness does exclude patients from driving certain public service vehicles, and after an admission for mania the patient may not drive for 6–12 months according to the UK Driver and Vehicle Licensing Agency (DVLA). The use of ECT in patients on lithium has been associated with prolonged confusional states, but a case control study did not find a higher frequency of adverse effects of ECT in patients on lithium (see chapter 40).

Cardiovascular effects

Lithium can produce benign reversible T-wave flattening or inversion, a pattern similar to that with hypokalaemia. Cardiac dysrhythmias are rare with therapeutic doses, especially in younger patients, but sinus node arrhythmias have been described (sick sinus syndrome) and caution should be exercised when using lithium in patients with cardiac failure and the elderly.

Skin

Lithium can produce or exacerbate acne and psoriasis. Tetracyclines should be used with caution because of their pharmacokinetic interaction with lithium, but retinoids can be used for acne. Hair loss and altered texture may occur.

Metabolic effects and weight gain

Patients tend to gain weight. The mechanism is unknown though increased consumption of sweet drinks may contribute; increased food intake and altered metabolism are also possible. Lithium produces subtle alterations in glucose and insulin metabolism and occasionally worsens control of diabetes. Fluid retention and oedema may occur with higher doses.

Parathyroid, bone and teeth

Lithium can produce mild increases in parathyroid hormone level and serum calcium and, rarely, hyperparathyroidism, with the risk of

THE DRUGS

secondary renal failure. No long-term effects on bone have been found in animals or adult humans. There is no direct effect of lithium upon the teeth but dry mouth or increased consumption of sweet drinks will lead to dental caries.

Sexual function

Impairment of sexual drive, arousal and ejaculation occurring in people with manic depression are rarely owing to lithium and more likely to the underlying condition or other drugs.

Neuromuscular junction

Lithium reduces acetylcholine release and potentiates neuromuscular blocking agents including succinylcholine; it exacerbates myasthenia gravis. Anaesthetists should be informed when patients are on lithium.

Blood and bone marrow

Lithium produces a benign reversible leucocytosis (without a leftward shift in cell precursors), probably by an effect on marrow growth factors.

LITHIUM TOXICITY

Clinical features

Lithium toxicity is indicated by the development of three groups of symptoms – gastrointestinal, motor (especially cerebellar) and cognitive (see Box 31.1). Nausea and diarrhoea progress to vomiting and incontinence. Marked fine tremor progresses to a coarse (cerebellar or Parkinsonian) tremor, giddiness, cerebellar ataxia, slurred speech and gross incoordination with choreiform movements and muscular twitching (myoclonus), upper motor neuron signs (spasticity and extensor plantar reflexes), EEG abnormalities and seizures. In mild toxicity there is impairment of concentration but this deteriorates into drowsiness and disorientation, and in more severe toxicity there is marked apathy and impaired consciousness leading to coma and death. Lithium toxicity can produce confusion, myoclonus and EEG

Box 31.1 Symptoms of lithium toxicity

Mild	Moderate	Severe
Nausea	Vomiting	Vomiting
Diarrhoea	Cerebellar ataxia	Incontinence
Severe fine tremor	Slurred speech	Choreiform/Parkinsonian movement
Poor concentration	Coarse tremor	General muscle twitching (myoclonus)
	Disorientation	Cerebellar dysfunction
	Drowsiness	Spasticity
		EEG abnormalities and seizures
		Apathy
		Coma

changes normally associated with Creutzfeldt-Jakob disease, but with lithium these are reversible.

Diagnosis of toxicity

Lithium toxicity should be assumed in patients on lithium with vomiting or cerebellar signs or disorientation. Other evidence of likely toxicity includes poor concentration. Muscle twitching and hypo-reflexia, convulsions and renal failure are serious signs of advanced toxicity. Lithium treatment should be stopped immediately, and serum lithium, urea and electrolyte levels measured. However, the severity of toxicity bears little relationship to serum lithium levels and neurotoxicity can occur with levels in the usual therapeutic range. Diagnosis should be based upon clinical judgement and not upon the blood level. Lithium should be restarted (at an adjusted dose) only when the patient's condition has improved, or an alternative cause of the symptoms has been found.

Treatment of lithium toxicity

Often cessation of lithium and provision of adequate salt and fluids, including saline infusions, will suffice. In patients with high serum levels (greater than 2 mmol/l) or coma, haemodialysis can speed the removal of lithium and reduce the risk of permanent neurological damage. It may have to be repeated.

Outcome

Patients who survive episodes of lithium toxicity will often make a full recovery. However, a proportion have persistent renal or neurological damage with cerebellar symptoms, spasticity and cognitive impairment. This outcome is more likely if patients are continued on lithium while showing signs of toxicity or during intercurrent physical illnesses. The signs of toxicity develop gradually over several days during continued lithium treatment, and in some cases continue to develop for days after treatment is stopped. Serum lithium levels can also continue to rise after treatment is stopped, probably through release of lithium from intracellular sites.

Factors predisposing to lithium toxicity

Conditions of salt depletion (diarrhoea, vomiting, excessive sweating during fever or in hot climates) can lead to lithium retention. Drugs that reduce the renal excretion of lithium include thiazide diuretics (but not frusemide or amiloride), certain non-steroidal anti-inflammatory drugs (NSAIDs; indomethacin, ibuprofen, piroxicam, naproxen, and phenylbutazone, but not aspirin, paracetamol or sulindac) and certain antibiotics (erythromycin, metronidazole and tetracycline) and angiotensin converting enzyme (ACE) inhibitors. These drugs should be avoided if possible. If they must be used, the dose of lithium should be reduced and blood levels monitored. The most common cause of lithium toxicity is the introduction of an NSAID or thiazide, especially in the elderly. Ibuprofen is rarely a cause in

THE DRUGS

Box 31.2 Lithium uses

Treatment of hypomania and mania

Prevention of recurrent affective episodes in bipolar illness and unipolar
  recurrent depression

In combination with antidepressants (augmentation therapy) for
  unipolar or bipolar depression

Treatment of irritability and aggression particularly in people with
  learning disability

As an adjunct to antipsychotics in schizophrenia

---

analgesic doses (below 1.2 g/day). Drugs that increase the risk of lithium toxicity at therapeutic doses include high doses of antipsychotics, calcium antagonists, carbamazepine and phenytoin (see chapter 12).

In patients with serious intercurrent illnesses, especially infections, lithium should be stopped or reduced in dose, and carefully monitored until the patient's condition is stable. Gastroenteritis and pneumonia are particularly liable to lead to toxicity.

In the elderly renal function is decreased, lower doses are required and toxicity can develop more readily.

Treatment of mania or aggression

The clinical uses of lithium are shown in Box 31.2. Because it is slow to act, lithium alone is not the first treatment of choice in manic illness, where an antipsychotic may be preferable. It has some value in hypomanic cases, especially out-patients, because it is not sedative and therefore acceptable to the patient, and should begin to show results within the week.

Many clinicians start with a dose of 400 mg at night, measure the blood level after 3 days, and increase the dose accordingly. This is usually well tolerated. A more rapid effect may be obtained by starting with 1200–1600 mg lithium carbonate daily in divided doses at 8 a.m. and 8 p.m., or 8 a.m., 4 p.m. and 10 p.m. (smaller daily intake for the elderly, or those with poor kidney function), and taking a timed blood sample at 3 days (and again at 7 days in the elderly or physically ill). Then adjust the dose up or down to reach the desired plasma level, generally between 0.8 and 1.2 mmol/l, and lower in the elderly. Blood level is measured again at 7 days. Doses can be altered every week with monitoring blood tests. Once it is clear the right plasma level has been reached, confirm its stability on the same dose by a monthly blood test until discharge to out-patients and then every 2–3 months until recovery. Monitoring of lithium levels should include reviewing the latest result alongside all previous levels. A chart helps. This will avoid inappropriate action based on a single spurious result and will indicate any long-term trends that might suggest renal impairment or drug interactions. For a comparison of results to be meaningful, the blood samples must be taken at the same time of day. The same procedure is appropriate for aggressive behaviour in those with learning disability.

Young patients may need and tolerate up to 2400 mg daily, although this is rare. Older people, on the other hand, achieve therapeutic levels at lower doses, and also experience both side-effects and therapeutic benefits at lower blood levels. Many elderly patients are treated effectively with 200 mg a day.

Prophylactic treatment of recurrent affective illness and other uses

In prophylaxis the effective plasma level is lower: 0.5–0.8 mmol/l, although, sometimes, a level of 1.0 or higher may be necessary. A daily intake of 800 mg lithium carbonate (20 mmol lithium) will be enough for most people. Again, adjust doses weekly to the desired stable plasma level and, provided circumstances do not change, 6-monthly follow-up tests will suffice. But make sure the patient understands about side-effects, toxic signs and the risk of mania with abrupt discontinuation.

If lithium is effective in prevention it will need to be continued indefinitely. Ten years without relapse is no guarantee of future health if lithium is then stopped. If it is stopped, it should be by gradual reduction (see chapter 12).

PREPARATION OF THE PATIENT

A physical examination and tests of the blood and urine should, if possible, precede drug treatment. Alternatively, in mania, obtain the samples soon after the patient is sedated, in order to elucidate any intercurrent physical illness, especially infection, and any causes of secondary mania (e.g. drugs), and to determine baseline renal, hepatic and thyroid function.

If abnormal renal function is suspected, urine should be tested and creatinine clearance should be measured, again as a baseline. The ability to excrete lithium in the urine can also be judged by the blood level achieved on regular dosing. If this creeps upwards, it may signify deteriorating renal function. If one suspects that a patient (e.g. an elderly person) may not have good renal function, start lithium cautiously, 400 mg daily, for example, and see the plasma concentration at 3 and 7 days later, adjusting the dose as before to get therapeutic levels.

Routine tests of renal, thyroid and cardiac function before and during lithium treatment in the absence of clinical evidence of disease are no substitute for the doctor clinically assessing patients in a thorough manner, looking for any side-effects or toxicity and if present, relating them to the dose and blood level. When tests are done regularly, a foolproof system of noting and filing results must be devised. Too often results go astray or float loosely in the case notes.

For people on lithium who become physically ill, the matter is quite different, and a physician's opinion can be helpful in judging the nature of the pathology.

All patients should be educated about the side-effects and signs of toxicity and given a standard information sheet supplied by the pharmacist. They should be aware of the possibility of interactions with other drugs and of changes during illness. All doctors should be

THE DRUGS

aware that it is safer to discontinue lithium for a few days during an intercurrent illness or suspected toxicity, than to continue it. Lithium monitoring is, in practice, often poorly done and continued vigilance is essential.

PREPARATIONS

Lithium is available as lithium carbonate tablets of 200, 250, 400 and 450 mg ('Camcolit', 'Priadel', 'Liskonum'), or lithium citrate liquid at 520 mg/5ml ('Priadel').

Note that 100 mg of lithium carbonate is 2.7 mmol lithium, 100 mg lithium citrate is 1.08 mmol lithium.

Individuals differ in the speed with which so-called slow or delayed-release preparations are absorbed.

FURTHER READING

Cookson, J. (1997) Lithium: balancing risks and benefits. *British Journal of Psychiatry*, **171**, 120–124.

Goodwin, G. M. (1994) Recurrence of mania after lithium withdrawal. Implications for the use of lithium in the treatment of bipolar affective disorder. *British Journal of Psychiatry*, **164**, 149–152.

Johnson, N. F. (1984) *The History of Lithium Therapy*. London: MacMillan.

—— (1988) *Depression and Mania: Modern Lithium Therapy*. Oxford: IRL.

Maj, M., Pirozzi, R., Magliano, L., *et al* (1998) Long-term outcome of lithium prophylaxis in bipolar disorder. 5-year prospective study of 402 patients a lithium clinic. *American Journal of Psychiatry*, **155**, 30–35.

Schou, M. (1979) Artistic productivity and lithium prophylaxis in manic–depressive illness. *British Journal of Psychiatry*, **135**, 97–103.

—— (1984) Long-lasting neurological sequelae after lithium intoxication. *Acta Psychiatrica Scandinavica*, **70**, 594–602.

—— (2002) Lithium at 52. *Journal of Affective Disorders*, in press.

Winter, M. E. (1993) *Basic Clinical Pharmacokinetics* (2nd edn). Vancouver, DC: Applied Therapeutics, Inc.

32. ANTICONVULSANTS FOR MOOD DISORDERS AND EPILEPSY

More than a third of patients with bipolar affective disorders do not respond satisfactorily to lithium in combination with antipsychotics or antidepressants. Furthermore, only a minority of bipolar patients tolerates lithium and gains significant benefits from it when followed up for 5 years. The discovery that certain anticonvulsants can be effective in mania and as prophylaxis for bipolar disorder, and that some are antidepressants, has led to their increasing use in bipolar patients.

HISTORY

The beneficial effects of these drugs on mood was first recognised when they were used in epilepsy and were found to have antimanic effects (carbamazepine) or antidepressant effects (lamotrigine). Valproic acid was used as a solvent for anticonvulsants before its own anticonvulsant properties were recognised. The French psychiatrist Lambert first described the use of valproate in bipolar disorder in 1966.

Ballenger and Post developed the theory that affective illness might involve a 'kindling' process in limbic brain areas, such as they had found with lidocaine-induced fits and cocaine-induced behavioural changes in animals. They speculated that anticonvulsants that help complex partial seizures (temporal lobe epilepsy), such as carbamazepine, might also be useful in bipolar disorder. They then confirmed the earlier discovery by Okuma and colleagues, in Japan, that carbamazepine is indeed useful both in mania and in prophylaxis.

MECHANISMS OF ACTION

Only a minority of patients in whom these drugs are effective show EEG abnormalities or evidence of structural abnormality in the brain. The primary mechanisms of action vary between drugs but include the following:

- alteration of ion channels in neural cell membranes, particularly those for sodium, potassium and calcium. This alters the electrical excitability and tends to diminish the size of action potentials and to curtail repetitive firing, and hence reduce release of transmitters
- enhancement of inhibitory transmitters, especially GABA
- reduction of excitatory transmitter release, particularly glutamate but also aspartate
- individual drugs may interact with particular

neurotransmitter receptors or reuptake mechanisms, for instance to enhance 5-HT transmission or to reduce dopamine transmission

- some effects are exerted, as with lithium, by interference with second-messenger systems.

THE USE OF ANTICONVULSANTS IN EPILEPSY

Classification of epilepsy

Anticonvulsants find their primary use as anti-epileptic drugs. Epilepsy is a condition that is characterised by recurrent seizures, which may be either primary generalised – if no focus is evident – or partial, if a focus is apparent. Partial seizures may be classified as either simple or complex, depending on whether consciousness is altered. Either type of partial seizure may also secondarily generalise and cause a convulsion (partial seizure with secondary generalisation). If a seizure is presumed to start out as being generalised (primary generalised), then it may be further classified into absence (brief staring episodes), generalised tonic–clonic or myoclonic. These classifications are important from the standpoint of drug therapy as some epilepsies respond preferentially to particular anti-epileptic drugs. There are also some specific syndromes within epilepsy that can be treated with some anti-epileptic drugs but are actually made worse by others. Juvenile myoclonic epilepsy – a very common type of epilepsy often mistaken for complex partial seizures with secondary generalisation – is treated well with valproate or lamotrigine, while carbamazepine (and sometimes other anti-epileptic drugs) exacerbates it markedly. Many of these patients go years or decades on anti-epileptic drugs that make them worse before the correct diagnosis is made.

Choice of drug

In general, lamotrigine and valproate are considered drugs of first choice in primary generalised epilepsies. Ethosuximide should be considered if the patient has absence seizures only and clonazepam or piracetam if myoclonic seizures are prominent. In the treatment of partial seizures with or without secondary generalisation, lamotrigine, carbamazepine, valproate and gabapentin are all possible choices. Phenobarbitone and phenytoin are still the most common drugs used worldwide, but are not used frequently as first-line therapy in the UK except as the intravenous form in the treatment of status epilepticus. Topiramate is useful for partial seizures that have been refractory to treatment with any of these anti-epileptic drugs. Clobazam is a useful adjunctive therapy for either primary generalised or partial onset seizures, particularly if they occur in clusters or are related temporally to the menses (catamenial seizures). Vigabatrin is still used occasionally (particularly for the treatment of infantile spasms), but it causes irreversible visual field deficits and should thus not be used routinely. The newer agent tiagabine has also been reported to cause irreversible field deficits and should not be used routinely until more data are made public about whether this is indeed a true side-effect of this drug. Levetiracetam will be available and is expected to be useful in a variety of epilepsy types.

Choice of anti-epileptic drug for an individual patient depends on the type of seizures, specific epilepsy syndrome, use of concomitant medications, previous experience with anti-epileptic drugs, gender, patient preference and consideration of adverse effects in a given individual. Anti-epileptic drugs should generally be started on low doses and titrated up gradually, using the lowest effective dose at all times. Gabapentin, valproate and phenytoin may be titrated up more quickly than others, while lamotrigine, carbamazepine and topiramate need to be started more slowly. All anti-epileptic drugs need to be weaned gradually. Consideration for weaning off anti-epileptic drugs needs to be assessed on an individual basis.

Combination treatment

Treatment of epilepsy with anti-epileptic drugs should ideally be limited to monotherapy whenever possible. If more than one agent is necessary, care should be given to potential drug interactions. Gabapentin and vigabatrin cause the fewest problems in this arena, while phenytoin is notorious for the many drugs it interacts with. Monitoring of serum levels in treatment is useful only for the older anti-epileptic drugs (phenytoin, phenobarbitone, primidone, carbamazepine and valproate). With primidone, it is also necessary to check phenobarbitone levels, and with carbamazepine, monitoring of the 10,11-epoxide metabolite can be a useful test if toxicity is suspected. Free levels may be more useful than total drug levels for those anti-epileptic drugs that are highly protein-bound (phenytoin and valproate). Serum levels are not clinically relevant for the newer agents (lamotrigine, gabapentin, tiagabine, vigabatrin, topiramate and levetiracetam) unless one is checking for compliance in a patient.

THE ANTICONVULSANT DRUGS AND THEIR USE IN MOOD DISORDERS

Absorption and metabolism

Anticonvulsants are generally lipid-soluble molecules; this usually means that they are well absorbed from the gut. In some cases, however, for instance gabapentin, they are so insoluble in water that their dissolution in the gut is slow; absorption is then very poor unless the tablet is specially formulated to speed dissolution. Carbamazepine and valproate are metabolised quickly and need to be taken more than once a day to maintain a therapeutic blood level, although levels in brain tissue and clinical effect may not fluctuate so rapidly as serum levels. Slow-release or modified-release preparations lead to reduced peak blood levels and are better tolerated, and less frequent doses are required. By contrast, phenytoin, phenobarbitone and primidone are metabolised slowly, and can be taken in a single daily dose.

Being highly lipid-soluble they are largely bound to proteins in blood plasma. The ratio of free to bound drug in the plasma is constant when one drug is taken. Measuring the total serum concentration will serve as an estimate of free drug, which is the pharmacologically

Table 32.1 Anticonvulsant pharmacokinetics

Drug name	Plasma protein binding (%)	Plasma half-life (hours)	Main metabolism	Enzyme induction	Enzyme inhibition
Carbamazepine	Variable 75–90	48 acute 7 long-term	IIIA4 IA2 (active metabolite)	+++	0
Valproate	10–12	8–20	Oxidation	None	+++
Lamotrigine	50	30 60 on valproate	Oxidation Glucuronide	0	0
Gabapentin	Low	5–9	Unchanged in urine	0	0
Topiramate	15	19–25	Renal	0	IIC19
Phenytoin	95	Variable	Oxidation	+++	0

0, none; +++, extensive.

active fraction, but when another drug is taken, there is competition for binding sites on plasma protein. For instance, carbamazepine may displace phenytoin. The total serum concentration of phenytoin may then appear to be low, while the free concentration is actually higher. Blood levels are, therefore, difficult to interpret when more than one such drug is being taken.

The anticonvulsants are metabolised mainly in the liver by the cytochrome P450 enzymes (see Table 32.1). Competitive inhibition can result in one drug causing a rise in the serum level of another. For instance, valproate inhibits enzymes that metabolise carbamazepine and lamotrigine and tends to raise their blood levels. Some anticonvulsants induce liver cytochrome enzymes, within 2 weeks. This occurs with barbiturates, phenytoin and carbamazepine. It leads to a reduction of the blood levels of the drugs themselves (in the case of carbamazepine and barbiturates) and of other drugs including lamotrigine and antipsychotics. Some drugs are relatively free of effects on liver enzymes; these include lamotrigine and gabapentin.

The neurochemical changes, which result from an anticonvulsant, or from altering the dose, including enzyme changes, take weeks to reach a steady state; clinical changes must therefore be judged over a lengthy period.

Enzymes induced by barbiturates and phenytoin include those that metabolise vitamin D. People with low dietary intake or lack of sunshine may develop vitamin D deficiency as a result. These drugs may also interfere with folate metabolism, resulting in a macrocytic anaemia. Peripheral neuropathy may result from pyridoxine (B6) deficiency in patients treated with phenytoin unless this vitamin is given as a supplement.

Forced normalisation

This is a phenomenon usually in severe epilepsy in which the reduction or cessation of seizures with a return towards normality of the EEG coincides with the development of psychosis or affective disorder. It has also been observed during treatment with older anticonvulsants, including barbiturates, phenytoin and carbamazepine. It makes the interpretation of psychotic episodes occurring during treatment with newer anticonvulsants, including vigabatrin, difficult. The situation is also called 'alternative psychosis'. But it may take the form of psychosis, depression, mania or anxiety states. In childhood, aggression and agitation are more common. In unmedicated patients the episode would last for days or weeks until a seizure occurs. When the condition results from drug treatment, discontinuation of the drug results in re-appearance of the seizures, but recovery from the abnormal mental state. Sometimes a temporary reduction of anticonvulsant therapy, allowing a fit to occur, can produce some improvement in the mental state.

Some anticonvulsants, for instance vigabatrin, can cause psychosis independent of their control of seizures.

Valproate

Valproate is a branched-chain fatty acid. It is also available as a dimer (two identical molecules joined together), called divalproex in the US ('Depakote', known in the UK as semi-sodium valproate), which was used in several clinical trials after the company was granted a patent separate from that for sodium valproate. It was marketed first in the US.

Uses

- All forms of epilepsy
- mania and the prophylaxis of bipolar disorder, especially mixed states and lithium non-responders (licensed for mania in the US and UK)
- in schizophrenia, as an adjunct to clozapine when the latter causes fits in therapeutic doses (see chapter 13)
- Prophylaxis of migraine (licensed in the US, but not the UK)

Valproate in acute mania

Valproate is effective in a proportion of patients with mania, including non-responders to antipsychotic drugs and lithium. Patients who respond to valproate do not necessarily respond to carbamazepine and vice versa. In the first large parallel-group placebo-controlled study (which included only patients who were unresponsive to or intolerant of lithium), 59% of patients on valproate improved compared to only 16% of those on placebo. Most of the improvement occurred within 1–4 days of achieving therapeutic levels. A second and larger study comparing divalproex to lithium or placebo in a 3-week parallel-group double-blind study is shown in chapter 5 (Table 5.1, p. 43–44). Half of the patients had been unresponsive to lithium previously. Valproate was as effective in rapid-cycling mania as in other patients with mania, and equally effective in the patients previously judged responders or non-responders to lithium. Subsequent analyses indicate that patients with mixed affective states may benefit more from valproate than from lithium. However, few patients in the study returned to normal functioning within 3 weeks. The place of valproate in routine practice seems likely – as in the case of lithium – to be in combination with antipsychotic drugs in mania, perhaps particularly in patients with a significant mixture of depressive symptoms, and as prophylaxis.

Valproate in prophylaxis

Valproate has been studied less conclusively in prophylaxis but it may be useful alone or as an adjunct in those who are resistant to lithium or carbamazepine (see chapter 12). The drug is effective in a large proportion of patients during the rapid-cycling periods of their illness; in one study, the efficacy against mania appeared greater than against depression in rapid cycling.

Mechanism of action

Valproate is thought to increase the function of the inhibitory transmitter GABA; there is little direct evidence for increased GABA levels but GABA-B receptors may be up-regulated by valproate. The drug may also enhance central serotonin activity, and may reduce adrenocorticotrophic hormone (ACTH) and cortisol levels.

Side-effects

Valproate is generally well tolerated, but side-effects include vomiting, tremor, ataxia, weight gain, rash, hair loss – usually transient – and, potentially, acute liver damage in children. The modified-release form is associated with fewer side-effects, such as nausea. A confusional state with asterixis (flapping tremor) occurs rarely, and high blood ammonia levels confirm the cause; liver damage is not involved. Pancreatitis has occasionally been reported, as has spontaneous bruising or bleeding. A foetal valproate syndrome has also been described with cardiac and other congenital abnormalities and with jitteriness and seizures in the neonate.

Pharmacokinetics

Valproate is metabolised in the liver and has a plasma half-life of 8–20 hours, which may be prolonged by cimetidine. It inhibits cytochrome enzymes and thereby tends to raise the blood levels of lamotrigine.

Practical aspects of treatment with valproate

Selection of patients

Patients with mania, who do not respond to lithium, or who cannot tolerate it, should be tried on valproate. Those with mixed affective disorders may be given valproate in preference to lithium. Those who have responded to valproate during mania may benefit from it as prophylaxis. The drug should be avoided during pregnancy.

Dosage

The starting dose of sodium valproate is ('Epilim') 200 mg two to three times daily, rising by 200 mg at 3-day intervals, towards 2000 mg daily according to clinical response. For more rapid control a starting dose of 20 mg/kg is used. The modified-release form ('Epilim Chrono') is started at 500 mg daily, and increased. Semisodium valproate ('Depakote') is started at 750 mg daily for mania, increasing to two times daily or three times daily.

Blood test monitoring

The recommended plasma concentration is in the range of 50–150 mg/l. In children and patients with a history of liver disease, liver function tests should be monitored before treatment and occasionally during the first 6 months.

Combination

Some patients benefit from the combination of lithium and valproate, having not responded to either drug alone. Although side-effects including weight gain, tremor and drowsiness may be greater, the combination is generally safe.

Carbamazepine

Carbamazepine is a dibenzazepine derivative with a tricyclic structure.

Uses

- All forms of epilepsy, except petit mal
- Mania (unlicensed in the UK)
- the prophylaxis of bipolar disorder (licensed for use in patients unresponsive to lithium)
- as an adjunct in depressive illness (unlicensed)
- trigeminal neuralgia
- for the reduction of aggression, for instance as an adjunct to antipsychotic drugs in schizophrenia (unlicensed).

Carbamazepine in mania

The use of carbamazepine in mania is discussed in chapter 12. There have been small placebo-controlled crossover studies but no large-scale placebo-controlled trial has been conducted. There have been several comparative trials with antipsychotic drugs or lithium. These suggest that 50–60% of patients show a good response to carbamazepine. Even for these, antipsychotic drugs are required in the first few weeks of treatment, while the dose of carbamazepine is gradually increased; there is some delay in its action, but less so than with lithium.

Controlled studies of carbamazepine prophylaxis

There is much less documented evidence for the efficacy of carbamazepine in prophylaxis than there is for lithium. Carbamazepine has been shown to be superior to placebo in one crossover study. Trials comparing carbamazepine and lithium suggest that, in general, lithium may be superior. Approximately 60% of bipolar patients show a good initial response to carbamazepine, but this may diminish over 2–3 years.

Depression

In one controlled study of treatment-resistant depression only about a third of patients showed some acute antidepressant response over 3–4 weeks. Its tricyclic structure may be relevant to its antidepressant effects.

Mechanism of action

An anti-kindling effect may underlie some of the actions of carbamazepine. However, the pharmacological mechanism of action in acute mania is unknown. Carbamazepine reduces L-type calcium channel activation by depolarisation, and may block the excitatory transmitter glutamate at NMDA-type receptors. It potentiates central 5-HT transmission in normal subjects, as judged by the prolactin response to l-tryptophan.

Side-effects

Most side-effects are dose-related and reversible. Treatment should, therefore, be initiated at low doses and gradually increased to allow tolerance to develop. The use of slow-release preparations, which can be given twice daily, can help to reduce side-effects.

The most common side-effects are nausea, dizziness, ataxia and diplopia. Other common side-effects include headache, drowsiness, and nystagmus. At higher doses confusion may occur. Hyponatremia and water intoxication can occur through potentiation of ADH, and lead to malaise, confusion and fits. Fluid retention may occur.

A maculopapular itchy rash develops within 2 weeks in up to 15% of patients; this requires great caution and usually cessation of the drug, and a full blood count should be performed. Carbamazepine must be discontinued if the rash worsens, the blood count is abnormal or other symptoms develop. This allergic side-effect seems more likely to occur if the dose is raised too quickly.

Serious toxic side-effects are agranulocytosis, aplastic anaemia, and Stevens-Johnson syndrome. Carbamazepine regularly lowers the white cell count by a pharmacological effect on the marrow. A moderate leucopenia occurs in 1–2% of patients, and often transiently at the start of treatment. Agranulocytosis and aplastic anaemia can develop suddenly, and occur in about eight patients per million treated.

Because of the possibility of foetal neural tube defects, carbamazepine should be avoided if possible in pregnancy; folate supplements are essential if it is continued.

Pharmacokinetics and drug interactions

Carbamazepine is metabolised by CYP IIIA4. A metabolite (carbamazepine 10,11-epoxide) has similar pharmacological activity.

Carbamazepine induces liver enzymes, and this results not only in the lowering of its own blood levels after 3 weeks of treatment, but also in increasing the metabolism of other drugs, including haloperidol, oral contraceptives, clonazepam, ethosuximide, valproate and TCAs. Its own plasma half-life may shorten from 48 to 7 hours during long-term treatment. The dose of oral contraceptives needs to be raised, or an alternative method of birth control should be used. The dose of warfarin may also need increasing.

Barbiturates and phenytoin induce enzymes and lower plasma levels of carbamazepine. On the other hand, the blood level of carbamazepine is increased by drugs including erythromycin, verapamil, dextropropoxyphene (in co-proxamol), cimetidine, valproate, some SSRIs (fluoxetine) and nefazodone. The metabolism of thyroid hormone is increased and blood levels lowered; particularly in combination with lithium, carbamazepine may precipitate hypothyroidism.

Being of tricyclic structure, carbamazepine should not be given in combination with an MAOI; serotonin syndrome is a potential risk.

Practical aspects of carbamazepine treatment

Selection of patients

A history of non-response to lithium does not reduce the chances of responding to carbamazepine. Patients who respond to carbamazepine are particularly those with dysphoric mania, severe mania or mixed states. Patients with no family history of mania and those with bipolar disorder secondary to brain damage have a greater chance of responding to carbamazepine than to lithium. In contrast to lithium, rapid-cycling patients benefit as much from carbamazepine as do other bipolar patients.

Dosage

The recommended starting dose is 100 mg twice daily, increasing by 200 mg every 2 or 3 days, up to 400 mg twice daily or more, depending on response in mania. For prophylaxis the increase should be at weekly intervals. Gradual introduction of the drug reduces the incidence of side-effects, including nausea, rashes and blood dyscrasias. For most people with mania 800–1200 mg is sufficient, but a few may require up to 1600 mg a day. For prophylaxis the range is usually 400–600 mg per day. Modified-release tablets (200 mg and 400 mg) are associated with reduced peak plasma levels and are taken once or twice daily at the same total daily dose as above. Patients should be warned of side-effects, and advised particularly to report any rashes, fevers or severe sore throats, which may herald agranulocytosis and require immediate discontinuation of the drug.

Blood tests

Serum levels are sometimes helpful in monitoring carbamazepine therapy but, as in epilepsy, clinical judgement is generally more useful in deciding on dose changes. No clear relationship between blood level and response in affective disorders has been found. A range of 15–30 mmol/l (5–10 mg/l) is generally cited in epilepsy. A target of above 7 mg/l provides some guidance in affective disorders but the dose should be determined mainly by clinical response and tolerance of side-effects.

THE DRUGS

The differential blood count and electrolyte levels should be monitored in the first few weeks. Hyponatremia requires a reduction of dose or discontinuation. Carbamazepine should be stopped immediately if the total white cell count is less than 3000 per mm³ or the neutrophil count is less than 1500.

Lithium and carbamazepine combination

Many patients appear to benefit more from the combination of lithium and carbamazepine than from either drug alone. Carbamazepine should, therefore, be considered as an addition to lithium, rather than simply as an alternative, although the combination may – as with antipsychotics – increase the risk of lithium toxicity.

Phenytoin

Uses

Phenytoin was widely used in all types of epilepsy except petit mal until newer drugs were developed. It has been shown to have antimanic action in combination with haloperidol, but is not licensed for this use.

Mechanisms of action

Phenytoin blocks fast sodium channels.

Doses

For adults, and children over 6 years, 100 mg daily in one or two doses increasing gradually to 600 mg daily depending on response.

Several days are required to reach a stable level after each dose increase because of the long half-life. Phenytoin has a narrow therapeutic index. A small increase in dose may produce a large and toxic increase in serum level and increase of dose should be linked with plasma monitoring. Because of saturation of the liver enzymes, aim for plasma levels of 10–20 mg/l (40–80 µmol/l). Patients sensitive to their facial appearance, adolescents especially, may not tolerate the facial coarsening, gum hyperplasia, acne and hirsutism.

Side-effects and interactions

Gastric upsets are common. At higher doses nystagmus, diplopia, vertigo, ataxic gait and other cerebellar signs may occur, also an acute brain syndrome, sometimes accompanied by dystonia and choreo-athetosis. Hyperplasia of gums develops in 20% of those on chronic treatment. Hirsutism, peripheral neuropathy, rash and rarely folate-deficiency anaemia may develop. The folate deficiency can be treated with folic acid, permitting continuation of phenytoin. Carbamazepine levels are lowered by concurrent prescription of phenytoin.

Lamotrigine

Lamotrigine, marketed in the UK since 1991 first as an adjunctive treatment for refractory epilepsy, has become widely accepted as a first-line treatment for epilepsy, and has been found to have beneficial effects on mood in epilepsy.

Use in unipolar depression and bipolar disorder

It has antidepressant effects in both unipolar and bipolar depression. The risk of inducing mania appears to be lower than with other antidepressants, but it appears not to have antimanic effects.

It has proved effective in rapid-cycling bipolar-II disorder, perhaps by virtue of its antidepressant effect. Its efficacy in the prophylaxis of bipolar-I disorder is promising, particularly in preventing depression.

Mechanism of action

Lamotrigine blocks fast sodium channels, thereby reducing the size of action potentials in nerve fibres, particularly during repetitive firing. It has also profound effects in reducing calcium currents. These actions are thought to reduce the release of neurotransmitters, especially the excitatory transmitter glutamate; this is released at cortical projections in the limbic areas of the ventral striatum, an area that also receives an inhibitory input from the mesolimbic dopamine pathway. At higher concentrations the release of aspartate is also reduced.

Side-effects

It is generally well tolerated, without weight gain or cognitive impairment, and with no reports of teratogenicity. The commonest side-effects are headache, nausea, diplopia, ataxia and dizziness. However, up to 10% of patients develop a rash, which usually subsides if the drug is stopped but is potentially serious, and can lead to Stevens-Johnson syndrome.

Interactions

Lamotrigine has no significant effect on cytochrome P450 enzymes, and is only 50% bound to plasma proteins. It is metabolised by oxidation and glucuronidation with no active metabolites. Its half-life is normally about 30 hours, but lengthened to 60 hours in patients on valproate, and shortened in those on carbamazepine, because of the effects of these drugs on hepatic enzymes.

A possible pharmacodynamic interaction with carbamazepine may potentiate neurotoxicity.

Doses

The risk of serious allergic reactions may be reduced by increasing the dose slowly in steps of 25 mg per week, to an average of 150 mg per day. In patients on valproate, the dose of lamotrigine should be halved. Dosing is complex and manufacturers' data should always be consulted.

Gabapentin

Gabapentin is structurally related to GABA. It is used as an adjunctive therapy for patients with resistant temporal lobe epilepsy. It is also used for neuropathic pain.

THE DRUGS

Effects on mood

When added to other treatments for epilepsy, some patients reported improvements in their sense of well-being, in contrast to other anticonvulsants. The development of hypomania has also been reported.

It has been recommended in combination therapy in patients in whom treatment with lithium, carbamazepine and valproate have not provided control, or as an alternative when these agents are not tolerated. However, a placebo-controlled crossover study found no efficacy in bipolar depression, and a large trial of its use as adjunctive treatment in mania showed gabapentin inferior to placebo.

The only psychiatric use established in a placebo-controlled trial is in social phobia, where its size of effect is small (see chapter 15).

Mechanism of action

It probably acts by interfering with calcium channels to alter transmitter release.

Side-effects

The most common are drowsiness, dizziness, ataxia, tremor and diplopia. These are usually mild and transient. Also reported have been weight gain, emotional lability and lowering of the white cell count.

Pharmacokinetics

It is not protein-bound or metabolised but is excreted unchanged in the urine, with a half-life of 5–9 hours. It has no known pharmacokinetic interactions with other drugs. Gabapentin is, therefore, easy to use in combination with other drugs.

Doses

At a dose of 1500–2400 mg per day it is usually well tolerated.

Topiramate

This is a fructose sulphamate anticonvulsant, of proven usefulness as adjunctive therapy in epilepsy. Preliminary studies in treatment-resistant bipolar disorder have been encouraging.

Mechanisms of action

These include reduction of sodium and calcium conductances, blocking excitatory (AMPA-kainate type) glutamate receptors, potentiation of GABA and inhibition of carbonic anhydrase.

Side-effects

CNS side-effects include concentration and memory difficulties, slowness and drowsiness, ataxia and paraesthesias. These are less troublesome if the dose is increased slowly and they usually subside within 8 weeks. Weight loss occurs, especially at higher doses and is appreciated by patients who have gained weight on other drugs. Kidney stones can develop, as with other carbonic anhydrase inhibitors.

Psychiatric side-effects in epilepsy have included depression and psychosis, mostly occurring in the first 3 months.

Pharmacokinetics

It has no active metabolites, has low plasma protein binding, and is largely excreted by the kidney, having a half-life of 19–25 hours in healthy people. It inhibits CYP-IIC19, and may thereby increase levels of phenytoin. The efficacy of oral contraceptives is reduced.

Vigabatrin

This is a structural analogue of GABA, developed as an inhibitor of the transaminase that breaks down GABA. It increases levels of GABA, but may also reduce glutamate release. Although it is effective in temporal lobe epilepsy, it can worsen absences and myoclonic seizures.

Vigabatrin was one of the first of the newer anticonvulsants. Unfortunately, depression and psychosis have been noted to develop in patients with epilepsy who use it, especially those with a previous psychiatric history. Forced normalisation may be involved in some cases (see p. 342). Another drawback is that monitoring of visual fields is required, because irreversible narrowing of visual fields has been reported.

ANTICONVULSANT COMBINATIONS IN MOOD DISORDERS

Although such approaches have previously been viewed as dangerous polypharmacy, there is a growing opinion that successful control of severe bipolar disorder may require combined treatment not only of antipsychotics and antidepressants with a mood stabiliser such as lithium, but also with combined mood stabilisers. Analogies with chemotherapy for malignancy, and adjunctive therapies for epilepsy, are stimulating clinical trials designed to prove the effectiveness of adding individual anticonvulsants to previous drugs in bipolar disorder (see p. 125).

The combination of two anticonvulsants poses special problems in monitoring, because of pharmacokinetic interactions. With the two most established drugs, carbamazepine induces enzymes including CYP3A, which metabolise itself, valproate and several antipsychotics, whereas valproate inhibits enzymes that metabolise carbamazepine and lamotrigine. Thus, metabolites accumulate that may compete for plasma protein binding. Lower plasma level targets are then appropriate, for instance 4–6 mg/l carbamazepine. The metabolites may also be pharmacologically active. There are reports of combining lamotrigine with carbamazepine or valproate.

FURTHER READING

Bowden, C. & Muller-Oerlinghausen, B. (1999) Carbamazepine and valproate: use in mood disorders. In *Schizophrenia and Mood Disorders: The New Drug Therapies in Clinical Practice* (eds J. Waddington & P. Buckley), pp. 179–189. Oxford: Butterworth Heinemann.

THE DRUGS

——, Brugger, A. M., Swann, A. C., *et al* (1994) Efficacy of divalproex vs lithium and placebo in the treatment of mania. *JAMA*, **271**, 918–924.

——, Calabrese, J. R., McElroy, S. L., *et al* (2000) A randomised, placebo-controlled 12-month trial of divalproex and lithium in treatment of outpatients with bipolar I disorder. *Archives of General Psychiatry*, **57**, 481–489.

Calabrese, J. R., Bowden, C. L., Sachs, G. S., *et al* (1999) A double blind placebo controlled study of lamotrigine monotherapy in outpatients with bipolar I depression. *Journal of Clinical Psychiatry*, **60**, 79–88.

Elferink, A. J. A. & van Zwieten-Boot, B. J. (1997) Analysis based on number needed to treat shows differences between drugs studied. *BMJ*, **314**, 603.

Ferrier, N. & Calabrese, J. (1999) Lamotrigine, gabapentin and the new anticonvulsants: efficacy in mood disorders. In *Schizophrenia and Mood Disorders: The New Drug Therapies in Clinical Practice* (eds J. Waddington & P. Buckley), pp. 190–198. Oxford: Butterworth Heinemann.

Greil, W. & Kleindienst, N. (1999) The comparative prophylactic efficacy of lithium and carbamazepine in patients with bipolar I disorder. *International Clinical Psychopharmacology*, **14**, 277–281.

Post, R. (1999) Psychopharmacology of mood stabilisers. In *Schizophrenia and Mood Disorders: The New Drug Therapies in Clinical Practice* (eds J. Waddington & P. Buckley), pp. 127–154. Oxford: Butterworth Heinemann.

33. DRUGS FOR DEMENTIA

As reviewed in chapter 16, the dementia syndrome (progressive global cognitive impairment) can be seen as a final common pathway for several distinct disease entities of which the most common are Alzheimer's disease, vascular dementia and dementia with Lewy bodies. Early studies of drug treatments for the dementias examined their efficacy in mixed cohorts. More recently specific putative treatments have been and are being evaluated for each of these common dementias, with particular emphasis being placed on possible treatments for Alzheimer's disease. Both for the dementias as a whole and for Alzheimer's disease in particular, treatment approaches can be classified as preventative, disease modifying and symptomatic.

DISEASE PREVENTATIVE APPROACHES IN ALZHEIMER'S DISEASE

The prevention of Alzheimer's disease can be attempted in several ways. The most direct approach is genetic. Further preventative strategies in Alzheimer's disease involve the use of antioxidants, anti-inflammatory drugs and hormones, and research on cholinesterase expression.

Genetic approaches

As our understanding of the genetic basis of the disease increases, the prospects for specific gene therapies improve. Several specific genetic markers for Alzheimer's disease have now been identified. Some are rare but occur in affected members of families with high rates of early-onset Alzheimer's disease; these may be regarded as causative. Others (most notably the E4 variant of the apolipoprotein E gene on chromosome 19) are commonly found in people with late-onset Alzheimer's disease and appear to reflect increased vulnerability. As yet no specific gene-modifying treatments have been evaluated.

Antioxidants

There is increasing evidence that Alzheimer's disease is associated with reduced activity within the brain of naturally occurring antioxidants (such as superoxide dismutase), resulting in increased vulnerability to oxidative damage to neurons. Several antioxidant chemicals have been suggested as potentially useful in protecting against or modifying Alzheimer's disease pathology. These include vitamin C, vitamin E, and the traditional Chinese remedy *Gingko Biloba*. There is some evidence that vitamin E postpones deterioration in established Alzheimer's disease and that *Gingko Biloba* may cause limited cognitive improvement. None of these substances is as yet licensed for the treatment or prevention of Alzheimer's disease.

Anti-inflammatories

The inflammatory process (both in the brain and peripherally) can induce the formation of amyloid peptides. Inflammation may thus be linked to the deposition of amyloid plaques, one of the characteristic pathological findings in the Alzheimer's disease brain. Naturalistic studies suggest that elderly people who regularly take non-steroidal anti-inflammatories have a reduced risk of developing Alzheimer's disease. No NSAID is as yet licensed for the treatment or prevention of Alzheimer's disease.

Hormones

Oestrogens have several actions that may be preventative or disease modifying in Alzheimer's disease. These include promotion of breakdown of amyloid precursor protein, antioxidant effects and facilitation of cholinergic neurotransmission. Several epidemiological studies suggest that women on hormone replacement therapy are at substantially (35–50%) reduced risk of developing Alzheimer's disease. There is also some evidence that oestrogens can improve cognitive function in women with established Alzheimer's disease. Higher doses (1.25 mg or more) may confer greater protection than lower (0.625 mg or less) doses. Co-administered progestins may reduce the protective effect. There are no comparative data on different oestrogen preparations and none suggesting therapeutic benefits for oestrogens in men. Oestrogens are not as yet licensed for the treatment or prevention of Alzheimer's disease.

Cholinesterase expression

This enzyme can be expressed in an abnormal form that leads to cell destruction, and research is targeted on drugs to alter this.

PREVENTING VASCULAR DEMENTIA

Preventative strategies for vascular dementia involve identifying those at high risk and attempting to modify specific risk factors. The risk factors for vascular dementia are essentially the same as risk factors for stroke and include hypertension, hyperlipidaemia, diabetes, smoking and obesity. Probably the best markers of high risk of vascular dementia are a history of stroke or of transient ischaemic attacks. Smoking cessation and optimal control of specific risk factors (all of which are common in old age) are effective both in preventing the establishment of vascular dementia and in slowing its progression. Statins, which lower blood lipids, may be useful in reducing risk of stroke (and by extension vascular dementia) even in the absence of clear-cut hyperlipidaemia. Detailed information on their use is beyond the scope of this chapter and the reader is advised to consult the *BNF*. The most widely used drug treatments for those at high risk of, or with established, vascular dementia are aspirin and dipyridamole, which exert an antithrombolytic effect by modifying platelet aggregation, adhesion and survival. The use of these antiplatelet agents is contraindicated in haemorrhagic stroke. Aspirin 75–150 mg/day is probably as effective as higher doses and carries less risk of inducing gastrointestinal bleeding. Dipyridamole may be used alone in patients in whom aspirin is contraindicated, or in conjunction with aspirin. It is thought that the effects of aspirin and dipyridamole on platelet activity are additive. The dose range for dipyridamole is between 300 and 600 mg day, in divided doses. A sustained-release formulation (200 mg twice daily) is also now available. Dipyridamole may increase the hypotensive effect of blood-pressure-lowering drugs and may reduce the activity of cholinesterase inhibitors.

DISEASE-MODIFYING TREATMENTS

Future developments for modifying the progression of Alzheimer's disease are likely to include modulators of protein processing – in particular preventing or removing deposits of amyloid and/or tau proteins (the main constituents of senile plaques and neurofibrillary tangles, respectively). Oestrogens and cholinesterase inhibitors may have limited activity in this area and more specific modulators are currently being developed.

Meanwhile, several drugs have been shown to have activity in protecting neurons against damage and/or to stimulate neuronal growth. These may be beneficial both in Alzheimer's disease and in vascular dementia.

These so-called nootropic drugs have been advocated for the treatment of Alzheimer's disease and other dementias such as vascular dementia. They were originally thought to exert their therapeutic action by inducing cerebral vasodilation. In this model, dementia is seen as being due to cerebrovascular insufficiency and thereby potentially treatable by inducing such cerebral vasodilation. Unfortunately, even in vascular dementia, vasodilation does not cause a beneficial redistribution of blood supply to ischaemic brain tissue. The longest established of this group of drugs are the ergot derivatives, of which the most widely used is co-dergocrine maleate ('Hydergine'). 'Hydergine' is currently classified as a metabolic enhancer and although there is little specific evidence for its efficacy, it may exert some neuroprotective effect both in Alzheimer's disease and in vascular dementia. The usual daily dose is 4.5 mg, in single or divided doses. Piracetam (800–100 mg daily) is another nootropic, though dementia is not as yet an indication for its use.

The MAO-B inhibitor selegiline has been shown significantly to postpone deterioration in established Alzheimer's disease. Selegiline at the usual dose of 10 mg/day is sufficiently MAO-B selective not to require a low tyramine diet. It is rapidly absorbed following oral administration and has several active metabolites including methamphetamine. Adverse interactions may occur with pethidine and with SSRIs. Alzheimer's disease and vascular dementia are not as yet recognised indications for the use of selegiline.

SYMPTOMATIC TREATMENTS

More recently interest has focused on Alzheimer's disease as a distinct disease entity, and within Alzheimer's disease research on drugs with specific activity on the cholinergic neurotransmitter system. These

THE DRUGS

355

have their basis in the observation that at neurotransmitter level the most pervasive deficit in Alzheimer's disease is reduction in levels of acetylcholine resulting from loss of cholinergic neurons (whose cell bodies are in the nucleus basalis of Meynert). Post-synaptic cholinergic receptors are relatively well preserved. It is important to remember, however, that many other neurotransmitter deficits (as well as gross neuronal loss and reduction in dendritic branching) are also found in Alzheimer's disease and that one would therefore not expect cholinergic boosting to reverse all the cognitive and behavioural deficits.

Initial trials of acetylcholine precursors (choline and lecithin) were disappointing. In contrast, cholinesterase inhibitors showed greater early promise that has been confirmed in several large clinical trials. As a result, four cholinesterase inhibitors (tacrine, donepezil, galantamine and rivastigmine) are currently licensed for the symptomatic treatment of mild to moderate Alzheimer's disease. Galantamine was originally extracted in the Ukraine from daffodils. Other such drugs have received extensive clinical trial evaluation: velnacrine, slow-release physostigmine and eptastigmine (a pro-drug of physostigmine). In general, cholinesterase inhibitors produce modest but statistically significant improvements or prevent deterioration in cognitive function, with some studies of some drugs also suggesting benefits in global functioning, daily living skills and carer burden. Degree of change varies greatly between individuals. In the light of this and of the nature of Alzheimer's disease as a chronically progressive condition, mean change scores in randomised controlled trials provide less clinically useful information than is usually the case. NNT analyses (see chapter 5), however, reveal NNTs of between 4 and 7 for several clinically meaningful indices of individual response and suggest that these drugs may be clinically useful and even cost-effective. Long-term data is still lacking but available evidence suggests that typical responses are of the order of a 6–12 month reversal or postponement of deterioration, with a minority of patients maintaining a more sustained improvement. There is also some suggestion that long-term use of cholinesterase inhibitors may delay disease progression in Alzheimer's disease.

There has to date been little formal study of symptomatic treatments in dementia with Lewy bodies. Cholinesterase inhibitors are probably effective, particularly in alleviating psychotic and behavioural symptoms. Dopaminergic treatments have proved disappointing.

Particularly during the first few years of clinical experience with these drugs, they should be prescribed within a locally agreed protocol. The main features of such a protocol are outlined below. Cholinesterase inhibitors should only be used in patients in whom there is a clear diagnosis of Alzheimer's disease with documentation that patients meet standard criteria such as those of ICD–10 or DSM–IV. The efficacy of this group of drugs has been shown only for the subgroup of Alzheimer's disease patients with mild to moderately severe Alzheimer's disease (Mini Mental State scores of 10–26 or, in the case of rivastigmine, which has been tested in a wider range of patients, 6–26). Patients and their carers should have the side-effects and possible benefits of the drugs explained to them and consider issues of consent and compliance (which may require carer support). Titration to optimal dose will require close initial monitoring. Clinician and carer (and where possible patients themselves) should monitor progress closely, with a decision taken after 3–6 months of treatment whether continuing the drug is justified. Such justification will usually involve improvement (or at least lack of deterioration) in at least two areas of functioning. Areas to be considered can include cognition, global functioning, mood, daily living skills, behaviour and carer burden. The initial prescription should be following specialist referral and assessment and specialist involvement in the decision to continue is also helpful. Rapid deterioration may occur following drug discontinuation (even where there has been little or no apparent benefit during treatment); this may be reversed following re-establishment of treatment.

Tacrine

Tacrine (tetrahydroaminoacridine) was the first cholinesterase inhibitor to complete the clinical trial process and be licensed. It produces similar cognitive changes to those found with other cholinesterase inhibitors but its clinical utility is severely limited by the high risk it carries of severe and sometimes irreversible hepatotoxicity. Tacrine is currently in use in the US and some other countries. Although licensed in the UK, it is not actively marketed and is unlikely to be widely used. Tacrine is 55% protein-bound and extensively metabolised in the liver via the cytochrome P450 IA2 enzyme system. Tacrine may increase blood theophylline levels and its own plasma levels may be elevated by concomitant cimetidine. The initial recommended dose of tacrine is 10 mg four times daily, increasing by 40 mg day (divided in four doses) every 6 weeks to a maximum of 40 mg four times daily. Liver function needs to be monitored carefully on patients taking tacrine and becomes abnormal in about 50% of patients on the drug. Weekly blood testing is necessary for the first 18 weeks, with further testing every 3 months if liver function remains normal. The drug should be discontinued if transaminase levels increase by more than three- to fivefold. The development of jaundice mandates immediate withdrawal of tacrine. Other tacrine side-effects are similar to those described for donepezil, below (but are more frequently observed). These side-effects reflect enhanced cholinergic function.

Donepezil

Donepezil is a specific and reversible inhibitor of acetylcholinesterase. It is well absorbed by mouth, with peak plasma concentrations after 3–4 hours. Donepezil has a half-life of about 3 days. Steady-state plasma concentrations are reached after 2–3 weeks. Donepezil is highly (95%) protein-bound, and is partly excreted intact in the urine and partly metabolised in the liver through the cytochrome P450 system. Donepezil is given in a single daily dose, preferably in the evening. The starting dose is 5 mg. Side-effects permitting, the dose can be increased after 4 weeks to 10 mg, with the possibility of increased efficacy but greater risk of side-effects. The most frequent side-effects seen are gastrointestinal (diarrhoea and muscle cramps). Other side-effects include fatigue, nausea, vomiting, insomnia and dizziness. No important drug interactions have been demonstrated, although there is potential for interference with anticholinergic medications (which should in any case be avoided in patients with Alzheimer's disease) and potentiation of depolarising neuromuscular blockers (such as suxamethonium) or cholinergic agonists. Overdosage may result in a cholinergic crisis characterised by nausea, vomiting, salivation, sweating, bradycardia, hypotension and respiratory collapse. Treatment is with atropine and supportive measures.

Rivastigmine

Rivastigmine is a carbamate derivative that binds to and temporarily inactivates acetylcholinesterase. Peak plasma concentrations occur 1 hour after oral ingestion. Rivastigmine is weakly (40%) protein-bound and is rapidly and extensively metabolised primarily via extrahepatic cholinesterase-mediated hydrolysis. Enzyme activity normalises about 9 hours after a single dose. Rivastigmine should be given twice daily. The initial recommended dose is 1.5 mg twice daily. If tolerated, this can be increased after 2 weeks to 3 mg twice daily and (after further 2-week periods) to 4.5 mg twice daily and thence to the maximum recommended dose of 6 mg twice daily. The main side-effects described are nausea, vomiting, abdominal pain, loss of appetite, asthenia and somnolence. Other side-effects (which are closely related to speed of dose titration) include sweating, malaise, weight loss and tremor. Unlike donepezil, rivastigmine clearance is not affected by impaired renal or hepatic function. Rivastigmine has a low propensity for adverse drug interactions. The management of rivastigmine overdosage is similar to that described for donepezil, above.

Galantamine

Galantamine is licensed as Reminyl. It is more selective for acetylcholinesterase than butyrylcholinesterase but produces greater enzyme inhibition in human erythrocytes than in human brain tissue. Preliminary results in patients with Alzheimer's disease have reported galantamine to be associated with a reduction in cognitive deterioration on some neuropsychiatric rating scales. Nausea and vomiting are the most commonly reported adverse effects; liver toxicity has not been reported to date. The dose is 4 mg twice daily, increasing to 8 mg twice daily after 4 weeks, and then if necessary to 12 mg twice daily.

FURTHER READING

Burns, A., Rossor, M., Hecker, J., *et al* (1999) The effects of donepezil in Alzheimer's disease – results from a multinational trial. *Dementia and Geriatric Cognitive Disorders*, **10**, 237–244.

Fulton, B. & Benfield, P. (1996) Galantamine. *Drugs and Ageing*, **9**, 60–65.

Livingston, G. & Katona, C. (2000) How useful are cholinesterase inhibitors in the treatment of Alzheimer's disease? A number Needed to treat analysis. *International Journal of Geriatric Psychiatry*, **15**, 203–207.

Rosler, M., Anand, R., Cicin-Sain, A., *et al* (1999) Efficacy and safety of rivastigmine in patients with Alzheimer's disease: international randomised controlled trial. *BMJ*, **318**, 633–638.

34. ANTI-ANXIETY DRUGS AND HYPNOTICS

BENZODIAZEPINES

Benzodiazepines are valuable hypnotics, anxiolytics or minor tranquillisers, and anticonvulsants. It is difficult to commit suicide with them in overdose when they alone are taken, and they can safely be taken with most other drugs without serious interactions.

Benzodiazepines work mainly by enhancing GABA transmission in the CNS, and do this by interacting allosterically with sites on GABA-A receptors (see chapter 7). CNS tolerance develops within days or weeks; the biochemical mechanism is unknown but dependence develops and unpleasant symptoms occur on withdrawal.

Benzodiazepine receptors may respond to as yet unknown endogenous substances that are blocked by benzodiazepines. The GABA-A and benzodiazepine receptors have multiple molecular subtypes, with variations in each of the five subunits (see p. 67). The subunits are from three families – α, β and γ. The benzodiazepine binding site straddles an α and a β subunit. Receptors with α-1 subunits predominate in the cerebral cortex, whereas those with α-5 subunits predominate in the hippocampus. Thus, benzodiazepine-1 receptors that have α-1 subunits mediate sedation, but anxiolytic actions may be more closely related to actions on α-2, 3 or 5 subunits. So, some drugs may be more sedative and others more anxiolytic.

Benzodiazepines are closely related compounds all with the same ring structure (Figure 34.1) to which atoms or radicals like -H, -OH, -CH$_3$, -Cl are attached at different points. In metabolism -CH$_3$ radicals can be removed (demethylation) and the active drug is turned into another active substance. Diazepam, medazepam, chlordiazepoxide and clorazepate all give rise to N-desmethyldiazepam (nordiazepam), and

---

Figure 34.1 The benzodiazepine structure

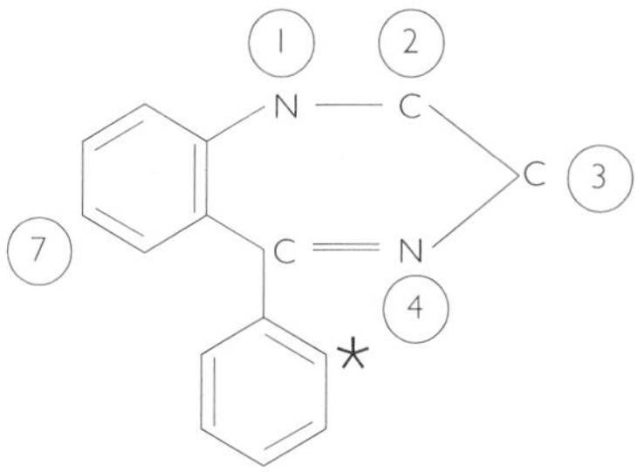

1-4, 7 and * are points to which atoms or radicals attach.

this metabolite itself will accumulate, having a half-life of several days. Diazepam, chlordiazepoxide and medazepam are all metabolised to oxazepam. Benzodiazepines differ among themselves chiefly in potency, and in speed of inactivation and excretion. Temazepam and oxazepam, for example, are quickly converted to inactive glucuronides and excreted by the kidney and are therefore short-acting, and useful as hypnotics. But diazepam is converted to nordiazepam, which is active and only slowly converted on to other substances that are inert, and lost. Temazepam capsules are liable to misuse and not available on NHS prescription; temazepam is classified as a controlled drug, but is not subject to additional prescribing requirements. It is now used less frequently.

Insomnia

Benzodiazepines are not harmless sedatives and hypnotics. They should be prescribed for a defined purpose within a plan of management. Prescribe for a finite period, for example 2 weeks, and then review their effects and only renew the prescription with justification. If treatment continues after dependence has begun to develop, the initial therapeutic effects are at least partly lost, and as each dose wears off the patient may experience a rebound exacerbation of the pre-existing condition to a more severe level than before. Attacks of panic may occur whenever a short-acting drug such as lorazepam is wearing off. Withdrawal reactions with longer-acting drugs (diazepam, nitrazepam) begin several days after stopping.

Difficulty in getting off to sleep can be treated with a rapid onset short-acting benzodiazepine such as lormetazepam, temazepam or loprazolam. After a good night's sedation the patient should wake fresh, without hangover, drowsiness or dysphoria. However, after a single dose there may be a rebound exacerbation of insomnia the following night. There is also a potential problem with ultra-short-acting drugs (such as triazolam, which is no longer licensed) that the person may awake early and in a confused state.

Effective doses of short-acting benzodiazepines cause tolerance in 3–14 days. On stopping treatment, 2 or 3 nights of insomnia will occur before natural sleep rhythm returns, and patients should be told this, otherwise they will ask for more drug. Be wary of using longer-acting benzodiazepines as night sedation, because the drugs accumulate and have effects the next day. Benzodiazepines are for short-term control of insomnia.

Anxiety

Episodes of acute anxiety can be prevented with a single dose of diazepam, which has both a rapid and a slow component of action. The patient must know the situations likely to provoke anxiety, and should practise once or twice before the situations occur in order to get the dose and timing right. For example, 2 mg or 5 mg of diazepam by mouth taken 1 hour before a stressful situation might be helpful.

Persistent anxiety can be controlled or made tolerable with a regular low dose of a longer-acting benzodiazepine such as chlordiazepoxide or diazepam. Although lower doses produce tolerance less quickly than larger doses, dependence is still a risk and treatment should not be longer than 4 weeks. Because chronic anxiety usually fluctuates in severity, intermittent use of these drugs, which is preferable to regular use, is a practical course. Even with intermittent use, prescribing for longer than a few months is not recommended.

Benzodiazepines in long-term use may increase the risk of depression and it is important to determine whether the patient's anxiety is one aspect of a depressive illness, and if so to treat that.

Anxiety is common in situations requiring adjustment, such as after a bereavement. Here the use of a benzodiazepine may impair the person's ability to grieve or make the necessary adjustment, and the drugs should be avoided.

Side-effects and interactions

Benzodiazepines cause impairment of mental ability, amnesia, decreased psychomotor reactions and coordination, and, in the elderly, ataxia. In some personalities they result, albeit very rarely, in disinhibition and even aggression. Avoid prescribing for personalities prone to dependency.

Cimetidine blocks benzodiazepine oxidation in the liver and so potentiates the effects. Inhibitors of the cytochrome CYP3A4 (e.g. fluoxetine, nefazodone) have a similar effect. Renal and liver disease increase sensitivity. Alcohol interacts with benzodiazepines centrally, and they potentiate one another, with increased incoordination, disinhibition and aggression. Benzodiazepines cause some respiratory depression, particularly in the elderly, and those with emphysema and bronchitis are made worse by them. In combination with opiates or other sedative drugs, the respiratory depression may be fatal at high doses.

Benzodiazepines still have a part to play in controlling human distress. Occasionally there will be circumstances where the evils of drug dependence are less than the disabling and painful symptoms of a psychiatric condition that cannot otherwise be ameliorated. A benzodiazepine may be better than alcohol, if that is the alternative for the patient. Patients should always be warned of the risks of dependence, the impairment of coordination and the interactions with alcohol, and advised not to drink.

Dependence

Abrupt withdrawal, after high doses or long use, can result in an acute brain syndrome with disorientation and delirium, rarely a paranoid psychosis and very rarely convulsions. Rapid withdrawal from low-dose treatment causes insomnia, anxiety, tremor and sweating – symptoms similar to those for which the benzodiazepine may have been first prescribed. Additional symptoms include nausea; heightened sensitivity to light and sound; a sense of imbalance, as on a rocking boat, which may impair mobility; peculiar and frightening sensory illusions; tinnitus; paraesthesia; depersonalisation; and derealisation. These can last for weeks and full recovery may take 1–2 years after long-term treatment. Here a careful plan of slow and phased withdrawal, using diazepam at an equivalent dose (for instance, 10 mg diazepam to 1 mg lorazepam), with concurrent support in a self-help group and relaxation classes, is helpful. Start by reducing the dose by a tenth every 2 weeks in

THE DRUGS

out-patients or every week in in-patients. Some patients will feel better as the dose is reduced, but be prepared to reduce more slowly in those who suffer withdrawal symptoms.

DIAZEPAM

Diazepam ('Diazemuls', 'Stesolid', 'Valium') is discussed in detail as a typical benzodiazepine. Other benzodiazepines are shown in Table 34.1. Diazepam may be used for:

- alleviation of anxiety
- treatment of insomnia associated with anxiety
- relief of delirium tremens
- tranquillisation in acute psychosis, including drug-induced states (see chapter 14)

Table 34.1 Other drugs

Generic name (proprietary name)	Method of delivery	Doses (mg except where stated)	Maximum daily dose (mg except where stated)
Anxiolytics			
Alprazolam[1] ('Xanax')	Tablets	0.25, 0.5 mg	3
Bromazepam[1] ('Lexotan')	Tablets	1.5, 3	18
Chlordiazepoxide[2] ('Librium')	Tablets	5, 10, 25	60–100
	Capsules	5, 10	
Clobazam[1] ('Frisium')	Capsules	10	30
Clorazepate[1] ('Tranxene')	Capsules	7.5, 15 mg	22.5
Lorazepam[2] ('Ativan')	Tablets	1, 2.5	4
	Injection[3]	4 mg/ml	9
Midazolam[2] ('Hypnovel')	Ampoules	1 mg/ml	
		2 mg/ml	
		5 mg/ml	
Oxazepam[2] ('Oxanid')	Tablets	10, 15, 30	90
Hypnotics			
Short acting			
Lormetazepam[1]	Tablets	0.5, 1	1.5
Temazepam[2] ('Normison')	Tablets	10, 20	40
	Capsules[1]	10, 15, 20, 30	30
	Elixir	10mg/5ml	
Loprazolam[2]	Tablet	1	2
Longer acting			
Nitrazepam[2] ('Mogadon')	Tablets	5	10
	Mixture	2.5mg/5ml	
Flunitrazepam[1] ('Rohypnol')	Tablets	1	1
Flurazepam[1] ('Dalmane')	Capsules	15, 30	30

1. Not available at NHS expense.
2. May only be prescribed under generic (not brand) name.
3. Withdrawal symptoms are common.

- abreaction (see chapter 40)
- control of status epilepticus.

A single oral dose of 5 or 10 mg, occasionally more, will dampen anxiety in ½–1 hour, or may be taken before an anxiety-provoking situation. This quick effect will wear off, in about 4 hours. The drug is metabolised to a less potent but more persistent anxiolytic. Repeated doses of 2 mg or more can be given on a regular schedule 2–3 times daily, when the main benefit will come from the accumulation of the less-potent metabolite nordiazepam, which builds over the course of 2 weeks and is slow to disappear when treatment is stopped. Prescribe the smallest dose that will relieve symptoms. Avoid giving more than 30 mg per day and review the dosage weekly.

Diazepam can be used for insomnia, particularly when the problem is getting off to sleep, but its metabolites may produce hangover effects next morning, especially when used on successive nights. Assess critically whether patients taking regular daytime diazepam need separate night sedation or, likewise, whether patients taking regular night sedation need daytime sedation. In acute stress, or to induce relaxation in a behavioural desensitisation programme, or in abreaction, 10 mg or even 20 mg can be given intravenously.

For delirium tremens and for acute tranquillisation, 10 mg or more diazepam is given intravenously until control is achieved, and then oral doses are used to maintain control until the acute state has remitted.

Chlordiazepoxide is also widely used in alcohol withdrawal. For moderately severe withdrawal, the dose starts with up to 120 mg on the first day (as 3–4 doses), reducing to 90 mg the second day, 50 mg the third day and by at least 25% daily until stopping after another 4–7 days. For withdrawal in a community setting, the dose starts at 25 mg three times daily, for 2 days, then twice daily for 2 more days and 25 mg and 10 mg on days 5 and 6. Diazepam 10 mg can be used in place of chlordiazepoxide 25 mg.

Diazepam is the treatment of choice for status epilepticus, by slow intravenous injection or, in infants, by rectal administration. Other benzodiazepines are not used in this way, but clonazepam can be a useful drug for epilepsy.

Side-effects

Tiredness or sleepiness may develop after some days, particularly on higher doses, or a morning hangover feeling. Ataxia and dizziness are less common. Nausea and headache have been reported in some cases. In a few patients irritability or aggressive behaviour appears. Benzodiazepines should be avoided in those with a history of personality disorder or drug or alcohol misuse. In some, anxiety may even be increased. Drug dependence develops on higher doses and withdrawal symptoms appear a week or so after the drug is stopped. Sudden withdrawal may occasionally provoke fits.

Diazepam is less suitable for the elderly because of the greater risk of mental confusion, ataxia or falls, or in the presence of cardio-respiratory disorders as respiration is depressed. It is available as tablets of 2 mg, 5 mg and 10 mg, capsules of 2 mg and 5 mg, a suspension of 2 mg/5 ml, an injection of 5 mg/ml (emulsion ('Diazemuls') is less likely to cause inflammation), and a rectal solution at 2 mg/ml and 4 mg/ml.

AZASPIRODECANEDIONES

Buspirone

This is a new class of drugs that act primarily as partial agonists at 5-HT-1A receptors both pre- and post-synaptically. They tend also to be antagonists at dopamine D_2 receptors.

Buspirone is the first available drug in this class and has mild anti-anxiety effects that develop within 1–2 weeks of treatment. The recommended dose is 5–10 mg three times daily. Claims are made for its uses as an adjunct to an MARI in depression and OCD but these remain to be proved. Tolerance and problematic withdrawal symptoms do not develop but the drug does not relieve benzodiazepine withdrawal symptoms. The side-effects include nausea, dizziness and headaches. It is available as tablets of 5 mg and 10 mg.

CYCLOPYRROLONES

Zopiclone

This group of compounds is structurally different from the benzodiazepines, but interact with the same part of the GABA-A receptor, and has similar properties to the benzodiazepines. Zopiclone is a sedative drug with a short half-life suitable for night sedation. It is metabolised by the CYP3A4 enzyme. It should be used with the same precautions as the benzodiazepines, should not be used for longer than 4 weeks, and should not be prescribed to those with a history of substance misuse or personality disorder, or those who are still drinking alcohol. The side-effects include a bitter taste, nausea and vomiting. Irritability, depression, amnesia and hallucinations have also been reported. One or two tablets are prescribed at night.

The dependence risk increases with long-term use and withdrawal problems include craving, anxiety, insomnia and derealisation, similar to benzodiazepine withdrawal. It is available as tablets of 3.7 mg and 7.5 mg.

IMIDAZOPYRIDINES

Zolpidem

Zolpidem is a non-benzodiazepine sedative that binds to the GABA-A receptor at the benzodiazepine-1 site. At sedative doses, zolpidem is not an anticonvulsant or muscle relaxant. Zolpidem begins to act in ½ –1 hour, with peak plasma levels occurring after 1–2 hours. Average plasma half-life is around 2½ hours. Its metabolism is largely controlled by the cytochrome enzyme CYP3A4. Plasma levels are increased by fluoxetine and decreased by rifampicin.

Zolpidem in doses of 5–10 mg is an effective hypnotic. Sleep architecture seems not to be grossly affected and hangover effects are very rare. Adverse effects are uncommon (light-headedness in 5% of patients). The drug appears to be safe in overdose and its effects are rapidly reversed by the benzodiazepine antagonist flumazenil. Tolerance and dependence have not been observed in short-term use. If prescribing is for 4 weeks or less, withdrawal reactions or rebound insomnia are not normally reported. As with all hypnotics, only short-term intermittent use is recommended. It is available as tablets of 5 mg and 10 mg.

PYRAZOLOPYRIMIDINE

Zaleplon

Zaleplon ('Sonata') is a pyrazolopyrimidine hypnotic that induces sleep via agonist activity at benzodiazepine-1 receptors.

Zaleplon is rapidly absorbed and short acting – its elimination half-life is around 1 hour. This short duration of action makes very unlikely any residual hangover effects the morning after taking the drug. Clinical studies of reaction times and other cognitive functions unequivocally support this supposition. Withdrawal symptoms and rebound insomnia seem not to occur after 28 days' continuous use.

The dose of zaleplon is 10 mg at night (5 mg for elderly patients). Co-administered drugs that affect the function of CYP IIIA4 are likely to alter plasma levels and elimination half-life of zaleplon. For example, cimetidine almost doubles zaleplon levels; rifampicin, an inducer, reduces levels by 75%.

CHLORAL HYDRATE

Uses

Chloral hydrate ('Noctec', 'Welldorm') is metabolised in the body to the chlorine-substituted alcohol, trichloroethanol. This is a safe hypnotic, with few side-effects. It is short acting and without hangover, and is particularly suitable for the elderly and physically frail. Because of the risk of dependency it should be prescribed with the same caution as the benzodiazpines. Only use short term and avoid if there is severe cardiac, renal or hepatic disease.

Taken in water, the mixture (0.5–2 gm for insomnia) can be unpleasant to swallow because of the taste and causes gastric irritation. Addition of milk may help, but a capsule ('Noctec') or tablet ('Welldorm' – chloral betaine) is better tolerated. It is available as tablets of 707 mg, which contains 414 mg chloral hydrate (in capsules this is 500 mg), a chloral mixture (oral solution) of 0.5 gm/5 ml and chloral elixir ('Elixir' – for paediatric use) at 143 mg/5ml. A related substance, triclofos sodium, is tasteless and causes less gastric irritation. The hypnotic dose is 1–2 gm. It is available as tablets of 500 mg and triclofos elixir oral solution at 500 mg/5 ml.

BARBITURATES

Barbiturates are used in psychiatry for ECT anaesthesia, to control epilepsy, sometimes for abreaction, occasionally in acute tranquillisation, but only rarely for symptom control, because they carry serious risks of drug dependence and toxicity in overdose.

The different members of the barbiturate group vary principally in the speed with which they are metabolised by the liver and excreted in the urine; the more slowly metabolised barbiturates are more likely to cause hangovers and to accumulate. Accumulation can cause a chronic brain syndrome – drowsiness, disorientation, muddled thinking, slurred speech and ataxia. The elderly are especially liable because their bodies deal more slowly with drugs.

When tolerance develops, the same dose no longer relieves the symptoms. The doctor then has to consider whether to increase the dose to achieve control of symptoms, bearing in mind the risk of dependence by step-wise increase of dose, or to stop barbiturates and use some other drug. In the dependent state the patient becomes irritable and moody whenever doses are not maintained. Cutting down the dose results in sleeplessness, agitation, complaints of tension, depression and even grand mal fits if the reduction is rapid. The drug must never be stopped abruptly but the dose reduced slowly over about 6 weeks, or as an in-patient over 2 weeks using chlormethiazole or chlordiazepoxide for cover, as with alcohol withdrawal.

Amylobarbitone sodium ('Sodium Amytal')

This drug is now used only rarely (and when antipsychotics have failed) to control severe emotional and behavioural disturbance and for short periods of a few days. Start with 400 mg or 600 mg orally and then 200 mg 4-hourly. More rapid control is gained by a single intramuscularly or slow intravenously dose of 250 mg or more (up to 0.5 gm intramuscularly or 1 gm intravenously), the dose being judged by its almost immediate effect and repeated in a revised dose when the effect begins to wear off. Combined barbiturate and antipsychotic can prove dramatically effective when the latter alone achieves little.

Side-effects and interactions

Be cautious if renal or liver disease is present because these two organs normally terminate barbiturate action. Barbiturates are powerful respiratory depressants and unsuitable in chronic bronchitis. Do not give to the elderly patient because of the risk of inducing disorientation.

Alcohol potentiates their effect and the two should never be taken together. The rare disease porphyria is exacerbated by them. Barbiturates induce liver enzymes, leading to increased metabolism of other drugs. In the blood they may displace other drugs binding to plasma albumin.

The prescribing of barbiturates, as outlined above, is exceptional: always remember the risks of drug dependence, of death from accidental poisoning, especially in the elderly, the ill and the alcoholic, and of suicide.

It is available as tablets of 60 mg and 200 mg, capsules of 60 mg and 200 mg, and injections of 250 mg and 500 mg powder in ampoules (for reconstitution).

Paraldehyde

This is a rapidly acting hypnotic and anticonvulsant that is safe in the presence of poor renal function because it is excreted predominantly in the breath.

Its use in the control of excitement is now obsolete because it is so unpleasant, and injection of more than 5 ml at one site can cause local necrosis and sterile abscess formation. It is now very occasionally used in rapid tranquillisation when all else has failed. Paraldehyde can also be used to control status epilepticus and delirium tremens, but other drugs are usually more appropriate.

People dislike its smell and taste. A rectal infusion, given as a 10% enema in saline, avoids this but may cause local irritation. A similar reaction can occur when the drug is taken orally. If giving it by deep intramuscular injection, beware of using plastic syringes, which it dissolves, and of damage to the sciatic nerve. Whichever method, the dose is 5–10 ml (not more than 5 ml at one injection site). Avoid if liver damage or lung disease is present. The drug interacts with disulfiram (see p. 377). It is available as an injection in 5 ml and 10 ml ampoules.

FURTHER READING

Guidelines

Committee on the Review of Medicines (1980) Systematic review of the benzodiazepines. Guidelines for data sheets. *BMJ*, **280**, 910–912.

Higgitt, A.C., Lader, M. H. & Fonagy, P. (1985) Clinical management of benzodiazepine dependence. *BMJ*, **291**, 688–690.

Montgomery, S. A. & Tyrer, P. J. (1988) Benzodiazepines: time to withdraw. *Journal of the Royal College of General Practitioners*, **38**, 146–147.

Priest, R. G. & Montgomery, S. A. (1988) Benzodiazepines and dependence: a College statement. *Bulletin of the Royal College of Psychiatrists*, **12**, 107–108.

Uses

Elie, R., Rüther, E., Farr, I., *et al* (1999) Sleep latency is shortened during 4 weeks of treatment with zaleplon, a novel nonbenzodiazepine hypnotic. *Journal of Clinical Psychiatry*, **60**, 536–544.

Jones, I. R. & Sullivan, G. (1998) Physical dependence on zopiclone: case reports. *BMJ*, **316**, 117.

Rickels, K., Schweizer, E., Case, G., *et al* (1990. Long term therapeutic use of benzodiazepines. 1. Effects of abrupt discontinuation. *Archives of General Psychiatry*, **47**, 899–907.

OPIATE SUBSTITUTE PRESCRIBING

Methadone ('Physeptone')

Methadone is a synthetic opiate licensed as an adjunct in the treatment of opioid dependence, as a substitute for heroin and other opiates. Controlled withdrawal is then easier to achieve using an oral drug with less acute withdrawal symptoms than the opiates.

It is a controlled drug with a high dependency potential and a low lethal dose. Prescribing should be considered only if:

- opioid drugs are being taken regularly (typically daily)
- there is convincing evidence of dependence; positive urine results, objective signs of withdrawal or general restlessness. Recent sites of injection may also be present.

Supervised daily consumption is recommended for new prescriptions, for a minimum of 3 months if possible. Alternatively, instalment prescriptions for daily dispensing and collection should be used. Certainly no more than 1 week's supply should be dispensed at one time, other than in exceptional circumstances.

Methadone should be prescribed in the oral liquid formulation. Tablets are likely to be crushed and inappropriately injected, and therefore should not be prescribed. It is important that all patients starting a methadone treatment programme be informed of the risks of toxicity and overdose, and the necessity for safe storage.

Dosage

The aim is to provide a dose that will prevent withdrawal symptoms, does not cause drowsiness and reduces or eliminates non-prescribed drug use (see chapter 21). Consideration must be given to the patient's tolerance, based on a history of the quantity, frequency and route of administration of opioids, and use of other drugs, including alcohol. It is imperative during the initial stages that the dose is carefully titrated against withdrawal symptoms and that the long half-life of methadone, time to achieve steady-state plasma levels and risk of cumulative toxicity are taken into account. The first 2 weeks of treatment with methadone are associated with a substantially increased risk of overdose mortality.

Initially 10–40 mg daily, increasing by 5–10 mg per day until there are no signs of withdrawal or intoxication (typically in the range of 30–60 mg). The plasma half-life is more than 24 hours and steady-state plasma levels should be achieved 5 days or more after the last dose increase. Most patients require once daily doses; a minority does better with divided twice daily doses.

Subsequent increases should not exceed 10 mg per week up to a total of 60–120 mg. Stabilisation is usually achieved within 6 weeks but may take longer.

Reduction regimes should be encouraged after a period of stabilisation and should be part of a negotiated treatment plan between doctor, keyworker and patient. There should be regular reviews and flexibility in the regime so that the client remains compliant and clinical improvements are apparent. The daily dose can be reduced by 5–10 mg every week or fortnight, until a stable dose is reached where the patient continues to abstain from illegal drug use.

Outcome

With methadone maintenance treatment, the majority of regular users of illicit opiates, seeking help from drugs services, can greatly reduce or discontinue their use of illicit opiates. Having done so on a stable basis, they can then attempt to reduce their use of methadone. However, methadone is itself highly addictive and only about 16% of those attempting to reduce gradually will succeed in discontinuing it and remain drug-free at 1 year.

Contraindications/precautions

Liver disease, renal disease, asthma, respiratory depression, obstructive airways disease and MAOI drugs are contraindications unless the reasons for long-term use are compelling. Hypertensive crises may occur with MAOI drugs.

Methadone must not be given to any patient showing signs of intoxication, owing to alcohol or other drugs. The risk of fatal overdose is greatly increased when methadone is taken concomitantly with alcohol and/or other respiratory depressant drugs, including benzodiazepines.

Pregnancy and breastfeeding

There is no evidence of an increase in congenital defects. It is important to minimise harmful activities associated with drug use, particularly non-prescribed drugs, and to avoid the patient going into a withdrawal state. Specialist advice should be obtained before prescribing, particularly with regard to the management and treatment plan during pregnancy.

Methadone is considered compatible with breastfeeding, with no adverse effects to nursing infant when the mother is consuming 20 mg/ 24 hours or less.

Side-effects

Methadone, with a longer duration of action than morphine, has similar effects but is not as sedative and produces less euphoria. Tolerance usually develops except to constipation and meiosis (pinpoint pupils).

Interactions

Methadone potentiates the CNS depressant effects of alcohol, opioid agonist analgesics, antidepressants, antipsychotics and other psychotropic drugs.

THE DRUGS

369

Naloxone and naltrexone block the effects of methadone and will precipitate withdrawal symptoms. Buprenorphine may precipitate withdrawal symptoms in methadone-dependent individuals. Rifampicin and phenytoin reduce the effect of methadone.

It is available as tablets of 5 mg, a mixture of 1 mg/ml, and an injection of 10mg/ml.

Buprenorphine ('Subutex')

Buprenorphine is a semi-synthetic opioid that resembles morphine, but has partial agonist activity at opiate μ- receptors. It binds strongly to the receptor site and will inhibit other μ-receptor agonists such as methadone, morphine and heroin, so that concurrent administration will not produce additional euphoric effects. The benefits of this are to eliminate or reduce the additional use of non-prescribed drugs and to reduce the risks of overdose. A high-dose formulation ('Subutex') is licensed for the management of opioid addiction and there is good evidence from overseas to support its usefulness as an alternative maintenance agent for individuals with lower levels of dependence, engaged in a well-supervised programme with specialist services. For example, patients whose dependence has resulted from therapeutic opiate use may be suitable.

Dosage

Buprenorphine undergoes extensive first-pass metabolism in the intestine and liver when administered orally. The tablets must be administered sublingually and allowed to completely dissolve in the mouth to bypass this effect and obtain therapeutic levels.

Buprenorphine may precipitate withdrawal symptoms in an opioid-dependent individual; therefore, initial doses should not be administered if methadone has been used in the preceding 24 hours or heroin in not less than 5 hours (recommend 8–12 hours). In any case there must be observable withdrawal symptoms prior to administration of buprenorphine and the dose should be carefully titrated initially until an adequate maintenance dose is achieved.

Dose

Initial starting dose 0.8–4 mg, increased in increments of 2–4 mg. Maintenance doses are usually in the range of 4–16 mg. All doses should be given as a single daily dose, including the initial titration phase. Individuals with high dependence (doses of methadone above 30 mg/day or equivalent) are more likely to experience withdrawal symptoms and buprenorphine may not be appropriate until their level of dependence is reduced. Reduction regimes should be based on the same principles as the methadone reduction programme.

Contraindications

Hypersensitivity to buprenorphine, severe respiratory or hepatic insufficiency, acute alcoholism or delirium tremens, pregnancy and breastfeeding.

Precautions

Concomitant use of any other CNS depressant drug, as may have additive effects; asthma or respiratory insufficiency; and hepatic or renal insufficiency.

Side-effects

Frequently constipation, headaches, insomnia, asthenia, drowsiness, nausea and vomiting, fainting and dizziness, orthostatic hypotension, and sweating and respiratory depression. Reports of hepatic necrosis, hepatitis with jaundice and hallucinations.

Interactions

Sedative drugs and alcohol may enhance CNS depressant effects. It also interacts with MAOIs.

It is available as sublingual tablets of 0.4 mg, 2 mg and 8 mg.

OPIATE WITHDRAWL AND DETOXIFICATION

Lofexidine

Lofexidine is a centrally acting α-2 adrenergic agonist, which inhibits neurotransmitter release. It has a similar action to clonidine, but with much less hypotension. It is effective at alleviating acute opiate withdrawal symptoms that are thought to be mediated by overactivity of central adrenergic neurons. It reduces anxiety, tremor and diarrhoea associated with opiate withdrawal. It is a non-opiate and therefore less liable to misuse and diversion.

Lofexidine has a role in the treatment of opiate-dependent individuals as part of a detoxification plan, and as an interim alternative to prescribing opiates to control withdrawal symptoms in an individual claiming to be dependent and without their medication/supply.

Dosage

Initially 200–400 μg twice daily, increased as necessary in steps of 200–400 μg daily, to a maximum of 2.4 mg daily. The recommended duration of treatment is 8–12 days for methadone cessation and then withdraw over 2–4 days or longer to prevent rebound hypertension. For assisted detoxification with naltrexone the duration of use is shorter (see below). The regime should be titrated against withdrawal symptoms and the initial dose may need to be increased in the early stages of opiate withdrawal.

Baseline blood pressure and pulse should be recorded and monitored regularly throughout treatment, particularly during the initial 2–3 days. If systolic blood pressure is below 90 mmHg, or 30 mmHg below baseline or pulse is less than 50 beats per minute, then the dose should be reduced or omitted.

Contraindications

Sensitivity to other imidazoline derivatives e.g. clonidine.

THE DRUGS

Precautions

Severe coronary insufficiency, recent myocardial infarction, bradycardia, cerebrovascular disease, chronic renal failure and pregnancy/lactation (limited data, safety not established).

Side-effects

Related to α-adrenergic effects, for example drowsiness and related symptoms and dryness of mouth, throat and nose. Hypotension and bradycardia may occur.

Interactions

Alcohol and other sedatives – lofexidine may enhance CNS depressant effects. TCAs may reduce the efficacy of lofexidine.

It is available as a tablet of 0.2 mg.

Clonidine ('Catapres', 'Dixarit')

It may be used as is lofexidine, but it produces a more significant drop in blood pressure. Clonidine is not licensed for use in opiate withdrawal.

Side-effects and interactions

The side-effects and interactions are drowsiness, dry mouth, oedema, bradycardia and depression. Lactation may be inhibited. Peripheral vascular diseases may be worsened, for example in Raynaud's disease. Hypertensive crises may occur on rapid withdrawal. Some MARIs lessen its hypotensive effect.

It is available as tablets of 0.1 mg and 0.3 mg, and capsules (sustained release) of 0.25 mg.

Naltrexone ('Nalorex')

Naltrexone is an orally active, centrally acting opiate receptor antagonist that blocks the effects of opioids, such as heroin, for up to 72 hours, and precipitates withdrawal symptoms in opioid-dependent individuals. It may also have anti-craving properties.

It has two main uses in treating addiction.It is licensed as an adjunctive treatment to prevent relapse in detoxified, formerly opioid-dependent, patients who have remained opioid free for at least 7–10 days. The intention is to deter future use by antagonising the effects of opiates drugs that may be taken. The patient must be well motivated with good psychosocial support and, ideally, arrangements should be made for supervised consumption to ensure compliance. Patients must also be warned that an attempt to overcome the block could result in acute opioid intoxication. However, in this use it has been found to be little or no better than placebo.

Second, it can aid detoxification. By competing for opiate receptors it displaces methadone and other opiate drugs, and thereby produces acute withdrawal symptoms of full intensity, which wane over the following 3–5 days.

In addition, although not licensed in the UK for this purpose, there is limited evidence to suggest that naltrexone may also be effective as an adjunct in the treatment of alcohol dependence. Two studies have shown that naltrexone improved abstinence, prevented relapse and decreased alcohol consumption over a 12-week treatment period, using a daily dose of 50 mg. However, other studies have not obtained similar findings. Further investigation is required to establish if naltrexone has an effective role in the treatment of alcohol dependence. Another opiate antagonist nalmefene, which has fewer side-effects, is also being investigated (see p. 210).

Dosage

For relapse prevention in opioid dependence it is important that the patient has cleared all opioids from their system (abstinent for 7–10 days), otherwise naltrexone will precipitate withdrawal symptoms.

Initially 25 mg, then 50 mg daily. Total weekly dose may be divided and given on 3 days of the week to improve compliance.

Administration of a single dose of naloxone, a short acting opiate antagonist for parenteral use only, prior to administering naltrexone, may be considered to establish the patient's opioid status and avoid prolonged withdrawal symptoms.

Assisted detoxification

Its use for detoxification should be as an in-patient with staff familiar with the treatment and after full explanation has been given to the patient (see p. 217). The patient should have already reduced his/her use of methadone to 30 mg daily or less. After observation for 24 hours without opiates the patient will show some withdrawal symptoms. He/she is commenced on lofexidine or clonidine. Two hours later he/she receives naltrexone, 1 mg orally. This intensifies the withdrawal symptoms within 15 minutes and further lofexidine or clonidine is given. Two hours after the first dose of naltrexone, if well tolerated, a further 2 mg is given, and 2 hours later 5 mg naltrexone. Should the withdrawal symptoms become too distressing, either naltrexone is withheld or diazepam is given up to 20 mg orally every 4 hours. On day 3 lofexidine is given, followed 1 hour later by naltrexone 12.5 mg twice daily. On day 4 naltrexone 50 mg may be given, and lofexidine used if necessary. Diazepam should no longer be needed then.

Insomnia may remain a problem, but hypnotics should be avoided if possible. Once on a full dose of 50 mg daily the patient may be discharged, to take 50 mg naltrexone daily for a further 2 weeks under out-patient supervision from specialist drugs workers.

Contraindications

Acute hepatitis or liver failure.

Precautions

Hepatic and renal impairment; liver function tests needed before and during treatment. Pregnancy and breastfeeding. Concomitant use of

THE DRUGS

opioid analgesics for pain control; high doses may be required, but monitor for opioid intoxication. Patients should carry a drug-warning card in case they need opiates for genuine pain relief.

Side-effects

Nausea and vomiting; abdominal pain; anxiety, nervousness, sleep, headache, reduced energy; joint and muscle pain; less frequently, loss of appetite, diarrhoea, constipation, increased thirst; chest pain; increased sweating and lacrimation; increased energy; feeling down, irritability, dizziness, chills; delayed ejaculation, decreased potency; rash; occasionally liver function abnormalities; and reversible idiopathic thrombocytopenia have been reported.

Interactions

Hypoglycaemic agents: insulin requirements may be increased. Thioridazine: extreme lethargy.

It is available as scored tablets of 50 mg.

ALCOHOL PROBLEMS: WITHDRAWAL AND DETOXIFICATION

The benzodiazepine chordiazepoxide is widely used (see chapter 20), but for in-patients an alternative is clormethiazole.

Clormethiazole

Clormethiazole ('Heminevrin') is a sedative drug; it is also used to control delirium tremens and alcohol-withdrawal symptoms, with close hospital supervision, usually as an in-patient, but always with daily monitoring. The dosage should be adjusted so that the patient is sedated but rousable. It may start with 9–12 capsules on the first day administered as three or four separate doses. This is followed by 6–8 capsules on the second day, 4–6 capsules on the third day, and a gradual reduction in dose until it is stopped altogether after a total of 7–9 days.

Side-effects

Addiction is the most serious problem and hence the drug should not be used for longer than 9 days. Sneezing, nasal tingling or burning and conjunctival irritation sometimes occur soon after starting treatment. These tend to improve with further doses and do not necessarily require cessation of treatment. Alcoholics who continue to drink while taking chlormethiazole risk fatal cardiorespiratory depression. Therefore, it should not be prescribed to alcoholics as out-patients except under daily supervision in a specialised clinic.

The drug is also used for short-term treatment of severe insomnia in the elderly in a dose of 1–2 capsules or 5–10 ml of syrup at night.

It is available as capsules of 192 mg chlormethizole base (equivalent to 5 ml syrup), syrup at 250 mg/5ml chlormethiazole edisylate and 0.8% infusion of 8 mg/ml chlormethiazole edisylate.

ALCOHOL PROBLEMS: RELAPSE PREVENTION

Acamprosate

Acamprosate is an anti-craving agent and is indicated for the maintenance of abstinence in alcohol withdrawal. It may act by stimulating GABA-ergic inhibitory neurotransmission and antagonising excitatory amino acids, particularly glutamate. Trial evidence suggests that acamprosate delays relapse into using alcohol, after detoxification, and increases the number of days abstention during a 1-year period of treatment and for 1 year following treatment. However, the overall effect does appear to reduce over this time. Treatment should be initiated as soon as possible after the withdrawal period once abstinence has been achieved. Treatment is recommended for 1 year and should be maintained if the patient relapses; however, continuous use of alcohol will negate the effects of acamprosate.

Prescribing of acamprosate must be used only as part of an integrated treatment plan that involves counselling and support.

Dosage

Subjects weighing 60 kg or more should take 2 tablets three times a day with meals. Subjects weighing less than 60 kg should take 4 tablets divided into three doses with meals.

Contraindications

Known hypersensitivity; pregnancy/breastfeeding (safety not established); renal insufficiency (serum creatinine above 120 mmol/l); and severe hepatic failure.

Side-effects

Tend to be mild and transient, generally gastrointestinal in nature or a rash.

Interactions

No reports of any to date.
It is available as a tablet of 333 mg.

Disulfiram ('Antabuse')

Disulfiram is an aversive agent that may be effective in helping some patients to maintain abstinence from alcohol. Disulfiram irreversibly inhibits enzymes, including aldehyde dehydrogenase, which results in greatly increased plasma levels of acetaldehyde if alcohol is ingested. Symptoms produced by this effect include facial flushing, pulsing headache, nausea, dizziness, weakness, orthostatic hypotension, arrhythmia, hypotension and even fatal collapse. The reaction may occur within 10 minutes and last for several hours.

Because of the potential severity of the reaction disulfiram is ideally restricted to the medically fit.

THE DRUGS

Patients must be fully informed of the nature of the treatment and the potential effects. The patient should be well motivated, have good psychosocial support and ideally arrangements should be made for daily supervised consumption of the drug.

Patients must be made aware that certain oral medications, tonics, remedies and foods may contain sufficient alcohol to induce a reaction. It is advisable for patients to carry a medical card stating their medication and appropriate warnings and advice.

Dosage

Disulfiram can be started with a challenge while medically supervised (see below), or without. In present practice the challenge tends to be dispensed with. Treatment should not be initiated without full assessment and careful monitoring. Patients must not consume alcohol for at least 24 hours prior to starting treatment, during treatment or for at least one week after cessation.

An initial dose of 800 mg as a single dose on the first day, reducing over 5 days to a maintenance dose of 100–200 mg daily should be administered; however, some individuals can tolerate doses of 500 mg. Compliance is improved by enlisting a family member or keyworker to help. Doses may be given on alternate days to facilitate supervised consumption.

The alternative approach, using a challenge, relies to some extent for its effectiveness on a strong aversive experience. Disulfiram is taken 1.0 g for the first 3 nights, thereafter 400 mg each morning. On the fifth morning, 1 hour after the last dose, give 150 ml of 95% alcohol diluted with the patient's favourite alcoholic drink. Within 2 hours the unpleasant experience should occur. The aim is to make a deep impression. If there is no adverse reaction, the dose can be increased and the challenge repeated. After the successful challenge continue disulfiram 400 mg daily for 3 weeks, and then reduce to 200 mg daily indefinitely.

Severe reaction may be ended with 1 g ascorbic acid orally or intravenously, and an intravenous injection of an antihistamine such as mepyramine maleate 25 mg or 50 mg.

The anti-alcohol effect lasts 2 days or more after the last dose of disulfiram.

Contraindications

Cardiac failure; coronary artery disease; previous history of cerebrovascular accident (CVA); hypertension; severe personality disorder; suicide risk or psychosis; and pregnancy/breastfeeding.

Precautions

Renal failure, hepatic/respiratory disease, diabetes mellitus and epilepsy.

Side-effects

Initially drowsiness and fatigue, nausea, vomiting, a garlic or metallic taste, smelly breath (halitosis), constipation and reduced libido. The drug can also cause depressive or hallucinatory symptoms, and rarely encephalopathy with confusion, neurological signs and abnormal EEG. Such reactions are less common since the recommended dose was reduced to 200 mg daily. Disulfiram can exacerbate schizophrenia, perhaps by its inhibition of dopamine β-hydroxylase, the enzyme that converts dopamine to noradrenalin.

Rarely allergic dermatitis, peripheral neuritis or hepatic cell damage occur.

Interactions

Disulfiram interferes with the metabolism of warfarin, antipyrine, phenytoin, chlordiazepoxide and diazepam to produce an increase in effect of these drugs. The effect of disulfiram may be reduced by amitriptyline and diazepam.

Disulfiram inhibits oxidation and renal excretion of rifampicin and there are reports of toxic reactions with metronidazole and isoniazid. Paraldehyde metabolism is blocked by disulfiram, yielding acetaldehyde, which produces a severe reaction.

It is available as a tablet of 200 mg.

FURTHER READING

Anton, R. F., Moak, D. H., Waid, R., *et al* (1999) Naltrexone and cognitive behavioural therapy for the treatment of outpatient alcoholics: results of a placebo-controlled trial. *American Journal of Psychiatry*, **156**, 1758–1764.

Buntwal, N., Bearn, J., Gossop, M., *et al* (2000) Naltrexone and lofexidine combination treatment compared with conventional lofexidine treatment for in-patient opiate detoxification. *Drug and Alcohol Dependence*, **59**, 183–188.

Farren, C. K. (1997) The use of naltrexone, an opiate antagonist, in the treatment of opiate addiction. *Journal Psychiatric Medicine*, **14**, 31–34.

Mayo-Smith, M. F., for the American Society of Addiction Medicine Working Group on Pharmacological Management of Alcohol Withdrawal (1997). Pharmacological management of alcohol withdrawal: a meta-analysis and evidence-based practice guidelines. *JAMA*, **278**, 144–151.Soyka, M. (1997) Relapse prevention in alcoholism: recent advances and future possibilities. *CNS Drugs*, **7**, 313–327.

Strang, J., Bearn, J. & Gossop, M. (1999) Lofexidine for opiate detoxification: review of recent randomised and open controlled trials. *The American Journal of Addictions*, **8**, 337–348.

Whitworth, A. B., Fischer, F., Lesch, O. M., *et al* (1996) Comparison of acamprosate and placebo in long-term treatment of alcohol dependence. *Lancet*, **347**, 1438–1442.

THE DRUGS

Beta-adrenergic receptors are of three types, β-1 in the heart, β-2 in the bronchi, skeletal muscle and liver, and β-3 in the adipose tissue. Some beta-blockers, such as propranolol, block all types. Others, such as atenolol, betaxolol and metoprolol are relatively selective for β-1 receptors and have less propensity to precipitate asthma than the others. The water-soluble drugs such as atenolol are less able to penetrate the brain and cause less sleep disturbance. Oxprenolol is a partial agonist and causes less slowing of the heart. The beneficial effects of beta-blockers in migraine are thought to be due to a separate action of blockade of 5-HT-1D receptors in cranial blood vessels.

Beta-blockers are widely used to treat hypertension and cardiac arrhythmias. They are also used to suppress somatic anxiety symptoms and to reduce akathisia. Pindolol has also been used as an adjunct to antidepressants.

PROPRANOLOL

Propranolol may be used for:

- bodily symptoms of anxiety
- fine tremor, as in anxiety, and familial tremor
- akathisia (not licensed).

Propranolol acts by blocking peripheral beta-adrenergic receptors and in this way relieves rapid pulse, palpitations, sweating and tremor. Anxious patients who are troubled mainly by the bodily symptoms of anxiety are therefore more likely to be helped by propranolol than those with mental symptoms of anxiety. Somatic symptoms arising from both acute panic attacks and chronic anxiety states can be relieved. The usual treatment is 10 mg, 20 mg or even 40 mg three or four times daily by mouth, beginning with the lower dose. Even higher doses may be tolerated. Beta-blockers are otherwise of limited value in panic disorder or social phobia.

High doses of up to 1000 mg were claimed to be helpful in treating schizophrenia, but this effect was due to a drug interaction, whereby propranolol inhibits the metabolism of chlorpromazine, raising its blood levels.

Propranolol is effective in familial tremor and other tremors not caused by anxiety, including lithium-induced tremor. On the other hand, β-2 agonists such as sulbutamol and terbutaline may cause tremor and feelings of muscular tension.

Propranolol (20–40 mg daily) is used to treat drug-induced akathisia. The non-selective pindolol (5 mg daily) is also used. The site of this action is thought to be central, since only the fat-soluble beta-blockers are effective, but the mechanism is unclear. Both specific β-1 and β-2 antagonists are effective. A more selective β-1 antagonist such as betaxolol (5–20 mg daily) or metoprolol is preferable, to reduce the risk of bronchospasm.

Table 36.1 Preparations of beta-blockers

Drug	Method of delivery	Dose (mg)
Propranolol	Tablets	10, 40, 80, 160
	Capsules (sustained release)	80, 160
Betaxolol	Tablet	20 (maximum 40 mg daily)
Metoprolol	Tablets	50, 100
	Modified release	200
Pindolol	Tablets	5, 15 (maximum 45 mg daily)

The beta-adrenergic blockade caused by propranolol reduces the pulse rate, but the rate should not be permitted to go below 55 beats per minute. Bradycardia can be reversed by 1–2 mg of atropine intravenously. Treatment with propranolol should be discontinued by gradual dose reduction and not abrupt withdrawal to avoid rebound tachycardia and hypertension (see Table 36.1 for preparations).

Side-effects and contraindications

Propranolol causes few side-effects in the physically healthy person. Light-headedness, visual and tactile hallucinations, tinnitus, erythematous skin rash and purpura have been reported. Propranolol can precipitate heart failure. If there is a history of cardiac disease, a cardiologist's advice should be sought before prescribing propranolol for anxiety. The drug interferes with the recognition of hypoglycaemia in the diabetic by preventing sweating and tachycardia. It may cause tiredness, insomnia with nightmares and depressive symptoms and coldness of the periphery.

Asthma and obstructive airways disease contraindicate its use because of the risk of acute bronchospasm.

PINDOLOL

This mixed beta-blocker and 5-HT-1A blocker has been used as a strategy to augment the effects of SSRIs in depression (see p. 253). However, the low doses generally used in order to minimise side-effects (2.5 mg three times a day), probably occupy the 5-HT-1A receptors insufficiently.

FURTHER READING

Dumon, J.-P., Catteau, J., Lanvin, F., *et al* (1992) Randomised, double-blind, crossover, placebo controlled comparison of propranolol and betaxolol in the treatment of neuroleptic-induced akathisia. *American Journal of Psychiatry*, **149**, 647–650.

Liebowitz, M. R., Schneier, F. Campeas, R., *et al* (1992) Phenelzine vs atenolol in social phobia. A placebo-controlled comparison. *Archives of General Psychiatry*, **49**, 290–300.

Rabiner, E. A., Bhagwagar, Z., Gunn, R. N., *et al* (2001) Pindolol augmentation of selective serotonin reuptake inhibitors: PET evidence that the dose used in clinical trials is too low. *American Journal of Psychiatry*, **158**, 2080–2082.

THE DRUGS

37. PSYCHOSTIMULANTS AND APPETITE SUPPRESSANTS

The amphetamines are a group of compounds related to D-alpha-methyl-phenylethylamine (D-amphetamine), which share an action to release dopamine, noradrenalin or 5-HT from neuronal stores. The mechanism by which they do this is unclear, but they may reverse the normal reuptake mechanism in the nerve endings and in the storage vesicles. They differ in the extent to which they release noradrenalin, dopamine or 5-HT, and at higher doses some are also MAOIs and block the reuptake of the transmitters. D-Amphetamine and methylphenidate act mainly upon dopamine and to a lesser extent noradrenalin release. They are psychostimulants and reduce appetite. Cocaine has similar effects, as well as being a local anaesthetic. Amphetamine increases growth hormone and cortisol release, by actions in the hypothalamus. Fenfluramine acts mainly upon 5-HT release, is sedative and reduces food take, increasing satiety, and increases prolactin release slightly. Modafinil is used in narcolepsy.

The stimulant amphetamines are of great interest to psychiatry because in low doses they produce euphoria similar to hypomania, but with reduced appetite; higher doses can produce a condition resembling paranoid schizophrenia, together with stereotyped behaviour similar to catatonic symptoms. They are also drugs of misuse and dependence.

DEXAMPHETAMINE

D-Amphetamine ('Dexedrine') is used for narcolepsy, ADHD, Kleine-Levin syndrome and for a time was used to counteract the sedative effects of anticonvulsants, as it raises the seizure threshold.

Amphetamines are used, often illegally, for their euphoriant action and for counteracting fatigue or for suppressing appetite. Tolerance for these effects, especially the euphoriant effect, develops rapidly. On withdrawal, lethargy and depression occur. There is, therefore, a serious risk of inducing dependence. For this reason, the prescription of amphetamine is controlled under Schedule 2 of the Misuse of Drugs Act. This stimulant should not be used to treat depression or as an appetite suppressant because of the risk of dependence, misuse and psychosis.

To treat narcolepsy or Kleine-Levin syndrome start with 10 mg in the morning and increase by 10 mg steps each week until control is achieved or a maximum of 50 mg per day reached. Clomipramine may be even more effective.

For children with ADHD start with 2.5 mg in the morning and increase by weekly steps of 2.5 mg to a maximum of 20 mg daily, divided into two or three doses daily.

The drug may cause insomnia, especially if taken late in the day. Misery and tearfulness can appear, usually transiently, in children taking therapeutic doses. Long-term use in high dosage may retard children's growth because of appetite suppression. Their height and weight must therefore be monitored.

High doses can cause perseveration of attention with consequent learning problems, so concentration must be monitored. Tics and stereotyped behaviours can be made worse. Agitation, excitement and even a paranoid psychosis with hallucinations can occur. Tachycardia, palpitations and a rise in blood pressure can all occur, so heart rate and blood pressure need to be examined regularly.

Beware of increasing tolerance and the development of psychological dependence. A depressive mood swing is to be expected on stopping.

The drug should not be given to people with a history of cardiovascular disease, hypertension, tics or drug dependence. It causes hypertensive and hyperpyrexial reactions if given with an MAOI. It is available as tablets of 5 mg.

METHYLPHENIDATE

The use of this drug in childhood ADHD is discussed in chapter 18. It may also be used in residual adult forms of the condition. It differs from amphetamine in producing little release of noradrenalin, but its effect on dopamine is also less. It is thought to interfere with only the vesicular uptake of dopamine.

In adults with residual ADHD it reduces the core symptoms in the majority of patients at a dose of 1 mg/kg daily. It is available as tablets ('Ritalin' or 'Equasym') of 5 mg, 10 mg and 20 mg.

MODAFINIL

Modafinil is licensed for use in narcolepsy. It is chemically and pharmacologically different from amphetamine. Its mechanism of action is not known but may involve noradrenalin, as it is attenuated by noradrenalin alpha-antagonists. It reduces daytime sleep in narcolepsy, without interfering with nocturnal sleep. Its effect is sustained for 40 weeks and discontinuation does not result in rebound hypersomnia, as is the case with amphetamine.

The most common side-effect is headache, but nervousness and nausea also occur. The dose is 200–400 mg daily and it is available as tablets ('Provigil') of 100 mg.

APPETITE SUPPRESSANTS

Most drugs marketed to assist in the treatment of obesity are stimulants such as phentermine ('Duromine') and should not be prescribed.

Fenfluramine, however, is sedative and carries much less risk of inducing dependence or psychosis, but it is no longer available for prescription following the occurrence of pulmonary hypertension. Depression could occur with abrupt cessation. It has been used as a neuroendocrine challenge to test 5-HT function, in depression and other conditions.

D-Flenfluramine was investigated in patients who became obese on antipsychotic drugs; weight loss occurred without deterioration in the mental state.

SIBUTRAMINE

As 'Reductil', sibutramine (capsules 10 mg and 15 mg) is marketed to aid weight reduction in people with a BMI over 30. It is sympathomimetic and enhances serotonin transmission, partly as a reuptake inhibitor. It should not be combined with other drugs that do so, such as MAOIs or SSRIs. It also stimulates energy expenditure. Side-effects include dry mouth, constipation, insomnia, nausea, tachycardia, raised blood pressure, anxiety and headache. There are several contraindications, including physical and psychiatric disorders. Blood pressure should be monitored every 2 weeks at first. The NICE concluded that it should not be given for more than a year. About 7% of initial weight is lost. A discontinuation syndrome has not been reported, but people regain most of the weight lost within 3 months. It is metabolised mainly by CYP3A4.

CAFFINE

Caffeine has stimulant but not euphoriant properties. It increases arousal and is an ingredient of certain compound tablets that would otherwise be sedative, for instance painkillers. Its alerting properties are thought to be due to its action as an antagonist of adenosine at receptors in the brain. It also inhibits phosphodiesterase, causing increased levels of cyclic-AMP, but this action appears at higher concentrations.

Caffeine has a half-life of about 5 hours. Hence, if consumed in the evening it can disturb sleep throughout the night; this effect is more noticeable with increasing age.

FURTHER READING

Chiarello, R. J. & Cole, J. O. (1987) The use of psychostimulants in general psychiatry. *Archives of General Psychiatry*, **44**, 286–295.

National Institute for Clinical Excellence (2001) Guidance on the use of sibutramine for the treatment of obesity in adults. *Technology Appraisal Guidance*, **31** (http:// http://www.nice.org.uk/pdf/SIBUTRAME%2031%20GUIDANCE.pdf).

Satel, S. L. & Nelson, J. C. (1989) Stimulants in the treatment of depression: a critical overview. *Journal of Clinical Psychiatry*, **59**, 241–249.

Spencer, T., Wilens, T., Biederman, J., *et al* (1995) A double-blind crossover comparison of methylphenidate and placebo in adults with childhood-onset attention-deficit hyperactivity disorder. *Archives of General Psychiatry*, **52**, 434–443.

Toone, B. K. & van der Linden, G. J. (1997) Attention deficit hyperactivity disorder or hyperkinetic disorder in adults. *British Journal of Psychiatry*, **170**, 489–491.

38. VITAMINS

Prescribing vitamins for psychiatric patients is justified only when a vitamin-deficiency state exists or there is strong suspicion that it does. Vitamin-deficiency states are uncommon in psychiatric patients but a diet of poor quality or quantity, over a lengthy period, can lead to deficiency in the B group, vitamin C, vitamin B_{12} and folic acid.

Such a state results from the unsupervised self-neglect that occurs with dementia, the elderly with mental illness, chronic schizophrenia and long-standing alcoholism, or from the deliberate self-starvation of anorexia nervosa and the extreme dietary practices resulting from delusional beliefs. An adequate diet, if the patient will have it, and vitamin supplements are all that are required to manage the deficiency in the short-term. A multiple vitamin preparation containing thiamine (vitamin B_1), riboflavine (vitamin B_2), nicotinamide (vitamin B_3), pyridoxine (vitamin B_6) and ascorbic acid (vitamin C) is often used. Folic acid may have to be prescribed if anaemia is present and this needs to be confirmed by a low red cell folate. Plasma folate levels indicate only current intake, not past deficiency. Dietary stores of vitamin B_{12} are usually large enough to withstand several years of poor diet. Excessive intake of a vitamin may result from a delusion and be harmful and occasionally life threatening, for example excessive amounts of carrot juice causing vitamin A poisoning.

Some psychiatric conditions result from vitamin deficiencies, though this is rare in Britain. Alcohol misuse and a poor diet may cause a thiamine deficiency, which, if not urgently treated, damages mid-brain structures, resulting in Wernicke's encephalopathy and subsequent Korsakoff's syndrome. Thiamine, given with other vitamins, prevents the syndrome from developing and probably shortens the delirium. Treatment is an urgent matter. Dietary deficiency of thiamine causes beriberi, with neurological (dry) symptoms and cardiovascular (wet) symptoms.

Pellagra is a rare consequence of nicotinamide deficiency; its main symptoms are diarrhoea, dermatitis and dementia (the three Ds) or psychosis. Dementia and cognitive impairment associated with vitamin B_{12} and folic acid deficiency may respond partially to replacement therapy. The vitamin deficiency may not be causal but may result from a poor diet brought about by a dementia. Folate deficiency does lead to depression and irritability.

Pyridoxine has been prescribed as a supplement to tryptophan, when that is used as an antidepressant, and also less successfully for pre-menstrual tension. But in neither case has its value been proved. In excess it causes peripheral neuropathy.

THIAMINE FUNCTION

Thiamine is a co-factor for crucial enzymes in carbohydrate metabolism (decarboxylating the keto amino acids pyruvate and ketoglutarate in Krebs' cycle, and transketolase or enolase in the pentose shunt).

THIAMINE REPLACEMENT

Thiamine deficiency has serious consequences, but thiamine replacement is frequently inadequate. There are two main problems. First, Wernicke's encephalopathy appears not to be well recognised in practice: post-mortem studies invariably show that brain lesions consistent with Wernicke's are found in a higher proportion of patients than that identified in clinical practice. Second, oral thiamine replacement may be inadequate to prevent Wernicke's encephalopathy. Absorption of thiamine from the gut is limited (unless it is in a polymeric form) to less than 10 mg in healthy individuals and substantially less than this in those with a history of alcohol misuse.

Parenteral thiamine replacement is therefore essential for all patients considered to be at risk of Wernicke's encephalopathy. The preparation 'Pabrinex' is commonly used in the UK. It contains 250 mg thiamine as well as riboflavin, ascorbic acid, pyridoxine and nicotinamide. Intravenous administration of a similar product, 'Parentrovite', was associated with a few reports of anaphylaxis. As a consequence, 'Pabrinex' is usually given by the intramuscular route. The optimal dosage has not been determined, but since the recommended daily intake of thiamine is 1.5 mg and it is essentially not stored in the body, a single daily dose of 'Pabrinex' intramuscularly is considered by many to be adequate therapy.

It is available as 'Pabrinex' for parenteral use and tablets of thiamine 25 mg, 50 mg and 100 mg.

FURTHER READING

Anon (1979) Wernicke's preventable encephalopathy (editorial). *Lancet*, **I**, 1122–1223.

Harper, C. (1983) The incidence of Wernicke's encephalopathy in Australia – a neuropathological study of 131 cases. *Journal of Neurological and Neurosurgical Psychiatry*, **46**, 593–598.

Thomson, A. D. & Leevy, C. M. (1972) Observations on the mechanism of thiamine hydrochloride absorption in man. *Clinical Science*, **43**, 153–163.

39. ANTI-ANDROGENS, OESTROGENS AND SILDENAFIL

DRUGS TO REDUCE SEXUAL DRIVE

Androgen secretion from the testes is controlled by luteinising hormone. Secretion of luteinising hormone from the pituitary is inhibited by progestogens. Drugs such as cyproterone and medroxy-progesterone act both to reduce testosterone levels, by reducing luteinising hormone secretion, and to block androgen receptors.

Cyproterone

Cyproterone acetate ('Androcur'), a powerful anti-androgen and progesterone-like compound, competitively blocks androgens at receptor sites, including those in the brain, and reduces secretion of luteinising hormone and testosterone. The reason for using the drug to control hypersexuality and deviant behaviour in the male is the assumption that such behaviour depends on androgen levels. The drug can be useful in helping the well-motivated male patient to control deviant sexual behaviour.

By reducing libido, cyproterone may improve the symptoms of paedophilia, exhibitionism, fetishism, other deviant behaviour and excessive demand for sexual intercourse if these practices are related to high sexual drive. Because of this, younger men are more likely to respond than older men are. A dose of 100 mg daily (range 50–200 mg) is recommended, but patients should be assessed after each dose change. Drug treatment should be combined with psychological treatment directed to encouraging motivation to change and altering sexual preoccupations.

The use of cyproterone raises ethical and legal problems because of its intended effect to control an important part of behaviour. The doctor should verify that the patient is fully informed of the side-effects and the nature of treatment. The MHA 1983 excludes sexual deviation as a recognised form of mental disorder, so that compulsory treatment cannot be given for this alone. When used to treat sexual aspects of mental illness in detained patients, cyproterone can be used without consent provided a second opinion under Section 58 gives approval, after 3 months of treatment for mental disorder.

Side-effects and interactions

Tiredness is the main unwanted side-effect and is usually transient, but gynaecomastia, which may be irreversible, occurs in 20% of those given the drug. Reversible infertility is common, with increased numbers of abnormal spermatozoa. Whether abnormal offspring are born to fathers taking cyproterone is unknown, but the patient should be warned.

Cyproterone may cause liver damage and so should not be used for patients with liver disease, and liver function should be checked.

Medroxy-progesterone acetate ('Depo-Provera') has also been used to reduce testosterone levels, and treat a variety of male sexual offenders with a high sex drive. However, it has side-effects and is not licensed for this use. The dose is 100–400 mg intramuscularly every 1–6 weeks. Testosterone levels can be monitored and fall within a day, remaining very low for a month.

Goserelin, a long-acting analogue of LH, reduces LH and testosterone levels for 1 month after a single injection. Its use is not restricted by Section 57 of the MHA. It is judged not to be a hormone, and a distinction is made between injections and implantation, according to a court ruling (Dyer, 1988).

Benperidol

Benperidol ('Anquil') can be used in place of haloperidol in disturbed psychotic states, especially when associated with disinhibition and hypersexuality. It is also used in people with personality disorders with sexual deviation or abnormal sexual preoccupations, but its effectiveness has not been established. Side-effects are as for butyrophenones and dosage varies from 0.25 mg to 1.5 mg daily in divided doses.

OESTROGEN TREATMENT

Oestrogen implants reduce male sex drive but cause side-effects, including feminisation. They are no longer used and would be restricted by Section 57 of the MHA 1983; this requires both consent and a second opinion from an approved doctor, for the implantation of hormones to reduce sexual drive.

Postnatal and perimenopausal depression

Oestrogens are not well absorbed by mouth, owing to first-pass metabolism. Transdermal oestrogen, administered as patches of 17β-oestradiol 200 μg daily, can improve postnatal depression, even in patients who have not responded to conventional antidepressants, but this is not a licensed indication. Depression in perimenopausal women is also improved, with 100 μg daily.

DRUGS FOR ERECTILE DYSFUNCTION

The discovery of the role of NO in penile erection (see chapter 22) was followed by the chance finding that a drug (sildenafil), being investigated as an anti-anginal agent, improved erectile function in some patients. This has dramatically changed the approach to treatment. About 10% of men suffer persistent erectile failure, and in men over 50 the majority have an organic cause, the most common being atherosclerosis. A much higher number suffer less complete dysfunction, for which there are many causes (see chapter 22).

Sildenafil

This is an inhibitor of a phosphodiesterase enzyme PDE-5, and prevents the breakdown of cyclic-GMP, thereby potentiating the effects of NO. It has weaker effects on PDE-6, which is present in the retina and involved in blue/green colour discrimination.

Sildenafil does not increase libido but promotes erections in response to sexual stimulation, for instance visual imagery. Patients with erectile dysfunction from a variety of causes (diabetes, neurological and psychogenic) benefit, with more frequent and more enduring erections, more successful intercourse and greater satisfaction for themselves and their partners. The effect is impressive, with NNT of less than 2 (see chapter 5). It is similarly effective in patients over 65, those on anti-hypertensives and those experiencing depression. Even patients with neurological disease and no residual erectile function benefit, but the greatest effects are in people with no known organic cause. Effects are maintained in the long term.

Sildenafil is rapidly absorbed with a peak effect after 1 hour, slightly longer if taken with food. It is metabolised mainly by CYP IIIA4, and has a plasma half-life of 3–5 hours.

The initial dose is 50 mg, taken not more than once a day, about an hour before attempted intercourse; the dose may be adjusted to between 25 and 100 mg, but doses higher than this confer no additional benefit and more side-effects.

Erythromycin increases blood levels of sildenafil by inhibiting IIIA4. Carbamazepine will have the opposite effect.

Side-effects and contraindications

The most common side-effects are headache, flushing, dyspepsia, nasal congestion and a colour tinge to vision. In a dose of 100 mg the blood pressure is transiently reduced, and this effect is likely to be potentiated if the patient is taking a nitrate drug for cardiac ischaemia. The ECG is not directly affected.

Many deaths have occurred in association with sildenafil, mostly in people with known risk factors (myocardial infarction, coronary artery disease, concomitant nitrate use).

Sildenafil is contraindicated in patients taking NO donors such as glyceryl trinitrate or other nitrates, in people for whom sexual activity carries a major cardiovascular risk (unstable angina, severe heart failure) and those with hypotension, or recent stroke or myocardial infarction. It should not be used in people with retinitis pigmentosa, and should be used with caution in those with bleeding disorders.

In a 28-day double-blind crossover studies on 44 men aged 18–70 with erectile dysfunction with no known organic cause (Eardley *et al*, 2001), sidenafil (25–75 mg up to once a day) was found to usually be effective. Side-effects included headaches (26%), flushing (9%) and dyspepsia (5%). No subjects discontinued because of side-effects. With the criterion of being satisfactory intercourse per tablet, 62% reported success, compared to 12% on placebo (ARR 50% and NNT 2 (CI 2–3)).

THE DRUGS

387

FURTHER READING

Treating sex offenders

Cooper, A. J. (1986) Progestogens in the treatment of male sexual offenders: a review. *Canadian Journal of Psychiatry*, **31**, 73–79.

Dyer, C. (1988) Mental Health Commission defeated over paedophile. *BMJ*, **296**, 1660–1661.

Gagne, P. (1981) Treatment of sex offenders with medroxy-progesterone acetate. *American Journal of Psychiatry*, **138**, 644–646.

Meyer, W. J., Cole, C. & Emory, E. (1992) Depo provera treatment for sex offending behaviour: an evaluation of outcome. *Bulletin of the American Academy of Psychiatry and Law*, **20**, 249–259.

Oestrogen in postnatal depression

Gregoire, A. J. P., Kumar, R., Everitt, B., *et al* (1996) Transdermal oestrogen for treatment of severe postnatal depression. *Lancet*, **347**, 930–933.

Sildenafil

Eardley, I., Morgan, R., Dinsmore, W., *et al* (2001) Efficacy and safety of sildenafil citrate in the treatment of men with mild to moderate erectile dysfunction. *British Journal of Psychiatry*, **178**, 325–330.

Langtry, H. D. & Markham, A. (1999) Sildenafil: a review of its use in erectile dysfunction. *Drugs*, **57**, 967–989.

Nurnberg, H. G., Lauriello, J., Hensley, P. L., *et al* (1999) Sildenafil for sexual dysfunction in women taking antidepressants. *American Journal of Psychiatry*, **156**, 1664.

——, Gelenberg, A., Hargreave, T. B., *et al* (2001) Efficacy of sildenafil citrate for the treatment of erectile dysfunction in men taking serotonin reuptake inhibitors. *American Journal of Psychiatry*, **158**, 1926–1928.

Seidman, S. N., Roose, S. P., Menza, M. A., *et al* (2001) Treatment of erectile dysfunction in men with depressive symptoms: results of a placebo-controlled trial with sildenafil citrate. *American Journal of Psychiatry*, **158**, 1623–1630.

Soares, C. N., Almeida, O. P., Joffe, H., *et al* (2001) Effect of estradiol for the treatment of depressive disorders in perimenopausal women: a double-blind, randomised, placebo-controlled trial. *Archives of General Psychiatry,* **58**, 537–538.

Drugs and ECT

Electroconvulsive therapy is a small but essential part of psychiatric practice, particularly important because of its greater efficacy and speed of onset than medication in severe depressive illness. Its effective use requires expertise and resources; legislation also has an influence on its utilisation, which tends to be less in more deprived centres. This chapter is concerned with the use of psychotropic medication in patients preparing for ECT, and concurrently in those receiving it.

The fit

It is the fit and not the electricity of ECT that is essential to the efficacy of ECT; fits induced by an intravenous drug like 'Metrazol' or an inhaled vapour – hexafluorodiethyl ether – are also therapeutic. Stimulation of a fit by brief pulses of current to the head is least unpleasant to the patient and most easily controlled. Effective treatment requires a current 50% or more above the threshold that is just sufficient to induce any seizure. The duration of the fit may not be of as great importance, but fits longer than 1 minute are associated with more confusion and memory loss. Cognitive effects after ECT are related also to the amount of electricity administered. The EEG shows greater predominance of δ activity after a course of ECT and this returns to baseline by about 30 days. The seizure is associated with a transient rise in intracranial pressure, through increased blood flow, and a transient disruption in the permeability of the blood–brain barrier.

Medication and ECT

Preparation

Electroconvulsive therapy activates the autonomic nervous system with increased parasympathetic tone at first, and sympathetic tone during the seizure. A second period of parasympathetic tone follows, before awakening. During the ECT procedure, pre-medication with an anticholinergic drug such as atropine or glycopyrrolate may be given (intravenously or intramuscularly) to reduce the bradycardia and bronchial secretions.

The tonic and clonic muscle contractions of a convulsion are unnecessary (and if violent may result in fractures), so they are suppressed by giving a small dose of a muscle relaxant acting at the motor end-plates. Commonly succinylcholine is used; it is normally quickly destroyed by pseudo-cholinesterase in the blood, so its action is brief. A non-depolarising muscle relaxant, such as atracurium, may be used as an alternative but this has longer durations of paralysis. The relaxant is usually given under cover of short-acting intravenous anaesthesia. Until recently the barbiturate methohexitone (0.75mg/kg) was widely used, but problems with availability have led to the use of alternatives, including etomidate, thiopental, propofol or ketamine. These vary in their effects upon seizure threshold and duration. Propofol shortens the seizure and may interfere with the efficacy of ECT. This is not a problem with etomidate. Ketamine has the potential to exacerbate psychosis (see p. 138), and this may be apparent in the post-ictal period.

Thresholds for fits vary. The threshold is raised by drugs with anticonvulsant properties, such as benzodiazepines, the anaesthetic agent propofol, or high doses of methohexitone (more than 1.5 mg/kg).

Seizures during ECT are now routinely monitored by EEG. If the duration is beyond 120 seconds, it should be terminated with an intravenous injection of the anaesthetic agent (for instance methohexital) or a benzodiazepine such as lorazepam 1–2 mg. The intervention should begin after 150–180 seconds.

Recovery to consciousness takes a few minutes, the time depending on the anaesthetic drug and its dose, other sedative drugs, age and state of health. Recovery of spontaneous breathing is sometimes delayed, either as a result of too much muscle-relaxant, or rarely because of pseudo-cholinesterase deficiency, an autosomal recessive. Artificial respiration will then have to be continued. Delayed recovery beyond 30 minutes is an anaesthetic emergency requiring intubation and transfer to intensive care.

Combining drugs and ECT

All medication being taken by the patient should be reviewed in conjunction with the anaesthetist before commencing a course of ECT. Psychotropic medication that should be considered for discontinuation before ECT includes mainly benzodiazepines and MAOIs, but also other antidepressants and mood-stabilisers.

Anticonvulsants and benzodiazepines

Patients with epilepsy should continue to receive their anticonvulsants during ECT, but the dose may be reduced if it is difficult to elicit adequate seizures. Anticonvulsants prescribed for psychiatric conditions may be tapered and discontinued until ECT is completed. Alternatively, the dose may be omitted for 24 hours before ECT is given. Benzodiazepines raise the seizure threshold and generally reduce the efficacy of ECT. They should be tapered and discontinued before ECT if possible.

Lithium

The co-administration of ECT with lithium has occasionally resulted in delirium or prolonged seizures. Although it is safe in most cases, consideration should be given to stopping lithium 36 hours before ECT and recommencing it 24 hours after the last treatment. Alternatively, the lithium dose may be withheld for 24–36 hours before each session of ECT.

Antidepressants

There is little evidence that continuing antidepressants during the course of ECT adds to its efficacy, although antidepressant medication is generally recommended after the course of ECT is completed. Many clinicians continue antidepressants while ECT is administered. There is concern about the cardiovascular effects of antidepressants in conjunction with ECT. Although the SSRIs would be safer in this respect, these drugs, particularly paroxetine, can lengthen the duration of seizures, and if this occurs excessively, the SSRI should be tapered and discontinued until the course of ECT is complete. The possibility of symptoms arising from discontinuation of antidepressants must be remembered.

Antipsychotics

These are the only drugs for which there is evidence of a beneficial effect in combination with ECT. There is less experience with the use of the atypical antipsychotics with ECT. Despite its effects on the EEG, clozapine has been used safely in combination with ECT.

MAOIs

Because of their potential interactions with other drugs, it is generally recommended that MAOIs be discontinued before elective surgery or ECT. However, routine ECT can be safely conducted in patients while taking MAOIs and doctors must weigh the risks and benefits of continuing or discontinuing MAOIs for ECT.

ABREACTION

A dose of anaesthetic insufficient to anaesthetise produces a state of altered consciousness, calm, relaxed, dreamy, inattentive to surroundings and more suggestible. This state induces freer, less guarded speech and can be used as a diagnostic aid for mute states or as an adjunct to psychotherapy. The technique has been called interview with sedation, or abreaction when accompanied by the display of strong emotion.

Mute states not due to neurological or medical causes are usually hysterical fugues or psychoses. An interview with sedation may enable the diagnosis, the forgotten identity being recalled or abnormal psychotic experiences and thinking being revealed. The discovery of delusions, abnormal thinking and abnormal experiences thus allows appropriate treatment for a depressive illness or schizophrenia.

In fugue states the recollection of identity may be accompanied by remembrance of unpleasant events preceding the memory loss, with emotional display and subsequent improvement. Persons of previously good personality whose symptoms began following a distressing event may re-experience the event. Emotions, allowed open expression and re-enactment, may lose their force, and clinical improvement may result.

A barbiturate or benzodiazepine by intravenous injection are the safest and easiest drugs to use. Sodium amytal 250 mg in 5 ml or 500 mg

THE DRUGS

in 10 ml is usually enough. The injection is given intravenously at the rate of 1 ml per minute while talking to the patient and noting respiration. Other drugs are 2.5% solution of sodium thiopentone, starting with 3 ml intravenously and then at the rate of 1 ml per minute up to 15 ml, or diazepam 10–20 mg intravenously over several minutes, although this tends to be less effective. It is best to have two doctors present, and an Ambu bag and oropharyngeal airway available, though these should not be required.

Talking may begin with suggestions of comfort and relaxation and asking about the effects of the injection; a heavy sigh is often the sign of the drug acting. Then proceed to ask about neutral matters of personal history, before moving on to incidents or topics of emotional concern. Do not give more drug than necessary to reach the relaxed state or the patient may go into a long sleep and forget. If important memories are recalled, keep the patient talking until the drug effect wears off, so that the recollection is maintained in full consciousness.

After recovery from the drug, discussion of the material uncovered helps to re-establish and re-integrate the forgotten material.

FURTHER READING

Jha, A. K., Stein, G. S. & Fenwick, P. (1996) Negative interaction between lithium and electroconvulsion therapy – a case-controlled study. *British Journal of Psychiatry*, **168**, 241–243.

Kellner, C. H. (1997) *Handbook of ECT*. Washington, DC & London: American Psychiatric Press.

Royal College of Psychiatrists (1995) *The ECT Handbook*. The Second Report of the Royal College of Psychiatrists' Special Committee on ECT. Council Report CR39. London: Royal College of Psychiatrists.

INDEX

INDEX OF DRUGS

Brand names are shown in *italics*; page numbers for main references in the text are shown in **bold** type.

Subject index

Page numbers for main references in the text are shown in **bold** type.